# The HEALTH ROBBERS

Consumer Health Library®
Series Editor: Stephen Barrett, M.D.
Technical Editor: Manfred Kroger, Ph.D.

Other titles in this series:

# *The* HEALTH ROBBERS

## *A Close Look at Quackery in America*

EDITED BY **STEPHEN BARRETT, M.D.**
AND **WILLIAM T. JARVIS, Ph.D.**

*Foreword by Ann Landers*

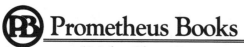 Prometheus Books

59 John Glenn Drive
Buffalo, New York 14228-2197

Published in 1993 by Prometheus Books

97   96   95   94   93      5   4   3   2   1

Library of Congress Cataloging-in-Publication Data

The Health robbers : a close look at quackery in America / edited by
    Stephen Barrett, M.D., and William T. Jarvis, Ph.D. ; foreword by
    Ann Landers.
        p.    cm. — (Consumer health library)
    Includes bibliographical references and index.
    ISBN 0-87975-855-4 (cloth)
    1. Quacks and quackery—United States. 2. Consumer protection—
United States.  I.  Barrett, Stephen, 1933–     .  II. Jarvis,
William T., 1935–     .  III. Series.
R730.H397   1993
615.8'56'0973--dc20                                          93-25357
                                                                  CIP

Printed in the United States of America on acid-free paper.

# Introduction

Day after day, we hear about our health. Advertisements bombard us. News is sensational. Health books abound.

Unfortunately, much of this information is false.

Health science has never had more to offer than it does today. Yet trust in doctors has fallen . . . and quackery is at an all-time high.

Some exploiters merely want our money. Others, perhaps more confused than crooked, seek converts to their misguided ideas.

- How can we tell experts from pretenders?
- How can we get reliable information?
- How can we communicate to get the best health care from our doctors?
- How effectively is our government protecting Americans from being cheated?

By exploring these questions, this book should help both your health and your pocketbook.

—Stephen Barrett, M.D.
William T. Jarvis, Ph.D.

# Foreword

P.T. Barnum was right. There's a sucker born every minute. And two to take him. How do I know? Because the victims write to me. And they have been writing to me every day for over thirty-five years.

Ann Landers receives approximately fourteen thousand letters a week from readers who represent every conceivable socioeconomic group. They live on suburban estates and in the city slums. My correspondents are from 6 to 110 years of age and include double-dome intellectuals as well as borderline morons. Almost half of the letters come from men.

Every bag of mail contains scores of inquiries that drive me up the wall. "How can they be so stupid?" I ask myself. And then I answer the question. It's not merely stupidity. It's desperation and wishful thinking that wipes out all reason and common sense. I become furious at the exploitation of these good people whose only crime is ignorance and vulnerability.

Here are some examples that have crossed my desk:

Dear Ann: Is it true that musk oil will turn a man on? My husband is 46 years old and sexually dead as a doornail. I've seen this musk oil advertised, but $11 is a lot of money for a little bottle. If you say it will help, I'll buy it.

Dear Ann: I'm a career girl, 28 years old, and haven't had more than three real dates in my life. The reason is because I am flat-chested. I mean I don't have any bust at all. All my life I've wanted to have nice round bosoms. Please tell me if this cream will help. (Advertisement enclosed.) As you can see, the "before" and "after" pictures are very convincing. What do you say?

Dear Ann: Is it true that cooking in aluminum will cause cancer? A man came to the door yesterday selling cookware. He scared the life out of me. His utensils cost $450 for the complete set. If what he says is true, about cancer, I mean, it sure would be worth it. But I hate to throw out these perfectly good pots and pans I've used for 10 years.

One after another the letters come—from the "exotic dancer" who wants to grow "georgeous nails in 20 days"—from the overweight housewife who will do anything to get thin except quit eating the things she loves. Then there are the females with bags under their eyes and extra chins who are sure they will look ten years younger if they use the enriched cream (secret formula) for thirty days. The trouble is—it's awfully expensive. "But it would be well worth the money if it works," writes Mrs. W. from Sheboygan. "Cheaper than a face lift. And no pain."

When men write and ask if the pomade and treatments guaranteed to grow hair will help, I often reply, "Yes. It will help the manufacturer and the man who sells it. They will get rich. As for you, it will help flatten your wallet, but it won't do anything for your bald head."

The letters from teenagers are especially pathetic: "My skin is such a mess of pimples and blackheads no girl would go out with me, so I don't even ask. Please don't suggest a doctor. I can't afford one. This soap and cream combination promises results within ten days. What do you think, Ann? And while I'm at it, Ann, maybe you can tell me if this mail-order speech course will help my brother. He stutters. His grades are awful. He's not dumb, he's just ashamed to speak up in class."

"Dear Ann: Our sex life is blah after 15 years. My husband wants to try a sex clinic, but some friends of ours went and you wouldn't believe the things they were asked to do. I don't go for that far-out stuff like changing partners. Frankly, I'm scared. What do you think?"

The saddest letters of all come from relatives of the desperately ill, those who are dying of cancer, or kidney disease. "Our family doctor said there was nothing more he could do, so we took mom to this wonderful chiropractor. She seems a little stronger today. Do you think, Ann, that we should have brought her to the chiropractor from the beginning and not wasted all that time and money on a specialist with a fancy diploma from Harvard hanging on his office wall?"

Every letter gets a personal reply in the mail, if there's a name and an address. I urge my readers to beware of quacks and phonies. I warn them against the charlatans and fakers. More often than I care to admit, I have received in return a seething reply: "How dare you take away our hope! I'll bet you are on the payroll of the American Medical Association. The medical doctor didn't do anything but send us big bills. Jesus Christ is the greatest healer of them all. Now that we have put our child in His hands, we know everything is going to be all right."

How can the public be protected against phonies, quacks, and unscrupulous money-grubbers who prey on the insecure, the frightened, and the sick? The answer is education. And that is what this book is all about.

Each chapter is written by a highly respected authority in his or her field. In the pages that follow, you will read the truth about a wide variety of food fads, worthless gadgets, pill pushers, and organized "health plans" designed to separate fools from their money. Ignorance is NOT bliss—and it never will be. Only the truth can set you free.

*Ann Landers*

# Contents

# Acknowledgments

The editors are grateful to the following individuals for their many helpful suggestions during the preparation of the manuscript:

Project manager    Eugene O'Connor, Associate Editor, Prometheus Books
Legal advisor      Michael Botts, Esq., Kansas City, Missouri
Technical editor   Manfred Kroger, Ph.D., Professor of Food Science,
                   The Pennsylvania State University

# Contributors

• Stephen Barrett, M.D., a retired psychiatrist, is a nationally renowned author, editor, and consumer advocate. He edited *Nutrition Forum* newsletter for nine years and has contributed frequently to *Priorities, Healthline,* and *Consumer Reports on Health.* He is a board member of the National Council Against Health Fraud and chairs its Task Force on Victim Redress. He is also a scientific and editorial advisor to the American Council on Science and Health. His thirty-five books include *Health Schemes, Scams, and Frauds*; *Vitamins and "Health" Foods: The Great American Hustle;* and the college textbook *Consumer Health—A Guide to Intelligent Decisions.* In 1984, he won the FDA Commissioner's Special Citation Award for Public Service in fighting nutrition quackery. In 1986, he was awarded honorary membership in the American Dietetic Association. In 1987, he began teaching health education at The Pennsylvania State University.

• William T. Jarvis, Ph.D., is an expert on the psychology and epidemiology of quackery. He is professor of health promotion and education at Loma Linda University, where he teaches courses dealing with controversial health practices. He founded and is president of the National Council Against Health Fraud. He is a scientific advisor to the American Council on Science and Health, an associate editor of *Nutrition Forum,* and co-chairman (with Dr. Barrett) of the paranormal health claims subcommittee of the Committee for the Scientific Investigation of Claims of the Paranormal (CSICOP). He is a member of the American Cancer Society's committee on questionable methods and wrote the society's booklets, "Questionable Methods of Cancer Management" and "Helping Your Patients Deal with Questionable Cancer Treatments." He has been a featured speaker at national health-fraud conferences and has testified in court and at government hearings on controversial health matters.

• Philip R. Alper, M.D., who practices internal medicine and endocrinology in Burlingame, California, is associate clinical professor of medicine at the University of California Medical Center in San Francisco. He is editor of the

*California Internist*, a contributing editor to *Medical Economics* magazine, and an editorial board member of the *Western Journal of Medicine.*

• Diana Benzaia is an award-winning journalist who also serves as a consultant to healthcare organizations.

• Mary Bernhardt, a freelance journalist who specializes in dental topics, is administrator of the Research and Education Foundation of the American Association of Endodontists. From 1968 to 1976, she was secretary of the American Dental Association's Council on Dental Health.

• John G. Clark, Jr., M.D., a retired psychiatrist, was associate clinical professor at Harvard Medical School and Massachusetts General Hospital. He was for many years a board member of the American Family Foundation, an educational organization that collects and disseminates information on cults and manipulative techniques of persuasion and control.

• Ellington Darden, Ph.D., was director of research for Nautilus Sports/ Medical Industries from 1973 to 1991 and continues to participate in seminars for the company. In 1989, he was selected as a Healthy American Fitness Leader by the President's Council on Physical Fitness and Sports. His forty-four books include the bestselling *Nautilus Book, High-Intensity Home Training, 32 Days to a 32-Inch Waist,* and *Soft Steps to a Hard Body.*

• The late Robert C. Derbyshire, M.D., a surgeon, was a leading authority on the licensing and discipline of physicians. He served as secretary-treasurer of the New Mexico Board of Medical Examiners and was president of the Federation of State Medical Boards of the United States.

• John E. Dodes, D.D.S., who practices general dentistry in Woodhaven, N.Y., lectures on quackery versus quality in dentistry. He is a board member of the National Council Against Health Fraud and president of its New York chapter. He also is a member of the Health Fraud Advisory Council of the New York State Department of Health.

• Victor Herbert, M.D., J.D., F.A.C.P., is professor of medicine at Mt. Sinai School of Medicine in New York City and chief of the Hematology and Nutrition Laboratory at the Sinai-affiliated Bronx VA Medical Center. He is a board member of the National Council Against Health Fraud and a member of the American Cancer Society's Committee on Questionable Methods. He has served on the Food and Nutrition Board of the National Academy of Sciences and its Recommended Dietary Allowances (RDA) Committee. He consults in nutrition to the World Health Organization (WHO), has been president of the American Society for Clinical Nutrition, and was chairman for five years of the American Bar Association's Committee on Life Sciences and the Law. He received the FDA Commissioner's Special Citation Award for Public Service in fighting nutrition quackery and is an honorary member of the American

Dietetic Association. He has written more than 650 scientific articles and received several national awards for his nutrition research. His books include *Nutrition Cultism: Facts and Fictions, Vitamins and "Health" Foods—the Great American Hustle, The Mount Sinai School of Medicine Complete Book of Nutrition,* and *Genetic Nutrition: Designing a Diet Based on Your Family Medical History.*

• Ray Hyman, Ph.D., is professor of psychology at the University of Oregon. He has written many professional papers about perception, creativity, and pseudopsychologies. He is co-author of *Water Witching U.S.A.,* a book about dowsing, and is author of *The Elusive Quarry,* a scientific appraisal of psychical research. A former professional magician, he is also a member of the executive council of the Committee for the Scientific Investigation of Claims of the Paranormal (CSICOP).

• Wallace F. Janssen, a former director of public information for the FDA, continues to serve as an FDA historian. He was responsible for the public warning that saved thousands of people from being victimized by the Hoxsey cancer treatment, and was an originator of several national congresses on quackery.

• Thomas H. Jukes, Ph.D. is professor of biophysics at the University of California, Berkeley. A distinguished biochemist, he has done nutritional research for many years. He is associate editor of *The Journal of Molecular Evolution* and has produced six books and more than five hundred articles in scientific journals.

• Reverend Lester Kinsolving, an Episcopal worker-priest, has had a lengthy career as a radio broadcaster and newspaper columnist. Currently he hosts a radio talk show on WCMB, Baltimore, and is editorial director of WPBC-AM in Washington, D.C.

• Ann Landers is a well-known personality whose syndicated column began in 1955 and now appears in more than 1,200 newspapers. Her foreword to this book is published with the kind permission of Ann Landers Creators Syndicate.

• Jacob Nevyas, Ph.D., Sc.D., now retired, taught biochemistry at the Pennsylvania College of Optometry and edited scientific publications.

• Jack Raso, M.S., R.D., who lives in New York City, is co-editor and publisher of *Nutrition Forum* newsletter and author of *Mystical Diets: Paranormal, Spiritual, and Occult Nutrition Practices.* He has taught at the undergraduate and graduate levels and is working with Drs. Barrett and Jarvis on an encyclopedia of paranormal healing.

• Bob Sprague, a newspaperman for twenty-one years, is an assistant professor of journalism at Emerson College in Boston.

• Wallace I. Sampson, M.D., F.A.C.P., who practices hematology and oncology in San Jose, California, is clinical professor of medicine at Stanford University School of Medicine and an associate editor of *Healthline* newsletter. He is a member of the Cancer Advisory Council for the State of California and board chairman of the National Council Against Health Fraud.

• Arthur Taub, M.D., Ph.D., is a neurologist whose specialty is the diagnosis and treatment of pain. He is also clinical professor of anesthesiology and a lecturer in neurology at Yale University School of Medicine.

• Varro E. Tyler, Ph.D., Sc.D., is the Lilly Distinguished Professor of Pharmacognosy (the science of medicines from natural sources) at Purdue University. A world-renowned authority on this subject, he has written *The Honest Herbal,* an evaluation of popular herbs, and is senior author of the textbook *Pharmacognosy.*

• Elizabeth M. Whelan, Sc.D., M.P.H., holds advanced degrees in epidemiology and public health from the Yale University School of Medicine and the Harvard School of Public Health. She is co-founder and president of the American Council on Science and Health (ACSH) and publisher of the council's quarterly magazine, *Priorities.* She has been a member of the U.S. Department of Agriculture's advisory committee on meat and poultry inspection, the Environmental Protection Agency's advisory committee on pesticides and toxics, and the American Cancer Society's national committee on cancer prevention and detection. She has moderated the nationally syndicated radio program "Healthline" and is a contributing editor to *American Baby, Mirabella,* and *Private Practice.* In 1986, she won the American Medical Writer's Association Walter Alvarez Award for excellence in medical communication. She is author or coauthor of twenty-three books, including: *Toxic Terror: The Truth Behind the Cancer Scare, Preventing Cancer, A Baby? Maybe, Panic in the Pantry,* and *A Smoking Gun: How the Cigarette Industry Gets Away with Murder.*

• Russell S. Worrall, O.D., who practices optometry in Colfax, California, is assistant clinical professor at the School of Optometry, University of California, Berkeley, and is a board member of the National Council Against Health Fraud.

• James Harvey Young, Ph.D., emeritus professor of history at Emory University, is a social historian whose special interest is the development of food and drug regulation in America. He has been a member of the FDA National Advisory Food and Drug Council. His books, *The Toadstool Millionaires, The Medical Messiahs,* and *American Health Quackery,* trace the history of quackery in America and government efforts to control it.

# 1

# How Quackery Sells

**William T. Jarvis, Ph.D.**
**Stephen Barrett, M.D.**

Modern health quacks are supersalespeople. They play on fear. They cater to hope. And once they have you, they'll keep you coming back for more . . . and more . . . and more. Seldom do their victims realize how often or how skillfully they are cheated.

Do viewers of an ad for a weight-loss "breakthrough" stop to think that a *real* breakthrough would be headlined in the news? Does the mother who feels good as she hands her child a vitamin pill think to ask herself whether it is really needed? Do buyers of "extra-strength pain relievers" wonder what's in them or whether an unadvertised brand might cost less? Do users of "herbal "energizers" realize that many herbs contain potent chemicals that may be harmful? Do subscribers to "health food" publications realize that articles are slanted to stimulate business for advertisers? Do people who hear testimonials stop to think that for every success there may have been dozens of failures? Do chiropractic patients who sign up for "preventive maintenance" know there is no scientific justification for such care? Do patients understand that the term "alternative medicine" refers to methods that have no proven value? Do survivors of cancer victims turn against the "alternative" purveyor who says "if only you had come to me earlier"? Do people who lobby for "health freedom" laws realize these are intended to excuse quacks from accountability rather than to improve consumer choice?

Not usually. Quackery confuses people with *doublespeak*—language that makes bad things sound good.

Most people think that quackery and health frauds are easy to spot. Some are, but most are not. Today's promoters wear the cloak of science. They use scientific terms and quote (or misquote) scientific references. On talk shows, they may be introduced as "scientists ahead of their time." The very word "quack" helps their camouflage by making us think of an outlandish character selling snake oil from the back of a covered wagon—and, of course, no intelligent people would buy snake oil nowadays, would they?

Well, maybe snake oil isn't selling so well. But acupuncture? "Organic" foods? Mouthwash? Hair analysis? The latest diet book? Megavitamins? "Stress" formulas? Chelation therapy? Cholesterol-lowering teas? Homeopathic remedies? AIDS cures? Or vitamin shots to pep you up? Business is booming for health quacks. Their annual take is in the *billions!* Spot-reducers, "immune boosters," water purifiers, "ergogenic aids," bust creams, spinal adjustments for "preventive maintenance," devices to increase manhood, systems to "balance body chemistry," cults to give life new meaning, special diets for arthritis. The list is endless.

What sells is not the quality of their goods and services, but their ability to influence their audience. To those in pain, they promise relief. To the incurable, they offer hope. To the nutrition-conscious, they say, "Make sure you have enough." To a public worried about pollution, they say, "Buy natural." To one and all, they promise better health and a longer life. Modern quacks can reach people emotionally, on the level that counts the most. This chapter shows how they do it.

## Appeals to Vanity

An attractive young airline stewardess once told a physician that she was taking more than twenty vitamin pills a day. "I used to feel rundown all the time," she said, "but now I feel really great!"

"Yes," the doctor replied, "but there is no scientific evidence that extra vitamins can do that. Why not take the pills one month on, one month off, to see whether they really help you or whether it's just a coincidence. After all, $300 a year is a lot of money to be wasting."

"Look, doctor," she said. "I don't care what you say. I KNOW the pills are helping me."

How was this bright young lady converted into a true believer? First, an appeal to her curiosity persuaded her to try and see. Then an appeal to her vanity convinced her to disregard scientific evidence in favor of personal experience—to *think for herself.* Supplementation is encouraged by a distorted concept of *biochemical individuality*—that everyone is unique enough to disregard the Recommended Dietary Allowances (RDAs). Quacks won't tell you that scientists deliberately set the RDAs high enough to allow for individual differences. A more dangerous appeal of this type is the suggestion that although a remedy for a serious disease has not been shown to work for other people, *it still might work for you. (You are extraordinary!)* Public awareness of psychosomatic effects strengthens the tendency toward empiricism. Many people reason that if faith in a treatment can result in improvement, anything might work for them.

A more subtle appeal to vanity underlies the message of the TV ad quack: *Do it yourself—be your own doctor.* "Anyone out there have 'tired blood'?" he used to wonder. (Don't bother to find out what's wrong with you, however. Just try my tonic.) "Troubled with irregularity?" he asks. (Pay no attention to the doctors who say you don't need a daily movement. Just use my laxative.) "Want to kill germs on contact?" (Never mind that mouthwash doesn't prevent colds.) "Trouble sleeping?" (Don't bother to solve the underlying problem. Just try my sedative.)

## Turning Customers into Salespeople

Most people who think they have been helped by an unconventional method enjoy sharing their "success story" with their friends. People who give such *testimonials* are usually motivated by a sincere wish to *help their fellow humans.* Rarely do they realize how difficult it is to evaluate a "health" product on the basis of personal experience. Like the airline stewardess, the average person who feels better after using a product will not be able to rule out coincidence—or the placebo effect (feeling better because he thinks he has taken a positive step). Since we tend to believe what others tell us of personal experiences, testimonials can be powerful persuaders. Despite their unreliability, they are the cornerstone of the quack's success.

Multilevel companies that sell nutritional products systematically turn their customers into salespeople. "When you share our products," said a sales manual of one such company, "you're not just selling. You're passing on news about products you believe in to people you care about. Make a list of people you know; you'll be surprised how long it will be. This list is your first source of potential customers."

Sharing a new way of life with your friends is rewarding, another company points out, but:

> Recruiting is the lifeblood of your business. If you believe that our company is the greatest in the world, if you believe your products are the finest products you have ever discovered or used, and if you believe

the opportunity is the greatest financial opportunity in the world—then your conviction, belief, and excitement will make you a good recruiter, providing you share your conviction with everyone you meet.

The more you sell, the more salesmen you recruit and supervise, the higher your profit percentages and bonuses. Topflight sales leaders can earn a free car and more than $100,000 a year while "working to benefit humanity." A sales leader from another company suggests, "Answer all objections with <u>testimonials</u>. That's the secret to <u>motivating</u> people!"

Don't be surprised if one of your friends or acquaintances tries to sell you vitamins or other health-related products. More than a million Americans have signed up as multilevel distributors. Like many drug addicts, they become suppliers to support their habit. A typical sales pitch goes like this: "How would you like to look better, feel better, and have more energy? Try my product(s) for a few weeks." People normally have ups and downs, and a friend's interest or suggestion, or the thought of taking a positive step, may actually make a person feel better. Many who sample their wares will mistakenly think they have been helped—and continue to buy them, usually at inflated prices.

Testimonials are sometimes faked or enhanced by fakery. An interesting example of this is described in *When Nature Speaks,* the biography of Forrest C. Shaklee, Sr., a retired chiropractor who founded Shaklee Corporation, one of the largest food-supplement companies. In 1912, when Shaklee was eighteen years old, he helped Bernarr Macfadden tour midwestern cities to spark interest in his courses in "physical culture." According to the book:

> Parades were held on the main street of each town, and consisted of a pride of muscular youths [including Shaklee], some musicians, and a flatbed wagon. . . . When enough of a crowd had been gathered around the flatbed, each of the youths was to exercise with a given piece of equipment. This was preceded by a discourse from Macfadden, extolling health through nature, diet and especially non-diet (he tended to look upon fasting as a blanket cure-all) and, of course, strenuous exercise. . . .
>
> The *pièce de résistance* of these outdoor displays was the lifting of an iron ball which appeared to weigh easily 500 pounds. Secured to the ball was a massive link chain, which one of the youths would grasp and which, with much concentration and apparent straining, he would raise gradually over his head. The crowds, watching in awed silence at the beginning of the feat, would break into cheers and applause when the ball was finally raised. When it was his turn at the ball, Forrest discovered that lifting it was easily accomplished; the ball was hollow!

*Faked endorsements* are being used to promote anti-aging products and other nostrums sold by mail. The literature, which resembles a newspaper page with an ad on one side and news on the other, contains what appears to be a handwritten note from a friend identified by first initial. "Dear Anne," it might say, "This really works. Try it! B." Although both the product and the "newspaper page" are fakes, many recipients wonder who among their acquaintances might have signed the note.

## The Use of Fear

The sale of vitamins has become so profitable that some otherwise reputable manufacturers are promoting them with misleading claims. For example, for many years, Lederle Laboratories (makers of *Stresstabs*) and Hoffmann-La Roche, two companies that sponsor many worthwhile scientific endeavors, advertised in major magazines that stress "robs" the body of vitamins and creates significant danger of vitamin deficiencies. There is no scientific support for these claims.

Another slick way for quackery to attract customers is the *invented disease.* Virtually everyone has symptoms of one sort or another—minor aches or pains, reactions to stress or hormone variations, effects of aging, etc. Labeling these ups and downs of life as symptoms of disease enables the quack to provide "treatment."

"Reactive hypoglycemia" is one such diagnosis. For decades, talk show "experts" and misguided physicians have preached that anxiety, headaches, weakness, dizziness, stomach upset, and other common reactions are often caused by "low blood sugar." But the facts are otherwise. Hypoglycemia is rare. Proper administration of blood sugar tests is required to make the diagnosis. A study of people who thought they had hypoglycemia showed that half of them reported symptoms during a glucose tolerance test even though their blood sugar levels remained normal.

"Yeast allergy" ("candidiasis hypersensitivity") is another favorite quack diagnosis. Here the symptoms are blamed on a "hidden" infection that is treated with antifungal drugs, special diets, and vitamin concoctions.

Some cancer quacks tell people that the true early signs of cancer include "gas" in the stomach or bowel, sudden weakness of the eyes, a tired feeling most of the time, muscle weakness and cramps, extreme mental depression, sudden change in hair texture, and the development of hernias. The diagnosis of cancer is then "confirmed" by the quack's own tests on urine, saliva, and/or blood samples. Since the cure rate for nonexistent cancer is 100 percent, the quack's treatment with diet, food supplements, and other wondrous substances can't possibly fail!

The following advertisement shows how the invented disease is employed by some chiropractors:

---

**TEN DANGER SIGNALS
THAT USUALLY INDICATE
THE NEED FOR CHIROPRACTIC**

1. Recurring headaches
2. Nervousness
3. Constipation
4. Backaches or leg pains
5. General weakness
6. Dizziness
7. Grating or popping noises when turning head
8. Neck pain or "crick"
9. Pain between the shoulder blades
10. General body muscle tension

---

Unlike the American Cancer Society's "Seven Warning Signs of Cancer," which have a scientific basis and are always the same, the lists used by chiropractors have no scientific basis and vary from one practitioner to another. They range from seven to sixteen supposed danger signals and may include more than forty different symptoms, many of which are insignificant and experienced by normal people. Most people who respond to such ads are told that their spine should be adjusted to relieve their symptoms and to prevent future trouble as well.

The *"Yet Disease"* is another chiropractic technique. It works like this: If a patient complains of pain in the left shoulder, the chiropractor asks, "Has the pain spread to the right shoulder . . . YET?" and then offers "preventive" spinal adjustments. When the pain fails to spread, the chiropractor takes the credit.

Interestingly, the same psychology can be used for almost any preventive measure, legitimate or not. "Don't smoke and you won't get lung cancer" and "Eat apricot pits and you won't get cancer" both use the same reasoning. If people can be convinced that a particular practice will prevent a disease, they will credit the practice if they don't get the disease. The fact that many people will not come down with the disease in a given time span will provide a large reservoir of testimonials for any preventive measure.

How can we differentiate between preventive measures that have value and the "Yet Disease" ploy used by quackery? The answer is scientific study. The fact that smokers have twenty times as much lung cancer as nonsmokers can be demonstrated, but apricot pits have not been proven to prevent cancer.

Food safety and environmental protection are important issues in our society. But rather than approach them logically, the food quacks exaggerate and oversimplify. To promote "organic" foods, they lump all additives into one class and attack them as "poisonous." They never mention that natural toxicants are prevented or destroyed by modern food technology. Nor do they let on that many additives are naturally occurring substances.

Sugar has been subject to particularly vicious attack, being (falsely) blamed for most of the world's ailments. But quacks do more than warn about imaginary ailments. They sell "antidotes" for real ones. Care for some vitamin C to reduce the danger of smoking? Or vitamin E to combat air pollutants? See your local supersalesperson.

Quack approaches to health care are even hawked for pets. Spinal manipulation, homeopathic remedies, acupuncture, anti-aging products, unnecessary vitamin supplements, and overpriced "natural" pet foods are promoted vigorously to pet owners.

One of quackery's most serious forms of fear-mongering has been its attack on public health measures. Although fluoridation's safety is established beyond scientific doubt, well-planned scare campaigns have persuaded thousands of communities not to adjust the fluoride content of their water to prevent cavities. Millions of innocent children have suffered as a result. Immunizations, pasteurization of milk, food irradiation, and modern advances in biotechnology also are targets of unfair attacks.

## Hope for Sale

Since ancient times, people have sought at least four different magic potions: the love potion, the fountain of youth, the cure-all, and the athletic superpill. Quackery has always been willing to cater to these desires. It used to offer unicorn horn, special elixirs, amulets, and magical brews. Today's products are vitamins, bee pollen, ginseng, Gerovital, pyramids, "glandular extracts," biorhythm charts, aromatherapy, and many more. Even reputable products are promoted as though they are potions. Toothpastes and colognes will improve our love life. Hair preparations and skin products will make us look "younger than our years." Olympic athletes tell us that breakfast cereals will make us champions. And youthful models reassure us that cigarette smokers are sexy and have fun.

False hope for the seriously ill is the cruelest form of quackery because it can lure victims away from effective treatment. Even when death is inevitable, however, false hope can do great damage. Experts who study the dying process tell us that while the initial reaction is shock and disbelief, most terminally ill patients will adjust very well as long as they do not feel abandoned. People who accept the reality of their fate not only die psychologically prepared, but also can put their affairs in order. On the other hand, those who buy false hope can get stuck in an attitude of denial. They waste not only financial resources but what little remaining time they have left.

The choice offered by the quack is not between hope and despair, but between false hope and a chance to adjust to reality. Yet hope springs eternal. The late Jerry Walsh was a severe arthritic who crusaded from coast to coast, debunking arthritis quackery on behalf of the Arthritis Foundation. Following a television appearance early in his career, he once received 5,700 letters. One hundred congratulated him for blasting the quacks, but 4,500 were from arthritis victims who asked where they could obtain the very fake products he was exposing!

## Clinical Tricks

The most important characteristic to which the success of quacks can be attributed is probably their ability to exude confidence. Even when they admit that a method is unproven, they can attempt to minimize this by mentioning how difficult and expensive it is to get something proven to the satisfaction of the FDA these days. If they exude *self-confidence* and enthusiasm, it is likely to be contagious and spread to patients and their loved ones.

Because people like the idea of making choices, quacks often refer to their methods as *alternatives.* Correctly used, the term can refer to aspirin and acetaminophen (Tylenol) as alternatives for the treatment of minor aches and pains. Both are proven safe and effective for this purpose. Lumpectomy can be an alternative to mastectomy for some breast cancers. Both procedures are backed by extensive scientific studies from which valid judgments can be drawn. Can a method that is unsafe, ineffective, or unproven be a genuine alternative to one that is proven? The answer is no.

Quacks don't always limit themselves to phony treatment. Sometimes they advise legitimate treatment as well—the quackery is promoted as *something extra.* One example is the "orthomolecular" treatment of mental disorders with high dosages of vitamins in addition to proven forms of treatment. Patients who receive the "extra" treatment often become convinced that they need to take vitamins for the rest of their lives. Such an outcome is inconsistent with one goal of good medical care, which is to discourage unnecessary treatment. Another example is the claim by some supplement manufacturers that their products can "support" whatever system of the body has a problem. Instead of making a direct therapeutic claim, they advise seeing a doctor but using their product(s) for "nutritional support" of the ailing body parts.

The *one-sided coin* is a related ploy. When patients on combined (orthodox and quack) treatment improve, the quack remedy (e.g., laetrile) gets the credit. If things go badly, the patient (and/or survivors) are told that they arrived too late, and conventional treatment gets the blame. Some quacks who mix proven and unproven treatment call their approach *complementary therapy.*

Quacks also capitalize on the natural healing powers of the body by *taking credit* whenever possible for improvement in a patient's condition. One multilevel company—anxious to avoid legal difficulty in marketing its herbal concoction—makes no health claims whatsoever. "You take the product," a spokesperson suggests on the company's introductory videotape, "and tell me what it does for you." An opposite tack—*shifting blame*—is used by many cancer quacks. If their treatment doesn't work, it's because radiation and/or chemotherapy have "knocked out the immune system." Emil J Freireich, M.D., of the M.D. Anderson Hospital and Tumor Institute in Houston, Texas, has combined these two ploys into a tongue-in-cheek plan for becoming a successful quack:

- Pick a disease that has natural variability.

- Apply the "treatment" when the patient's disease is getting progressively worse.

- If the patient's condition improves or stabilizes, take credit. Then stop the treatment or decrease the dosage.

- If the patient's condition worsens, say that the dosage must be increased or that the treatment was stopped too soon.

- If the patient dies, say that the treatment was applied too late.

The "secret" of this method's success is to take credit for any improvement but blame worsening in the patient's condition on something else.

To promote their ideas, quacks often use a trick where they bypass an all-important basic question and *ask a second question* which, by itself, is not valid. An example of a "second question" is "Why don't the people of Hunza get cancer?" The quack's answer is "because they eat apricot pits" (or some other claim). The first question should have been "Do the people of Hunza get cancer?" The answer is yes! Every group of people on earth gets cancer. So do virtually all animals (vegetarians and meat-eaters alike) and many types of plants. Moreover, it is a myth that Hunzas live especially long. Another common gambit is the question, "Do you believe in vitamins?" The real question should be, "Does the average person eating a well-balanced diet need to take supplements ?" The answer is no.

Another selling trick is the use of *weasel words.* Quacks often use this technique to suggest that one or more items on a list is reason to suspect that you *may* have a vitamin deficiency, a yeast infection, or whatever else they are offering to fix. A tabloid ad for "Hair Vitamins" provides a blatant example: "If your falling or thinning hair is directly attributable to vitamin deficiencies," the ad suggested, "then that very same hair may literally thrive when those vitamin deficiencies are finally remedied!" The weasel words are "if" and "may." Unless someone is starving to death, the likelihood that hair loss is due to dietary deficiency is probably zero.

The *money-back guarantee* is a favorite trick of mail-order quacks. Most have no intention of returning any money—but even those who are willing know that few people will bother to return the product.

Another powerful persuader—*something for nothing*—is standard in ads promising effortless weight loss. It is also the hook of the telemarketer who promises a "valuable free prize" as a bonus for buying a water purifier, a six-month supply of vitamins, or some other health or nutrition product. Those who bite receive either nothing or items worth far less than their cost. Credit card customers may also find unauthorized charges to their account.

The willingness to believe that a stranger can supply unique and valuable "inside" information—such as a tip on a horse race or the stock market—seems to be a universal human quirk. Quacks take full advantage of this trait in their promotion of *secret cures.* The gadget quack, for example, will swear you to secrecy before giving treatment with his little black electrical box. He wants you to feel privileged to obtain his cure—but he also wants to prevent you from arousing the suspicions of your less gullible friends. Quacks really have good reason for secrecy. They want their work kept secret from legal authorities who would prosecute their misdeeds. True scientists do not keep their breakthroughs secret; they share them with all humankind. If this were not so, we would still be going to private clinics for the vaccines and other medications used to conquer smallpox, polio, tuberculosis, and other serious diseases.

## Seductive Tactics

The practice of healing involves both art and science. The art includes all that is done for the patient psychologically. The science involves what is done about the disease itself. If a disease is psychosomatic, art may be all that is needed. Old-time doctors didn't have much science in their little black bags, so they relied more upon the art (called "bedside manner") and everyone loved them. Today, there is a great deal of science in the bag, but the art has been relatively neglected.

In a contest for patient satisfaction, art will beat science nearly every time. Quacks are masters at the *art* of delivering care. The secret to this art is to make patients believe they are cared about as people. To do this, quacks *lather love lavishly.* One way this is done is by having receptionists make notes on patients' interests and concerns in order to recall them during future visits. This makes each patient feel special in a very personal way. Some quacks even send birthday cards to every patient.

Chiropractors have developed a systematic approach to enhance the power of suggestion. A leading practice-building manual includes the following comments which can be made during the first ten visits:

Visit #1: "That adjustment took well."

Visit #2: "What's better?" If patient states that nothing is better . . . say, "but the adjustment took so well yesterday that some improvement should have been noticed. Think hard now . . . isn't something better?" If patient tells of conditions that are better, say, "Wonderful! Great! Good for you! I'm proud of you! I appreciate your getting well!" Give patients (a) attention, (b) acceptance, (c) approval, (d) recognition.

Visit #3: "What's better? Your eyes are brighter."

Visit #4: "What's better? I hope you're feeling as good as you look."

Visit #5: "What's better? You're getting a spring in your step."

Visit #6: "What's better? You're getting in fighting trim."

Visit #7: "What's better? Your body and mind are getting more rest in each hour of sleep than ever before."

Visit #8: "What's better? Did you know you'll live longer as a result of these adjustments?"

Visit #9: "What's better? Did you you know you'll have fewer colds, sore throats, etc., as a result of these adjustments?"

Visit #10: "What's better? Did you know you'll do better work during the time you are having these adjustments?"

Although seductive tactics of this sort may give patients a powerful psychological lift, they may also encourage over-reliance on an inappropriate therapy.

By the way, the discussions of chiropractic in this chapter are not meant to imply that all chiropractors are quacks or that chiropractors never help people. The reason we make so many references to chiropractors is that much of their quackery is so well-defined and organized that there are actually written documents that describe it in detail. We regard acquisition of some of their practice-building texts (which are not intended for public eyes) as one of the most significant accomplishments of our twenty-five-year investigation of quackery.

## Handling the Opposition

Quacks are involved in a constant struggle with legitimate health care providers, mainstream scientists, government regulatory agencies, and consumer-protection groups. Despite the strength of this science-based opposition, quackery manages to flourish. To maintain their credibility, quacks use a variety of clever propaganda ploys. Here are some favorites:

*"They persecuted Galileo!"* The history of science is laced with instances where great pioneers and their discoveries were met with resistance. William Harvey (nature of blood circulation), Joseph Lister (antiseptic technique), and Louis Pasteur (germ theory) are notable examples. Today's quacks boldly assert that they are further examples of people ahead of their time. Close examination, however, will show how unlikely this is. First of all, the early pioneers who were persecuted lived during times that were much less scientific. In some cases, opposition to their ideas stemmed from religious forces. Second, it is a basic principle of the scientific method that the burden of proof belongs to the proponent of a claim. The ideas of Galileo, Harvey, Lister, and Pasteur overcame their opposition because their soundness could be demonstrated.

A related ploy, which is a favorite with cancer quacks, is the *"conspiracy"* charge. How can we be sure that the AMA, the FDA, the American Cancer Society, and others are not involved in some monstrous plot to withhold a cancer cure from the public? To begin with, history reveals no such practice in the past. The elimination of serious diseases is not a threat to the medical profession—doctors prosper by curing diseases, not by keeping people sick. It should also be apparent that modern technology has not altered the zeal of scientists to eliminate disease. When polio was conquered, iron lungs became virtually obsolete, but nobody resisted this advancement because it would force hospitals to change. Neither will medical scientists mourn the eventual defeat of cancer.

Moreover, how could a conspiracy to withhold a cancer cure hope to be successful? Many physicians die of cancer each year. Do you believe that the vast majority of them would conspire to withhold a cure for a disease that equally affects them, their colleagues, and their loved ones? To be effective, a conspiracy would have to be worldwide. If laetrile, for example, really worked, many other nations' scientists would soon realize it.

Many quacks claim to offer an alternative to "allopathic medicine." The term "allopathic" was created by Samuel Hahnemann, the founder of homeopathy, to characterize the prescientific physicians of his day who based their practices on the humoral theory derived from ancient Greek cosmology. The concept of allopathy was to treat symptoms with opposites—e.g., to cool the feverish, produce diarrhea in the constipated, and constipate those with diarrhea. Some proper therapies fit this rationale even today. But to the ancient Greeks, fever meant an excess of the "blood humor" because the patient was flushed, and the allopathic remedy was to bleed the patient in an attempt to balance the humors. As science overtook medicine, it displaced both allopathy and homeopathy, but the term "allopath" still is used to refer to scientific physicians.

Quacks also refer to scientific health care as "traditional medicine," implying that it is closed-minded. *Webster's Dictionary* defines tradition as "the handing down of information, beliefs, and customs by word of mouth or by example from one generation to another." Traditional systems still cling to fanciful notions—like "energy meridians" and heavenly influences on behavior—that are thousands of years old. Closed-mindedness seems to be a virtue in these systems. Modern medicine actually is iconoclastic (anti-traditional).

Organized quackery poses its opposition to medical science as a philosophical conflict rather than a conflict about proven versus unproven or fraudulent methods. This creates the illusion of a "holy war" rather than a conflict that could be resolved by examining the facts.

Quacks like to charge that *"Science doesn't have all the answers."* That's true, but it doesn't claim to have them. Rather, it is a rational and responsible process that can answer many questions—including whether procedures are safe and effective for their intended purpose. It is quackery that constantly claims to have answers for incurable diseases. The idea that people should turn to quack remedies when frustrated by science's inability to control a disease is irrational. Science may not have all the answers, but quackery has no answers at all! It will take your money and break your heart.

To discredit scientists as "eggheads," quacks sometimes claim that a group of scientists once got together and determined that bumblebees violate the scientific laws of aerodynamics and therefore should not be able to fly. Northrop Aviation engineers grew so tired of hearing this bit of folklore during World War II that they caught bumblebees and actually worked out the scientific formulas whereby they took off and maintained flight.

Another ploy is the claim that in 1978 the Office of Technology Assessment reported that only 10 to 20 percent of medically accepted treatments had been demonstrated to work by controlled trials. Although controlled trials are important, many scientific truths are derived from other types of careful observation acknowledged in the report.

Many treatments advanced by the scientific community are later shown to be unsafe or worthless. Such failures become grist for organized quackery's public relations mill in its ongoing attack on science. Actually, "failures" reflect a key element of science: its willingness to test its methods and beliefs and abandon those shown to be invalid. True medical scientists have no philosophical commitment to particular treatment approaches, only a commitment to develop and use methods that are safe and effective for an intended purpose.

When placed on the defensive, quacks sometimes pretend that *ignorance is a virtue.* A self-proclaimed "psychic healer" who had only a fifth-grade education employed this tactic. Admitting her ignorance of medical matters, she suggested that "emptyheadedness" made it easier for "otherworldly sources" to get messages through to her, since her head wasn't cluttered up with information.

Chiropractors use this same form of argument by saying they are "too busy making sick people well" to find out how their treatment works. In reality, the first thing science wants to determine is not *how* a treatment works but *if* it works. Chiropractors claim that the fact that their profession has survived for nearly a hundred years is proof enough; but this is faulty reasoning. Astrology has survived for thousands of years without proof of its validity. Ignorance is neither a virtue nor an excuse to ply one's trade with sick people.

Some proponents of quackery clamor to have their methods tested—by others, of course. If the scientific community refuses to set up clinical trials (which is likely because scientists don't like to waste their limited resources testing methods that appear worthless), quacks claim they are being *suppressed.* If a clinical trial is launched, quacks trumpet to the world that their method is being tested. The longer the test takes, of course, the greater the opportunity to milk this type of publicity.

When a quack remedy flunks a scientific test, its proponents merely reject the test. Science writer John J. Fried provides a classic description of this in his book *Vitamin Politics:*

> Because vitamin enthusiasts believe in publicity more than they believe in accurate scientific investigation, they use the media to perpetuate their faulty ideas without ever having to face up to the fallacies of their nonsensical theories. They announce to the world that horse manure, liberally rubbed into the scalp, will cure, oh, brain tumors. Researchers from the establishment side, under pressure to verify the claims, will run experiments and find that the claim is wrong.

The enthusiasts will not retire to their laboratories to rethink their position. Not at all. They will announce to the world that the establishment wasn't using enough horse manure, or that it didn't use the horse manure long enough, or that it used horse manure from the wrong kind of horses. The process is never-ending. . . . The public is the ultimate loser in this charade.

Promoters of laetrile were notorious for shifting their claims. First they claimed that laetrile could cure cancer. Then they said it couldn't cure, but could prevent or control cancer. Then they said laetrile was a vitamin and cancer a vitamin-deficiency disease. Nowadays they say that laetrile alone is not enough—it is part of "metabolic therapy," which includes special diet, supplement concoctions, and other modalities that vary from practitioner to practitioner.

The *disclaimer* is a related tactic. Instead of promising to cure your specific disease, some quacks will offer to "cleanse" or "detoxify" your body, balance its chemistry, release its "nerve energy," bring it in harmony with nature, stimulate its "vital force," or do other things to "help the body to heal itself." This type of disclaimer serves two purposes. Since it is impossible to measure the processes they describe, it is difficult to prove them wrong. In addition, if the quack is not a physician, the use of nonmedical terminology may help to avoid prosecution for practicing medicine without a license.

Books espousing unscientific practices commonly suggest that the reader consult a doctor before following their advice. This disclaimer is intended to protect the author and publisher from legal responsibility for any dangerous ideas contained in the book. The disclaimer also implies confidence that the advice can survive medical scrutiny. Both author and publisher know full well, however, that most people won't ask their doctor. If they wanted medical advice, they probably wouldn't be reading the book in the first place.

Sometimes the quack will say, "You may have come to me too late, but I will try my best to help you." That way, if the treatment fails, you have only yourself to blame. Patients who see the light and abandon quack treatment may also be blamed for stopping too soon.

An unlicensed naturopath made such a claim in the case of Ruth Conrad, a middle-aged Idaho woman who had consulted him for a sore shoulder. When she also complained about a bump on her nose, the naturopath stated that it was cancerous and gave her a black herbal salve to apply directly. Within a few days, Mrs. Conrad's face became very painful and she developed red streaks that ran down her cheeks. When she telephoned, the naturopath said that the presence of the lines was a good sign because they "resemble a crab, and cancer is a crab." He also advised her to apply more of the black salve. Within a week, a large part of Mrs. Conrad's face, including her nose, came off. It took three years and seventeen plastic surgical operations to reconstruct her face. When questioned during a deposition, the naturopath insisted that if Mrs. Conrad had completed treatment with him, her face would have healed with no disfigurement except for "a slight dimple where the tissue healed."

Curiously, the disclaimers made by quacks are rarely strong enough to discourage the purchase of what they are selling.

## "Health Freedom"

If quacks can't win by playing according to the rules, they try to change them by switching from the scientific to the political arena. In science, a medical claim is treated as false until proven beyond a reasonable doubt. But in politics, a medical claim may be accepted until proven false or harmful. This is why proponents of laetrile, chiropractic, orthomolecular psychiatry, chelation therapy, and the like, take their case to legislators rather than scientific groups.

Quacks use the concept of *"health freedom"* to divert attention away from themselves and toward victims of disease with whom we are naturally sympathetic. "These poor folks should have the freedom to choose whatever treatments they want," cry the quacks—with crocodile tears. They want us to overlook two things. First, no one wants to be cheated, especially in matters of life and health. Victims of disease don't demand quack treatments because they want to exercise their "rights," but because they have been deceived into thinking that they offer hope. Second, the laws against worthless nostrums are not directed against the victims of disease but at the promoters who attempt to exploit them.

Any threat to freedom strikes deeply into American cultural values. But we must also realize that complete freedom is appropriate only in a society in which everyone is perfectly trustworthy—and no such society exists. Experience has taught us that quackery can even lead people to poison themselves, their children, and their friends.

Consumer protection laws have been passed to protect desperately ill people who are vulnerable. These laws simply require that products offered in the health marketplace be both safe and effective. If only safety were required, any substance that would not kill you on the spot could be hawked to the gullible.

Some people claim we have too much government regulation. But the issue should be one of quality not quantity. Good regulatory laws are very important. Our opposition should be to bad regulations that stifle our economy or cramp our lifestyles unnecessarily. Consumer protection laws should be preserved.

Unfortunately, some politicians seem oblivious to these basic principles and expound the "health freedom" concept as though they are doing their constituents a favor. In reality, "health freedom" constitutes a hunting license for quackery, with open season declared on the sick, the frightened, the alienated, and the desperate. It represents a return to the law of the jungle in which the strong feed upon the weak.

**Common Misconceptions**

Although most Americans are harmed by quackery, few perceive it as a serious problem and even fewer are interested in trying to do anything about it. Many misconceptions appear to contribute to this situation:

• *Misconception #1: Quackery is easy to spot.* Quackery is far more difficult to spot than most people realize. Modern promoters use scientific jargon that can fool people not familiar with the concepts being discussed. Even health professionals can have difficulty in separating fact from fiction in fields unrelated to their expertise.

• *Misconception #2: Personal experience is the best way to tell whether something works.* When you feel better after having used a product or procedure, it is natural to give credit to whatever you have done. This can be misleading, however, because most ailments resolve themselves and those that don't can have variable symptoms. Even serious conditions can have sufficient day-to-day variation to enable quack methods to gain large followings. In addition, taking action often produces temporary relief of symptoms (a placebo effect). For these reasons, controlled scientific studies are usually necessary to establish whether health methods actually work.

• *Misconception #3: Most victims of quackery are easy to fool.* Individuals who buy one diet book or "magic" diet pill after another are indeed gullible. And so are many people who follow whatever fads are in vogue. But the majority of quackery's victims are merely unsuspecting. People tend to believe what they hear the most. And quack ideas—particularly regarding nutrition—are everywhere. Another large group of quackery's victims is composed of individuals who have serious or chronic diseases that make them feel desperate enough to try anything that offers hope. Alienated people—many of whom are paranoid—form another victim group. These people tend to believe that our food supply is unsafe; that drugs do more harm than good; and that doctors, drug companies, large food companies, and government agencies are not interested in protecting the public. Such beliefs make them vulnerable to those who offer foods and healing approaches alleged to be "natural."

• *Misconception #4: Quackery's victims deserve what they get.* This is based on the idea that people who are gullible should "know better" and therefore deserve whatever they get. This feeling is a major reason why journalists, enforcement officials, judges, and legislators seldom give priority to combating quackery. Even doctors asked to testify as expert witnesses in quackery cases often refuse to do so because they have no sympathy for the victims. As noted above, however, most victims are not gullible. Nor do people deserve to suffer or die because of ignorance or desperation.

• *Misconception #5: Quacks are frauds and crooks.* Quackery is often discussed as though all of its promoters are engaged in deliberate deception. This is untrue. Promoters of mail-order quackery are almost always hit-and-run artists who know their products are fakes but hope to profit before the Postal Service shuts them down. But most other promoters of quackery seem to be true believers, zealots, and devotees whose problem is lack of criticism—a failure to apply skepticism to the favored therapy, very much like a religious person who blindly accepts "the faith." The FDA defines "health fraud" as "promotion of an unproven product for profit." This, too, can cause confusion because in ordinary usage—and in the courts—the word "fraud" connotes deliberate deception.

• *Misconception #6: Most quackery is promoted by quacks.* Most people think of quackery as being promoted by quacks and charlatans who deliberately take advantage of their victims. Actually, most people promoting quackery are its victims who share misinformation and personal experiences with others. For example, many customers of multilevel companies that sell overpriced vitamin supplements are friends, relatives, or neighbors of those already using them. Quackery is involved, but no "quacks." Pharmacists also profit from the sale of nutrition supplements that few of their customers need. In most cases pharmacists don't promote them but simply profit from the propaganda of others. Much quackery is involved in telling people something is bad for them (such as food additives) and selling them a substitute (such as "organic" or "natural" food). Quackery is also involved in misleading advertising of foods, nutrition supplements, and nonprescription drugs. Again, no "quack" is involved—just hype from an advertising agency. Many ads for foods fit into this category by mentioning some biochemical fact about the nutrients they contain even though there is no reason to be concerned about the particular nutrient. A recent example is an ad suggesting that Florida orange juice is good for children because "It has more potassium—a mineral that's important for normal muscle functioning." There is no reason why parents need to pay the slightest attention to the potassium content of their children's diet. Potassium is sufficiently widespread in foods that children will get enough no matter what foods they consume.

To make matters even more complicated, quackery is not all-or-nothing. A practitioner may be scientific in many respects and only minimally involved in unscientific practices. And products can be useful for some purposes but worthless for others.

Dictionaries define quackery as "the practices or pretensions of a quack" and define a quack as "a pretender to medical skill." We think it is better to define quackery as "promotion of false or unproven health claims for profit." This covers the broadest possible spectrum of quackery and avoids implying that its promoters intend to deceive. The profit does not have to be financial; it also could involve one's status or sense of worth.

• *Misconception #7: Most quackery is dangerous.* Quackery can seriously harm or kill people by inducing them to abandon or delay effective treatment for serious conditions. It can also wreck the life of people who are so thoroughly misled that they devote themselves to promoting the methods and welfare of the quack. Although the number of people harmed in these ways cannot be determined, it is not large enough or obvious enough to arouse a general public outcry. Most victims of quackery are harmed economically rather than physically. Moreover, many people believe that an unscientific method has helped them. In most cases, they have confused cause-and-effect and coincidence. But sometimes an unproven approach actually relieves emotionally related symptoms by lowering the person's tension level.

Statements condemning quackery rarely arouse indignation in people who have not been personally affected. Thus it is probably unrealistic to believe that opposition to quackery will become a high-priority issue for the general public. It is perceived as a serious problem by professionals who are offended by the audacity of quacks who defile science and hurt the public. But most professionals feel too busy to get involved.

• *Misconception #8: "Minor" forms of quackery are harmless.* Quackery involving small sums of money and no physical harm is often viewed as harmless. Examples are "nutrition insurance" with vitamin pills and wearing a copper bracelet for arthritis. But their use indicates confusion on the part of the user and vulnerability to more serious forms of quackery. There is also harm to society. Money wasted on quackery would be better spent for research, but much of it goes into the pockets of people (such as vitamin pushers) who are spreading misinformation and trying to weaken consumer protection laws.

The Feingold diet is an example of quackery whose potential harm is underestimated. Although the diet itself is harmless, it is probably harmful to teach children that the way they behave depends upon what they eat rather than on what they feel. Also, social development can be jeopardized if eating habits subject children to ridicule or lead them to avoid group activities where forbidden foods are served.

• *Misconception #9: The media are trustworthy.* Most people seem to think that statements about health issues "wouldn't be allowed" if they weren't true. Radio and television talk shows abound with promoters of nutrition quackery. Some promoters have their own publications and a few even have their own radio or TV talk shows. Some media outlets do achieve great accuracy, but most are willing to publish sensational viewpoints which they believe are newsworthy and will increase their audience. Even exposés of questionable methods are often "balanced" by including testimonials from satisfied customers. Money can also affect the flow of health information. Magazines that carry cigarette ads are notorious for ignoring the dangers of cigarette smoking. General magazines that carry vitamin ads almost never publish articles advising readers not to waste their money on vitamins.

• *Misconception #10: Advertising outlets are ethical.* There is a widespread public belief that if something isn't legitimate, publications and broadcast outlets would not allow it to be advertised. While most outlets have some limitations, most do not limit ads for health products. Standards are quite variable. All bust developers, sex enhancers, sauna belts, sauna suits, and spot-reducers are fakes; but their promoters have little difficulty in obtaining advertising outlets. Publishers and advertising managers sometimes claim they have no practical way to determine whether proposed ads are legitimate and that they must protect freedom of speech. Both positions are baloney. Ads can be checked quickly and easily by consulting a trusted authority; and freedom of speech does not include a right to defraud people.

• *Misconception #11: Education is the answer.* Education can help unsuspecting people learn to recognize quackery. However, many who are desperate, gullible, or alienated are difficult if not impossible to educate. Law enforcement is necessary to protect them.

• *Misconception #12: Government protects us.* Although various government agencies are involved in fighting quackery, most don't give it sufficient priority to be effective. Moreover, the agencies involved lack a coordinated plan to maximize their effectiveness.

• *Misconception #13: Quackery's success represents medicine's failure.* It is often suggested that people turn to quacks when doctors are brusque with them, and that if doctors were more attentive, their patients would not turn to quacks. It is true that this sometimes happens, but most quackery does not involve medical care. Doctors should pay attention to the emotions of their patients and make a special effort to explain things to them. But blaming medicine for quackery is like considering the success of astrology the fault of astronomy. Some people's needs exceed what ethical, scientific health care can provide. The main reason for quackery's success is its ability to seduce unsuspecting people. Several years ago a survey done in New Zealand found that most cancer patients who used "alternative" therapies were satisfied with their medical care and regarded "alternative" care only as a supplement.

• *Misconception #14: Quackery is medicine's responsibility.* Many people think that medical doctors have a special ability to recognize quackery, a special ability to combat it, and a special duty to do so. It is true that medical training enables most doctors to identify quackery readily. (Unfortunately, a small percentage are quacks.) But it is clear that the medical profession cannot do the job alone. Effective control of quackery will require concerted effort by educators, writers, editors, publishers, advertising managers, talk show producers, legislators, law enforcement officials, and defrauded victims.

• *Misconception #15: The AMA has the power to stop quackery.* Many people (including some physicians) seem to think that the American Medical Association has some magical power to stop quackery. In fact, the quacks often accuse the AMA of "conspiring to destroy alternative medicine" even though it is minimally involved. For many years the AMA maintained a department that was active against many types of quackery. But in 1975 it was shut down, and so was the AMA's quackery committee. Quacks cry "conspiracy" in an attempt to gain support by portraying themselves as underdogs. Their real enemy is not the AMA but consumer protection laws based on the principles of science.

• *Misconception #16: Fighting quackery is hopeless.* It is often reasoned that: (1) most victims of quackery are looking for magic; (2) such people cannot be protected from their own follies; and, therefore, (3) quackery cannot be controlled. This reasoning has two flaws. First, as explained above, most victims of quackery are not looking for magic. Second, effective law enforcement can limit quackery's toll.

Alienated individuals who are "true believers" in quack methods can also arouse the feeling that fighting quackery is hopeless. These individuals are usually beyond help, but they constitute only a small proportion of quackery's victims. Effective law enforcement can protect many of them, too. The best strategy for professionals confronted by "true believers" is to avoid wasting time with them.

Quackery's persistence causes many people to feel there is no point in trying to combat it. We disagree. Think about death and disease. No matter how much disease is cured, death still comes. But no one suggests that we stop fighting disease. Our goal should be to limit quackery as much as possible. Although the problem can never be eradicated, it can be greatly reduced if more people work on it.

### How to Avoid Being Tricked

The best way to avoid being tricked is to stay away from tricksters. Unfortunately, in health matters, this is no simple task. Quackery is not sold with a warning label. Moreover, the dividing line between what is quackery and what is not is by no means clearly drawn. A product that is effective in one situation may be part of a quack scheme in another. (Quackery lies more in the promise than in the product.) Practitioners who use effective methods may also use ineffective ones. For example, they may mix valuable advice to stop smoking with unsound advice to take vitamins. Even outright quacks may relieve some psychosomatic ailments with their reassuring manner.

This book illustrates how adept quacks are at selling themselves. Sad to say, in most contests between quacks and ordinary people, the quacks still are likely to win.

# 2

# Vitamin Pushers and Food Quacks

## Victor Herbert, M.D., J.D., F.A.C.P.

We remain in the midst of a vitamin craze. Nutrition hustlers are cleaning up by stoking our fears and stroking our hopes. With their deceptive credentials, they dominate air waves and publications. Talk show hosts love them because their false promises of superhealth draw huge audiences. The situation now appears even worse than it was more than twenty-five years ago, when FDA Commissioner George P. Larrick stated:

> The most widespread and expensive type of quackery in the United States today is the promotion of vitamin products, special dietary foods, and food supplements. Millions of consumers are being misled concerning the need for such products. Complicating this problem is a vast and growing "folklore" or "mythology" of nutrition which is being built up by pseudoscientific literature in books, pamphlets, and periodicals. As a result, millions of people are attempting self-medication for imaginary and real illnesses with a multitude of more or less irrational food items. Food quackery today can only be compared to the patent medicine craze which reached its height in the last century.

"Health food" rackets cost Americans billions of dollars a year. The major victims of this waste are the elderly, the pregnant, the sick, and the poor.

## The Fundamentals of Good Nutrition

Have you been brainwashed by vitamin pushers? Do you believe you should supplement your diet with extra nutrients? Do you believe that, "If some is good,

23

more is better"? Or that "extra nutrients can't hurt"? Or that they provide "nutrition insurance"? If you believe any of these things, you have been misled.

The fundamentals of good nutrition are simple: To get the amounts and kinds of nutrients your body needs, eat moderate amounts of food from each of the food groups designated by the U.S. Department of Agriculture's Daily Food Guide. You should eat a wide variety within each category. Your daily average should include:

| | |
|---|---|
| Bread, Cereal, Rice, & Pasta Group | 6 to 11 servings |
| Vegetable Group | 3 to 5  servings |
| Fruit Group | 2 to 4  servings |
| Milk, Yogurt, & Cheese Group | 2 to 3  servings |
| Meat, Poultry, Fish, Dry Beans, Eggs, & Nuts Group | 2 to 3  servings |

Except for the milk group, the number of recommended servings depends on the individual's age, gender, size, and activity level, with the lower numbers for people needing about 1,600 calories daily and the higher ones for those needing about 2,800 calories. (For detailed instructions send $1 for USDA's *Food Guide Pyramid* booklet [Publication No. HG 249] to the Consumer Information Center, Pueblo, CO 81009.) These portions provide adequate quantities of all vitamins, minerals, protein components, and dietary fiber. In fact, normal people eating a balanced variety of foods are likely to consume *more* nutrients than they need. Of course, health hucksters won't tell you this because their income depends upon withholding that truth. Unlike responsible practitioners, they do not make their living by trying to keep you healthy, but rather by tempting you with false claims. These claims raise their personal appearance fees, sell their books and magazine articles, and promote the products of companies in which (unknown to you) they may have a financial interest.

### The Dangers of Excess Vitamins

When on the defensive, quacks are quick to demand, "How do you know it doesn't help?" The reply to this is, "How do you know it doesn't *harm*?" Many substances that are harmless in small or moderate doses can be harmful either in large doses or by gradual build-up over many years. Just because a substance (such as a vitamin) is found naturally in food does not mean it is harmless in large doses. In fact, the National Academy of Sciences has published an entire book on this subject called *Toxicants Occurring Naturally in Foods*.

When scientists speak of "excess" vitamins, they mean dosages in excess of the "Recommended Dietary Allowances (RDAs)" set by the Food and Nutrition Board of the National Research Council, National Academy of Sciences. The RDAs are the "levels of intake of essential nutrients considered, in the judgment of the Food and Nutrition Board on the basis of available scientific knowledge, to be adequate to meet the known nutritional needs of practically all healthy persons."

RDAs should not be confused with "requirements." They are more than most people require. They are set not only to meet body needs, but to allow substantial storage to cover periods of reduced intake or increased need. Amounts higher than the RDAs serve no vitamin function in the body. They should be considered *drugs* and can be an invitation to trouble.

Too much vitamin A can cause lack of appetite, retarded growth in children, drying and cracking of the skin, enlarged liver and spleen, increased intracranial pressure, loss of hair, migratory joint pains, menstrual difficulty, bone pain, irritability, and headaches.

Excess vitamin $B_6$ can cause symptoms resembling those of multiple sclerosis, including numbness and tingling of the hands, difficulty in walking, and electric shocks shooting down the spine. Over a hundred cases have been reported during the past few years. Although all the afflicted individuals improved greatly when they stopped taking the vitamin, a few did not recover completely. Some of them had been taking less than 50 mg/day. (The RDA is about 2 mg.) In light of these cases, supplementation with high dosages of vitamin $B_6$ appears inadvisable.

Prolonged excessive intake of vitamin D can cause loss of appetite, nausea, weakness, weight loss, polyuria (excessive urination), constipation, vague aches, stiffness, kidney stones, calcifying of tissues, high blood pressure, acidosis, and kidney failure that can lead to death.

Large doses of niacin, recommended by purveyors of "orthomolecular psychiatry," can cause severe flushing, itching, liver damage, skin disorders, gout, ulcers, and blood sugar disorders. Sustained-release niacin produces less flushing than ordinary (crystalline) niacin, but is far more likely to cause liver toxicity. In drug doses, niacin can play a valuable role in the treatment of abnormal blood cholesterol levels. But it should *never* be used for this purpose without medical supervision.

Excess vitamin E can cause headaches, nausea, fatigue, giddiness, inflammation of the mouth, chapped lips, gastrointestinal disturbances, muscle weakness, low blood sugar, and increased bleeding tendency. By antagonizing the action of vitamin A, large doses of vitamin E can also cause blurred vision. Vitamin E can also reduce sexual organ function—despite the claim that the vitamin *heightens* sexual potency. (This claim is based on experiments with rats. Quacks don't tell you that what may be true with rats may be just the opposite with humans!)

Another way to look for health trouble is with ascorbic acid—vitamin C. Excess vitamin C may damage growing bone, cause diarrhea (making it particularly dangerous for AIDS patients), produce "rebound scurvy" in newborn infants whose mothers took such dosage, lead to adverse effects in pregnancy, cause kidney stones, and result in false urine tests for sugar in diabetics. By increasing iron absorption from food, large doses can also increase the risk of iron-overload disease in susceptible individuals.

There are two situations in which the use of vitamins in excess of the RDAs is legitimate. The first is the treatment of *medically diagnosed* deficiency states—conditions that are rare except among alcoholics, persons with intestinal malabsorption defects, and the poor, especially those who are pregnant or elderly. The other use is in the treatment of certain conditions in which vitamins are used for their chemical (nonvitamin) actions. None of these situations is suitable for self-treatment.

## Vitamin Pushers Are Usually Charlatans and Quacks

The *Random House Unabridged Dictionary of the English Language* says that a charlatan is "one who pretends to more knowledge or skill than he possesses; quack." It then defines quack as:

> (1) a fraudulent or ignorant pretender to medical skill; (2) a person who pretends, professionally or publicly, to skill, knowledge, or qualification which he does not possess; a charlatan; (3) being a quack: a quack psychologist who complicates everyone's problems; (4) presented falsely as having curative powers: quack medicine; (5) to advertise or sell with fraudulent claims.

The pretense to greater knowledge or skill comes in various forms, some quite subtle. It may involve impressive-sounding but bogus credentials. When a quack and a responsible scientist are brought together as guests, talk show hosts may remark: "You both have such excellent credentials, and yet you make diametrically opposed statements. What is the layman to think?" What the audience *should* think is that one of the "experts" is very likely a quack.

Talk show quacks sometimes support their case by quoting the findings of a "great scientist" (another quack) who has "published many studies in scientific journals." Be cautious. They may be publications that do not have review systems to screen out garbage and will publish almost anything they receive. Laypersons may not know this. Quacks don't care about the quality of their information. They merely accept any findings that appear supportive and reject all evidence that contradicts their ideas.

Some quacks have a more modest-seeming approach: "I have published a few papers on this—maybe it takes more papers to convince some people." Don't let this fool you. Scientific truth is not determined by the number of papers but by the quality of published reports. One thousand poorly designed studies are one thousand pieces of junk. One well-designed study is worth its weight in gold. (Or as the prominent debunker James Randi has pointed out, one intact balloon is worth far more than ten thousand balloons with holes in them.) Quacks hate well-designed "controlled" studies and rarely attempt to do them. When quacks refer to their own "research," they often mean their unscientific combination of thoughts, including ideas taken out of context from the writings of others.

How can you identify promoters of unscientific or fraudulent ideas about nutrition? The following behavior should make you suspicious.

### *They use anecdotes and testimonials to support their claims*

We all tend to believe what others tell us about personal experiences. But separating cause and effect from coincidence can be difficult. If people tell you that product X has cured their cancer, arthritis, or whatever, be skeptical. They may not actually have had the condition. If they did, their recovery most likely would have occurred without the help of product X. Most single episodes of disease end with just the passage of time, and most chronic ailments have symptom-free periods. Establishing medical truths requires careful and repeated investigation—with well-designed experiments, not reports of coincidences misperceived as cause-and-effect. That's why testimonial evidence is forbidden in scientific articles and is usually inadmissible in court.

Never underestimate the extent to which people can be fooled by a worthless remedy. During the early 1940s, many thousands of people became convinced that "glyoxylide" could cure cancer. Yet analysis showed that it was simply distilled water!

Symptoms that are psychosomatic (bodily reactions to tension) are often relieved by anything taken with a suggestion that it will work. Tiredness and other minor aches and pains may respond to any enthusiastically recommended nostrum. For these problems, even physicians may prescribe a placebo. A placebo is a substance that has no pharmacological effect on the condition for which it is used, but is given to satisfy a patient who supposes it to be a medicine. Vitamins (such as B$_{12}$) are commonly used in this way.

Placebos act by suggestion. Unfortunately, some doctors swallow the advertising hype or become confused by their own observations and "believe in vitamins" beyond those supplied by a good diet. Those who share such false beliefs do so because they confuse coincidence or placebo action with cause and effect. Homeopathic believers make the same error.

Talk show hosts give quacks a boost when they ask, "What do all the vitamins you take do for you personally?" Then thousands or even millions of viewers are treated to the quack's talk of improved health, vigor, and vitality—with the implicit point: "It did this for me. It will do the same for you." A most revealing testimonial experience was described during a major network show that featured several of the world's most prominent promoters of nutritional faddism. While the host was boasting that his new eating program had cured his "hypoglycemia," he mentioned in passing that he was no longer drinking twenty to thirty cups of coffee a day. Neither the host nor any of his "experts" had the good sense to tell their audience how dangerous it can be to drink so much coffee. Nor did any of them recognize that the host's original symptoms were probably caused by excess caffeine.

### They promise quick, dramatic, miraculous cures

Often the promises are subtle or couched in "weasel words" that create an illusion of a promise, so promoters can deny making them when the fed close in. False promises of cure are the quacks' most immoral practice. They don't seem to care how many people they break financially or in spirit—by elation over their expected good fortune followed by deep depression when the "treatment" fails. Nor do quacks keep count—while they fill their bank accounts—of how many people they lure away from effective medical care into disability or death.

### They use disclaimers couched in pseudomedical jargon

Instead of promising to cure your disease, some quacks will promise to "detoxify" your body, "balance" its chemistry, release its "nerve energy," bring it in harmony with nature, "stimulate" or "strengthen" your immune system, or "support" various organs in your body. (Of course, they never identify or make valid before-and-after measurements of any of these processes.) These disclaimers serve two purposes. First, since it is impossible to measure the processes quacks allege, it may be difficult to prove them wrong. Moreover, if a quack is not a physician, the use of nonmedical terminology may help to avoid prosecution for practicing medicine without a license—although it shouldn't.

### They display credentials not recognized by responsible scientists or educators

The backbone of educational integrity in America is a system of accreditation by agencies recognized by the U.S. Secretary of Education and/or the Council on Postsecondary Accreditation. "Degrees" from nonaccredited schools are rarely worth the paper they are printed on. In the health field, there is no such thing as a reliable school that is not accredited.

Since quacks operate outside of the scientific community, they also tend to form their own "professional" organizations. In some cases, the only membership requirement is payment of a fee. My office wall displays fancy "professional member" certificates for Charlie Herbert (a cat) and Sassafras Herbert (a dog). Each was acquired simply by submitting the pet's name, our address, and a check for $50. Don't assume that all groups with scientific-sounding names are respectable. Find out whether their views are scientifically based.

Unfortunately, possession of an accredited degree does not guarantee reliability. Some schools that teach unscientific methods (chiropractic, naturopathy, and acupuncture) have achieved accreditation. Worse yet, a small percentage of individuals trained in reputable institutions (such as medical or dental schools or accredited universities) have strayed from scientific thought.

Some quacks are promoted with superlatives like "the world's foremost nutritionist" or "America's leading nutrition expert." There is no law against this tactic, just as there is none against calling oneself the "World's Foremost Lover." However, the scientific community recognizes no such title.

### They encourage patients to lend political support to their treatment methods

A century ago, before scientific methodology was generally accepted, valid new ideas were hard to evaluate and were sometimes rejected by a majority of the medical community, only to be upheld later. But today, treatments demonstrated as effective are welcomed by scientific practitioners and do not need a group to crusade for them. *Quacks seek political endorsement because they can't prove that their methods work.* Instead, they may seek to legalize their treatment and force insurance companies to pay for it. Judges and legislators who believe in *caveat emptor* (let the buyer beware) are natural allies for quacks.

### They say that most disease is due to faulty diet and can be treated with "nutritional" methods

This simply isn't so. Consult your doctor or any recognized textbook of medicine. They will tell you that although diet is a factor in some diseases (most notably coronary heart disease), most diseases have little or nothing to do with diet. Common symptoms like malaise (feeling poorly), fatigue, lack of pep, aches (including headaches) or pains, insomnia, and similar complaints are usually the body's reaction to emotional stress. The persistence of such symptoms is a signal to see a doctor to be evaluated for possible physical illness. It is not a reason to take vitamin pills.

Some quacks seem to specialize in the diagnosis and treatment of problems considered rare or even nonexistent by responsible practitioners. Years ago hypothyroidism and adrenal insufficiency were in vogue. Today's "fad" diagnoses are "hypoglycemia," "mercury amalgam toxicity," "candidiasis hypersensitivity," and "environmental illness." Quacks are also jumping on the allergy bandwagon, falsely claiming that huge numbers of Americans are suffering from undiagnosed allergies, "diagnosing" them with worthless tests, and prescribing worthless "nutritional" treatments.

### They recommend a wide variety of substances similar to those found in your body

The underlying idea—like the wishful thinking or sympathetic magic of primitive tribes—is that taking these substances will strengthen or rejuvenate the corresponding body parts. For example, according to a "health food" store brochure:

> Raw glandular therapy, or "cellular therapy" . . . seems almost too simple to be true. It consists of giving in supplement form (intravenous or oral) those specific tissues from animals that correspond to the "weakened" areas of the human body. In other words, if a person has a weak pancreas, give him raw pancreas substance; if the heart is weak, give raw heart, etc.

Vitamins and other nutrients may be added to the various preparations to make them more marketable. When taken by mouth, such concoctions are no better than placebos. They usually don't do direct harm, but their allure may steer people away from competent professional care. Injections of raw animal tissues, however, can cause severe allergic reactions to their proteins. Some preparations have also caused serious infections.

Proponents of "tissue salts" allege that the basic cause of disease is mineral deficiency—correction of which will enable the body to heal itself. Thus, they claim, one or more of twelve salts are useful against a wide variety of diseases, including appendicitis (ruptured or not), baldness, deafness, insomnia, and worms. Development of this method is attributed to a nineteenth-century physician named W.H. Schuessler.

Enzymes for oral use are another rip-off. They supposedly can aid digestion and "support" many other functions within the body. The fact is, however, that enzymes taken by mouth are digested into their component amino acids by the stomach and intestines and therefore do not function as enzymes within the body. Oral pancreatic enzymes have legitimate medical use in diseases involving decreased secretion of one's own pancreatic enzymes. Anyone who actually has a pancreatic enzyme deficiency probably has a serious underlying disease requiring competent medical diagnosis and treatment.

## When talking about nutrients, they tell only part of the story

Quacks tell you all the wonderful things that vitamins and minerals do in your body and/or all the horrible things that can happen if you don't get enough. But they conveniently neglect to tell you that a balanced diet can provide all the nutrients you need, and that the USDA food-group system makes balancing your diet simple. Unfortunately, it is legal to lie in a publication or lecture or on a talk show as long as the claims are not connected to selling a specific product. Many supplement manufacturers use subtle approaches. Some simply say: "Buy our product X. It contains nutrients that help promote healthy eyes (or hair, or whatever organ you happen to be concerned about)." Others distribute charts telling what each nutrient does and the signs and symptoms of deficiency disease. This encourages supplementation with the hope of enhancing body functions and/or avoiding the troubles described.

Another type of fraudulent concealment is the promotion of "supplements" and herbal extracts based on incomplete information. Many health-food industry products are marketed with claims based on faulty extrapolations of animal research and/or unconfirmed studies on humans. The most notorious such product was L-tryptophan, an amino acid. For many years it was promoted for insomnia, depression, premenstrual syndrome, and overweight, even though it had not been proven safe or effective for any of these purposes. In 1989, it triggered an outbreak of eosinophilia-myalgia syndrome, a rare disorder characterized by severe muscle and joint pain, weakness, swelling of the arms and legs, fever, skin rash, and an increase of eosinophils (certain white blood cells) in the blood. Over the next year, more than 1,500 cases and twenty-eight deaths were reported. The outbreak was traced to a manufacturing problem at the plant of a wholesale supplier. The naked truth is that L-tryptophan should not have been marketed to the public in the first place because—like most single-ingredient amino acids—it had not been proven safe and effective for medicinal use. In fact, the FDA issued a ban in 1973 but did not enforce it.

### They claim that most Americans are poorly nourished

This is an appeal to fear that is not only untrue, but ignores the fact that the main forms of bad nourishment in the United States are undernourishment among the poverty-stricken and overweight in the population at large, particularly the poor. Poor people can ill afford to waste money on unnecessary vitamin pills. Their food money should be spent on nourishing food.

With one exception, food-group diets contain all the nutrients that people need. The exception involves the mineral iron. The average American diet contains barely enough iron to meet the needs of infants, fertile women, and, especially, pregnant women. This problem can be solved by cooking in a "Dutch oven" or any iron pot or eating iron-rich foods such as soy beans, liver, and veal muscle. Iron supplements should be used only under competent medical supervision. However, about 10 percent of Americans are genetically predisposed toward iron-overload disease, which means that supplementation may cause them to accumulate harmful amounts of iron in body tissues.

It is falsely alleged that Americans are so addicted to "junk" foods that an adequate diet is exceptional rather than usual. While it is true that some snack foods are mainly "naked calories" (sugars and/or fats without other nutrients), it is not necessary for every morsel of food we eat to be loaded with nutrients. In fact, no normal person following the USDA food-group principles is in any danger of vitamin deficiency.

### They tell you that if you eat badly, you'll be OK if you take supplements

This is the "Nutrition Insurance Gambit." The statement is not only untrue but encourages careless eating habits. The remedy for eating badly is a well-balanced diet. If in doubt about the adequacy of your diet, write down what you eat for several days and see whether your daily average is in line with the USDA's guidelines. If you can't do this yourself, your doctor or a registered dietitian can do it for you.

### They allege that modern processing methods and storage remove all nutritive value from our food

It is true that food processing can change the nutrient content of foods. But the changes are not so drastic as the quack, who wants you to buy supplements, would like you to believe. While some processing methods destroy some nutrients, others add them. A balanced variety of foods will provide all the nourishment you need.

Quacks distort and oversimplify. When they say that milling removes B-vitamins, they don't bother to tell you that enrichment puts them back. When they tell you that cooking destroys nutrients, they omit the fact that only a few nutrients are sensitive to heat. Nor do they tell you that these few nutrients are easily obtained from a portion of fresh uncooked fruit, vegetable, or fresh or frozen fruit juice each day.

### They claim that fluoridation is dangerous

Curiously, quacks are not always interested in real deficiencies. Fluoride is necessary to build decay-resistant teeth and strong bones. The best way to obtain adequate amounts of this essential nutrient is to augment community water supplies so their fluoride concentration is about one part fluoride for every million parts of water. But quacks are usually opposed to water fluoridation, and some advocate water filters that remove fluoride. It seems that when they cannot profit from something, they may try to make money by opposing it.

### They oppose pasteurization of milk

One of the strangest aspects of nutrition quackery is its embrace of "raw" (unpasteurized) milk. Public health authorities advocate pasteurization to destroy any disease-producing bacteria that may be present. Health faddists and quacks claim that it destroys essential nutrients. Although about 10 percent of the heat-sensitive vitamins (vitamin C and thiamine) are destroyed during pasteurization, milk would not be a significant source of these nutrients anyway. Raw milk, whether "certified" or not, can be a source of harmful bacteria that cause dysentery and tuberculosis. The FDA has banned the interstate sale of raw milk and raw-milk products packaged for human consumption. In 1989, a

California Superior Court judge ordered the nation's largest raw-milk producer to stop advertising that its raw-milk products are safe and healthier than pasteurized milk and to label its products with a conspicuous warning.

### *They claim that soil depletion and the use of "chemical" fertilizers result in less nourishing food*

These claims are used to promote the sale of so-called "organically grown" foods. If an essential nutrient is missing from the soil, a plant simply doesn't grow. Chemical fertilizers counteract the effects of soil depletion. Plants do vary in mineral content, but this is not significant in the American diet. Quacks also lie when they claim that plants grown with natural fertilizers (such as manure) are nutritionally superior to those grown with synthetic fertilizers. Before they can use them, plants convert natural fertilizers into the same chemicals that synthetic fertilizers supply.

### *They claim that under stress, and in certain diseases, your need for nutrients is increased*

Many vitamin manufacturers have advertised that "stress robs the body of vitamins." One company has asserted that, "if you smoke, diet, or happen to be sick, you may be robbing your body of vitamins." Another has warned that "stress can deplete your body of water-soluble vitamins . . . and daily replacement is necessary." Other products are touted to fill the "special needs of athletes."

While it is true that the need for vitamins may rise slightly under physical stress and in certain diseases, this type of advertising is fraudulent. The average American—stressed or not—is not in danger of vitamin deficiency. The increased needs to which the ads refer almost never rise above the RDAs and can be met by proper eating. Someone who is really in danger of deficiency due to an illness would be *very* sick and would need medical care, probably in a hospital. But these promotions are aimed at average Americans who certainly don't need vitamin supplements to survive the common cold, a round of golf, or a jog around the neighborhood! Athletes get more than enough vitamins when they eat the food needed to meet their caloric requirements.

Many vitamin pushers suggest that smokers need vitamin C supplements. Although it is true that smokers in North America have somewhat lower blood levels of this vitamin, these levels are still far above deficiency levels. In America, cigarette smoking is the leading cause of death preventable by self-discipline. Rather than seeking false comfort by taking vitamin C, smokers who are concerned about their health should stop smoking. Moreover, since doses of vitamin C high enough to acidify the urine speed up excretion of nicotine, they may even cause some smokers to smoke more to avoid symptoms of nicotine withdrawal. Suggestions that "stress vitamins" are helpful against emotional stress are also fraudulent.

### They claim you are in danger of being "poisoned" by ordinary food additives and preservatives

This is a scare tactic designed to undermine your confidence in food scientists and government protection agencies. Quacks want you to think they are out to protect you. They hope that if you trust them, you will buy what they recommend. The fact is that the tiny amounts of additives used in food pose no threat to human health. Some actually protect our health by preventing spoilage, rancidity, and mold growth.

Two examples illustrate how ridiculous quacks can get about food additives, especially those found naturally in food. Calcium propionate is used to preserve bread and occurs naturally in Swiss cheese. Quacks who would steer you toward (higher-priced) bread made without preservatives are careful not to tell you that a one-ounce slice of "natural" Swiss cheese contains the same amount of calcium propionate used to retard spoilage in two one-pound loaves of bread. Similarly, those who warn about monosodium glutamate (MSG) don't tell you that the wheat germ they hustle as a "health food" is a major natural source of this substance.

Also curious is their failure to warn that many plant substances marketed as "herbs" are potentially toxic and can cause discomfort, disability, or even death. The April 6, 1979, *Medical Letter* listed more than thirty such products sold in "health food" stores, most used for making herbal teas.

### They push you to buy a water purifier

Although contaminants have been reported in some water supplies, most households have no cause to worry. But fraudulent sellers who offer "free home water testing" suggest otherwise. Some add tablets or drops to your tap water, claiming that particle formation or a color change signifies contamination. When the change occurs (due to *normal* chemical reactions), they claim your water is polluted and may cause cancer. Some sellers say that our government recommends widespread use of purification systems, has approved their testing method, or has approved or licensed their equipment. Such claims are false.

Offers for free home testing of tap water are almost always part of a sales promotion. Nor can home-testing provide the in-depth analysis required to determine whether water actually needs treatment or what type of system would be best. If worried about your water supply, call the Environmental Protection Agency's Safe Drinking Water Hotline (800-426-4791) or consult your local or state health department or a state-certified laboratory.

### They claim that "natural" vitamins are better than "synthetic" ones

This claim is a flat lie. Each vitamin is a chain of atoms strung together as a molecule. Molecules made in the "factories" of nature are identical to those made in the factories of chemical companies. Does it makes sense to pay extra for vitamins extracted from foods when you can get all you need from the foods themselves?

### They claim that sugar is a deadly poison

Many vitamin pushers would have us believe that sugar is "the killer on the breakfast table" and is the underlying cause of everything from heart disease to hypoglycemia. The fact is, however, that when sugar is used in moderation as part of a normal, balanced diet, it is a perfectly safe source of calories and eating pleasure. In fact, if you ate no sugar, your liver would make it from protein and fat because your brain needs it.

### They recommend that everybody take vitamins or "health foods" or both

Food quacks belittle normal foods and ridicule the food-group systems of good nutrition. They may not tell you that they earn their living from such pronouncements—via public appearance fees, product endorsements, sale of publications, or financial interests in vitamin companies, health food stores, or organic farms.

The very term "health food" is a deceptive slogan. All food is health food in moderation; any food is junk food in excess. Did you ever stop to think that your corner grocery, fruit market, meat market, and supermarket are also health-food stores? They are—and they generally charge less than stores that use the slogan.

Many vitamin pushers make misleading claims for bioflavonoids, rutin, inositol, paraaminobenzoic acid (PABA), and other such food substances. These substances are not needed in the diet, and the FDA forbids nutritional claims for them on product labels.

By the way, have you ever wondered why people who eat lots of "health foods" still feel they must load themselves up with vitamin supplements?

### They offer phony "vitamins"

Since vitamins are so popular, why not invent some new ones. Ernst T. Krebs, M.D., and his son Ernst T. Krebs, Jr., invented two of them. In 1949, they patented a substance that they later named pangamate and trade-named "vitamin B-15." The Krebses also developed the quack cancer remedy, laetrile, which was marketed as "vitamin B-17."

To be properly called a vitamin, a substance must be an organic nutrient that is necessary in the diet, and deficiency of the substance must be shown to cause a specific disease. Neither pangamate nor laetrile is a vitamin. Pangamate is not even a single substance; different sellers put different synthetic ingredients in the bottle. Laetrile contains six percent of cyanide by weight and has actually poisoned people.

### They suggest that hair analysis can be used to determine the body's nutritional state

"Health food" stores and various unscientific practitioners suggest this test. For $25 to $40 plus a lock of your hair, you can get an elaborate computer printout of vitamins and minerals you supposedly need. Hair analysis has limited value (mainly in forensic medicine) in the diagnosis of heavy metal poisoning, but it is worthless as a screening device to detect nutritional problems. In fact, a deficiency in the body may be accompanied by an *elevated* hair level. If a hair analysis laboratory recommends supplements, you can be sure that its computers are programmed to recommend them to everyone.

Several years ago, Dr. Stephen Barrett sent hair samples from two healthy teenagers under different assumed names to thirteen commercial hair analysis laboratories. The reported levels of most minerals varied considerably between identical samples sent to the same laboratory and from laboratory to laboratory. The labs also disagreed about what was "normal" or "usual" for many of the minerals. So even if hair analysis could be useful in nutritional practice, there's no assurance that commercial laboratories perform it accurately.

*They suggest that a questionnaire can be used
to indicate whether you need dietary supplements*

No questionnaire can do this. A few entrepreneurs have devised lengthy computer-scored questionnaires with questions about symptoms that could be present if a vitamin deficiency exists. But such symptoms occur much more frequently in conditions unrelated to nutrition. Even when a deficiency actually exists, the tests don't provide enough information to discover the cause so that suitable treatment can be recommended. That requires a physical examination and appropriate laboratory tests. Many responsible nutritionists use a computer to help evaluate their clients' diet. But this is done to make *dietary* recommendations, such as reducing fat content or increasing fiber content. Supplements are seldom useful unless the person is unable (or unwilling) to consume an adequate diet.

Be wary, too, of brief questionnaires purported to provide a basis for determining whether supplements may be needed. Responsible questionnaires compare the individual's average daily consumption with the recommended numbers of servings from each food group. The safest and best way to get nutrients is generally from food, not pills. So even if a diet is deficient, the most prudent action is usually diet modification rather than supplementation with pills.

*They say it is easy to lose weight*

Diet quacks would like you to believe that special pills or food combinations can cause "effortless" weight loss. But the only way to lose weight is to burn off more calories than you eat. This requires self-discipline: eating less, exercising more, or preferably doing both. There are 3,500 calories in a pound of body weight. To lose one pound a week (a safe amount), you must eat an average of 500 fewer calories per day than you burn up. The most sensible diet for losing weight is one that is nutritionally balanced in carbohydrates, fats, and proteins. Most fad diets "work" by producing temporary weight loss—as a result of calorie restriction. But they are invariably too monotonous and are often too dangerous for long-term use. Unless a dieter develops and maintains better eating and exercise habits, weight lost on a diet will soon return.

*They warn you not to trust your doctor*

Quacks, who want you to trust them, suggest that most doctors are "butchers" and "poisoners." For the same reason, quacks also claim that doctors are nutrition illiterates. This, too, is untrue. The principles of nutrition are those of human biochemistry and physiology, courses required in every medical school. Some medical schools don't teach a separate required course labeled "Nutrition" because the subject is included in other courses at the points where it is most relevant. For example, nutrition in growth and development is taught in pediatrics, nutrition in wound healing is taught in surgery, and nutrition in pregnancy is covered in obstetrics. In addition, many medical schools do offer separate instruction in nutrition.

A physician's training, of course, does not end on the day of graduation from medical school or completion of specialty training. The medical profession advocates lifelong education, and some states require it for license renewal. Physicians can further their knowledge of nutrition by reading medical journals and textbooks, discussing cases with colleagues, and attending continuing education courses. Most doctors know what nutrients can and cannot do and can tell the difference between a real nutritional discovery and a piece of quack nonsense. Those who are unable to answer questions about dietetics (meal planning) can refer patients to someone who can—usually a registered dietitian.

Like all human beings, doctors sometimes make mistakes. However, quacks deliver mistreatment most of the time.

### They claim they are being persecuted by orthodox medicine and that their work is being suppressed because it's controversial

Quacks may also claim that the American Medical Association is against them because their cures would cut into the incomes that doctors make by keeping people sick. Don't fall for such nonsense! Reputable physicians are plenty busy. Moreover, many doctors engaged in prepaid health plans, group practice, full-time teaching, and government service receive the same salary whether or not their patients are sick—so keeping their patients healthy reduces their workload, not their income.

Quacks claim there is a "controversy" about facts between themselves and "the bureaucrats," organized medicine, or "the establishment." They clamor for medical examination of their claims, but ignore any evidence that refutes them.

Any physician who found a vitamin or other preparation that could cure sterility, heart disease, arthritis, cancer, or the like, could make an enormous fortune. Patients would flock to such a doctor (as they now do to those who *falsely* claim to cure such problems), and colleagues would shower the doctor with awards—including the $1,000,000+ Nobel Prize! And don't forget, doctors get sick, too. Do you believe they would conspire to suppress cures for diseases that also afflict them and their loved ones?

### They sue to intimidate their critics

The majority of "nutrition experts" who appear on TV talk shows and whose publications dominate the "health" sections in bookstores and health food stores are quacks and charlatans. Why are they not labeled as such? Many years ago, investigative reporter Ralph Lee Smith answered this question in an exposé of Carlton Fredericks. Smith said it is the "question of libel":

> A reputation for being legally belligerent can sometimes go far to insulate one from critical publicity. And if an attack does appear in print, a threat of legal action will sometimes bring a full retraction.

Smith noted that the threat of legal action can be particularly effective when made against scientific publications, especially those sponsored by universities or publicly supported organizations.

Many people assume that scientists will speak out against nutrition quacks because they have nothing to fear from a libel suit by a quack. Nothing to fear? Defending against a phony libel suit can be lengthy and cost tens of thousands of dollars. We need "Good Samaritan" laws to cover the cost of defending libel actions brought by quacks. We also need vigorous use of legal procedures against malicious lawsuits. Any critic sued by a quack should consider a countersuit for malicious harassment, abuse of process, and barratry.

Lawsuits have been used not only against critics, but also against insurance companies who refuse to pay for quack treatments. In some cases, courts have ruled that the company must pay because the language of the insurance policy did not specifically exclude the treatment in question or because the court gave undeserved credibility to claims that the treatment worked. A recent article in the *Journal of the American Medical Association* advised insurance companies to revise their contracts and urged the courts to base their judgments on peer-reviewed scientific literature and opinions from impartial court-appointed experts.

### More Public Protection Is Needed

The doctrines of freedom of speech and freedom of the press give quacks great leeway in deceiving the public. It is perfectly legal to give false or misleading advice as long as the person giving it is not selling the touted product or providing a service at the same time.

Quacks project an aura of sincerity and public interest. They spout (unprovable) "case histories" and glowing tales of personal experience. They cite sloppy and worthless "research" as "the great work of great men." Their deceptions dominate the media.

Can the Federal Communications Commission (FCC) or the Federal Trade Commission (FTC) attack nutrition misinformation via laws that require broadcasters to operate in the public interest as well as laws that require "truth in advertising"? However, the FCC usually acts only after receiving complaints, and *a public that does not know it is being misinformed cannot complain.* The FTC appears to tackle the grossest forms of advertising deception or deceptive trade practice. It seldom acts against subtle forms of misleading information, and many complaints it receives are shelved for "lack of agency manpower." Purveying misinformation for profit is a deceptive trade practice. The FTC is empowered to move against those who profit from public appearances in which they purvey such information, but it rarely does so.

Why don't the state attorneys general act? Presenting misleading nutrition information perpetrates a fraud on the consuming public. The First Amendment does not protect smut speech and writings that are alleged to injure mental health. Why then should it protect misleading nutrition communications that can harm both mental and physical health?

Few preachers of nutrition gospel ever mention the negative potential of their advice—for example, that excess vitamins or unproven remedies can harm people. I believe that this failure is prosecutable as fraudulent concealment or negligence chargeable not only to the huckster but also to the station or publisher that provides a forum. The states and/or their courts should revise or interpret their "reckless endangerment" statutes to include reckless endangerment of public health by promotion of dangerous "nutritional" remedies. I also wonder whether the more dangerous of the quack's misrepresentations could be enjoined as a public nuisance. Perhaps a public-spirited prosecutor will try these approaches someday.

Under our civil laws, it may be possible for a private citizen to recover substantial damages if harm results from reliance on the misinformation purveyed by a quack. The victim would need to establish that the purveyer had a duty not to mislead. When doctors recommend a remedy, they have a duty both to use care in selecting it and to warn of complications. Patients who are harmed because their doctor fails to do either one of these can sue for negligence. Quacks, too, should be held responsible for the harm *they* do.

A California case has created a precedent that can be cited by anyone who has been harmed by following the advice of a nutrition quack when given in a broadcast, and possibly in a book. In *Weirum vs. RKO General, Inc.,* the

Supreme Court of California upheld a jury verdict of $300,000 against a radio station that had offered a cash prize to the first person who could locate a traveling disc jockey. Two teenagers spotted the disc jockey and tried to follow him to a contest stopping point; but during the pursuit, one of the cars was forced off the road, killing its driver. The jury found that the broadcast had created a foreseeable risk to motorists because its contest conditions could stimulate accidents. Members of the National Council Against Health Fraud have informed many radio and television producers and book publishers that their quackery-promoting activities create unreasonable and foreseeable risks. Thus warned, they might have serious difficulty defending themselves against suits by injured parties.

When products are falsely promoted by an individual who is also selling them directly to a consumer, the illegality is clearly defined by state laws. For example, many health-food retailers, multilevel distributors, and bogus "nutritionists" advise clients to take products for specific health problems. In most such cases, the person giving the advice could be prosecuted for practicing medicine without a license, theft by deception, or other charges related to consumer fraud.

**The FDA Is under Attack**

Under current laws, it is illegal for manufacturers to make therapeutic claims that are not recognized by the scientific community. Many manufacturers circumvent these laws by marketing vitamins, minerals, amino acids, herbs, and various other products as "dietary supplements," even though they are really intended for therapeutic use. In 1991, the FDA established a Dietary Supplements Task Force to explore whether these products should be more tightly regulated.

Antiquackery leaders would like the term "dietary supplements" restricted to products composed of one or more essential nutrients that may be usefully added to the diet. Under this definition, modest doses of vitamins and minerals would qualify as ingredients. Single amino acids, even the essential ones, would not, because isolated amino acid deficiencies do not occur. Nor would the word "dietary supplement" be legal for herbal products and the large number of nutrient concoctions whose real purpose is intended to be therapeutic.

In 1992, the "health food" industry and its allies launched a massive letter-writing campaign to prevent the FDA from narrowing the definition of "dietary supplements." The centerpiece of this campaign is legislation spearheaded by Senator Orrin Hatch (R-UT) and Representative Bill Richardson (D-NM).

The 1993 versions of their bills are titled the Dietary Supplement and Health Education Act. Hatch's bill (S. 784) defines "dietary supplements" as vitamins, minerals, herbs, amino acids, and other substances intended "to supplement the diet by increasing the total diet intake." (This definition covers everything the health-food industry would like to call a supplement.) The bill would also (1) prevent the FDA from classifying such products as drugs, regulating their dosage, or making them available only by prescription; (2) permit manufacturers to make therapeutic claims based on flimsy evidence; and (3) stall most FDA regulatory actions by permitting manufacturers who receive a warning letter to protest to the Department of Health and Human Services or seek court review. Richardson's version (H.R. 1709) is similar but not quite as restrictive. If either bill passes, the FDA's ability to protect consumers from quack "nutrition" products will be severely weakened.

In June 1993, the Dietary Supplements Task Force issued twenty recommendations related to safety and honest labeling. These included: (1) the FDA should determine safe levels of daily intake for each vitamin and mineral; (2) capsules and tablets of individual amino acids should be regulated as drugs; (3) other types of "supplements" should be regulated as food additives, which would mean that if a substance has no known nutritive value, the label must say so; (4) the FDA should act against misleading "name claims," including brand names that imply therapeutic benefit; and (5) the FDA should continue to bring actions against "supplements" that are illegally marketed as drugs (intended for unproven therapeutic uses). The task force also urged the agency to establish and implement an educational campaign to provide the public with scientifically objective information about the safety, proper use, benefits, and risks of products. The Hatch/Richardson bills, of course, are intended to block implementation of some of these recommendations.

**Back-Door "Recognition"**

In 1991, former Congressman Berkley Bedell spearheaded passage of a law ordering the National Institutes of Health (NIH) to establish an office (now called the Office of Alternative Medicine) to foster research into unconventional practices. In various interviews, Bedell acknowledged that he had undergone unconventional treatment "to replenish nitrogen" for a suspected recurrence of prostate cancer. Early in 1992, NIH appointed an ad hoc advisory panel that included Bedell and leading advocates of acupuncture, energy medicine, homeopathy, Ayurvedic medicine, and several types of "alternative" cancer therapies. A few qualified researchers were placed on the panel, but they had little influence over subsequent events. In June 1992, the panel met to discuss research principles and to hear testimony from more than fifty assorted practitioners. In addition to promoting their own approach to health care, many panelists and testifiers praised NIH for its "openness" and commented to the press that the event "legitimized" unconventional medicine itself. The resultant publicity was massive. It remains to be seen whether the NIH Office of Alternative Medicine will actually foster useful research. Even if it does, any such benefit is unlikely to outweigh the harm caused by the publicity given to quack methods.

Hatch's and Richardson's bills would establish an NIH Office of Dietary Supplements, to coordinate and promote research on "the benefits of dietary supplements in maintaining health and preventing chronic disease and other health-related conditions" and to advise the FDA on dietary supplement issues. You can be sure that vitamin pushers would trumpet such an office as government "recognition" that their products are important.

## The Bottom Line

Vitamin pushers and food quacks benefit only themselves. Their victims are not only milked financially (for billions of dollars each year), but may also suffer serious harm from vitamin overdosage and from seduction away from proper medical care.

There is nutritional deficiency in this country, but it is found primarily among the poor, particularly among those who are elderly, pregnant, or young children. Their problems will not be solved by the phony panaceas of hucksters but by better dietary practices. The best way to get vitamins and minerals is in the packages provided by nature: foods that are part of a balanced and varied diet. If humans needed to eat pills for nutrition, pills would grow on trees.

The basic rule of good nutrition is moderation in all things. Contrary to the claim that "It may help," the advice of food quacks may harm—both your health and your pocketbook. They will continue to cheat the American public, however, until the communications industries develop sufficient concern for the public interest to attack their quackery instead of promoting it. And if the media cannot develop adequate social conscience on their own, they should be forced to do so by stronger laws and more vigorous law enforcement. Stronger regulation of "dietary supplements" is also essential.

I don't mean to imply that everyone who promotes quack ideas is deliberately trying to mislead people. One reason why quackery is so difficult to spot is that most people who spread health misinformation are quite sincere in their beliefs. For them nutrition is not a science but a religion—with quacks as their gurus. But where health is concerned, sincerity is not enough!

# 3

# The Make-Believe Doctors

## Robert C. Derbyshire, M.D.

Let me tell you a true story. Freddie Brant was born in Louisiana in 1926 and was forty-three years old at the time of my tale. Reared in poverty, he quit school after the fifth grade. After four years in the Army during World War II he found that jobs were scarce for a man with only a fifth grade education, so he joined the paratroops. In 1949, along with a fellow paratrooper, Brant was sentenced to seven years in the penitentiary for bank robbery. He began his "medical education" working in the prison hospital. After he was released, Brant continued his education by working for four years as a laboratory and x-ray technician for Dr. Reid L. Brown of Chattanooga, Tennessee. There he picked up not only more medical lore but also the diplomas of his employer.

Brant was now ready to begin the practice of medicine. Assuming the identity of Dr. Reid L. Brown, he moved to Texas where he obtained a license by endorsement and served for three years on the staff of the State Hospital at Terrell. He then resigned and took his wife on a vacation trip. Stopping for a Coca Cola in the small village of Groveton, Texas, Brant treated the injured leg of a child. He found that Groveton had long been without a doctor and its people were clamoring for medical care. "Dr. Brown" soon became established as the town physician and as a community leader.

Freddie Brant, alias Reid L. Brown, M.D., might still be carrying on his thriving practice in Groveton, Texas, had he not run afoul of a computer. By coincidence he ordered drugs from the same pharmaceutical firm in Louisiana that was used by the real Dr. Reid Brown. The computer gagged when it discovered orders on the same day from physicians with identical names in

Groveton and Chattanooga. Following an investigation, Freddie Brant was charged with forgery and with false testimony that he was a doctor.

The exposure of Freddie Brant caused great consternation in Groveton, but its citizens still rallied around their "doctor." Many were the testimonials to his skill. According to one news report, the list of his patients included some of Groveton's leading citizens as well as farmers, loggers, and welfare patients. The druggist said that many cases of hardship were caused by the Freddie's arrest. A particularly glowing testimonial came from a farmer who said:

> My wife has been sick for fourteen years. We've been to doctors in Lufkin, Crockett, and Trinity, and he did her more good than any of 'em. She was all drawed up, bent over, you ought to have seen her. He's brought her up and now she's milking cows and everything.

The citizens of Groveton remained loyal to Brant, and a grand jury refused to indict him. Authorities then brought him to trial in another county for perjury, but the case ended in a hung jury with eight members voting for acquittal. *Chicago's American* reported that justice was thwarted because of a "lava flow of testimonials from Groveton and Terrell to the effect that Freddie Brant was a prince of a medical man, license or no license." In an unkind cut, the report stated that the people of Groveton should have known that Reid Brown was not a doctor because he did too many things wrong. For example, he made house calls for five dollars and charged only three dollars for an office visit. He approved of Medicare and would drive for miles to visit a patient, often without fee if the patient was poor. Besides, his handwriting was legible.

What were the secrets of Freddie Brant's success as an impersonator? They were many, but the main ones were his readiness to refer any potentially complicated case to nearby towns, a personality which inspired confidence, and a willingness to take time to listen to his patients.

From 1969 through 1978, I found forty-seven impostors who were "successful" enough to be worthy of study. This figure did not include fly-by-night impersonators who pretended to be physicians in order to cash worthless checks or engage in confidence games. Most of these are exposed within a few hours or days.

Let us take a look at the typical successful impostor. His medical background might consist of a tour of duty as a medical corpsman in the Army or as a pharmacist's mate in the Navy. He might have served as a hospital orderly or as a laboratory technician. He might have obtained his medical education as a patient in a mental hospital. The sole medical background of one was service as a hospital elevator operator. By associating with physicians, the impostor learns enough medical jargon to fool the unwary. He must also have a good memory and a persuasive manner. Curiously, I have found no records of women medical impostors.

A surprising number of impostors had no medical background whatever. Anthony Vecchiarello and his brother, Louis, were two such practitioners. Together with Marino J. Maturo, they operated a thriving clinic in Washington, D.C., for five years before the authorities finally caught up with them. Anthony had been a mechanic. Louis, among other things, had sold burglar alarms. Maturo, having dropped out of the University of Miami after failing chemistry, zoology, mathematics, and Italian, had worked as an x-ray technician in Florida. All three had obtained full medical licenses using forged Mexican credentials that had never been checked by the authorities. Two of them had also been admitted to membership in the district medical society, which soon began to refer patients to them.

**State Hospital Opportunities**

State hospitals have provided a pathway to fraudulent medical practice. One of the most fascinating examples is that of Oscar Monte Levy, a man with no medical background who was hired as superintendent of a state mental hospital in West Virginia. Levy's credentials were based solely upon a diploma stolen from a Dr. Menendez, a graduate of the University of Havana Medical School. This man might have enjoyed a long and profitable career as a hospital administrator. But he resigned after nine months and moved to another region where he obtained a position as staff psychiatrist in a state hospital mainly on the basis of recommendations from the first state. However, his second career was cut short when his new colleagues became suspicious of his manner and exposed him. Obviously Levy committed a grave error by resigning his high position as a hospital superintendent. I could not learn his reasons for doing so. Possibly he became tired of administrative duties and yearned to practice clinical psychiatry.

Whatever mild amusement I derived from the story of "Dr. Menendez" soon turned to dismay as I read on. The director of the Department of Health in the state where Menendez was first employed, whose duty it was to check the credentials of this impostor, said that the state hospital was hiring certain foreign doctors on a temporary basis. Obviously, the director's examination of credentials had been entirely superficial.

When Levy was finally exposed, he was sentenced to three years in prison—not for impersonating a doctor, but for what the authorities considered a more serious crime. He had been so indiscreet as to marry a West Virginia girl while still wed to a woman from New York, and was therefore guilty of bigamy.

While the authorities in neither state should have been taken in by "Dr. Menendez," there might have been extenuating circumstances, all too familiar to members of boards of medical examiners. During the 1970s, there were pressures in this country to resettle foreign physicians, particularly those who were thought to be fugitives from communism. Second, a shortage of qualified applicants for staff positions at state hospitals resulted in standards being lowered to permit physicians unqualified for regular licenses to fill these positions. Third, highly placed politicians often interceded for them. These three factors combined to place such pressure on boards of medical examiners that it is remarkable that they resisted as effectively as they did.

Despite these problems, I was able to find only six impostors who had entered practice by way of state hospitals. No doubt others had gone undetected.

## Length of Practice

How long do impostors flourish? At least twenty-two are known to have practiced for more than a year. There were two whose hoaxes lasted for twenty years. Perhaps the all-time champion was "Dr. J.D. Phillips," who practiced medicine in various places for thirty years. According to an article in *Coronet* (August, 1953), he fooled not only patients in eleven states, but also the United States government; several county and state health departments; and dozens of respectable physicians, nurses, and administrators in various hospitals. According to *Coronet,* "Rarely has a faker been unmasked more often and less permanently. Certainly no one has gone to so much trouble to remain loyal to his profession." His medical knowledge was gained from the doctor in his home town with whom he made rounds. Said "Dr. Phillips" without undue modesty: "I went around with him and absorbed it all. I have a photographic memory and am not exactly dumb."

"Dr. Phillips" served time in various penitentiaries for passing bad checks and for defrauding hotels. He used these periods to study in the prison libraries. Finally his background was so firm that he was entrusted with surgery at the Maryland State House of Correction. According to the physician in charge, Phillips was "literally a good resident." At some time during this period he was able to steal a medical license from a physician long inactive because of illness. He then had the nerve to send an affidavit to his adopted medical school that he had lost his M.D. diploma. He was promptly sent a duplicate.

The downfall of "Dr. Phillips" was finally brought about by his greed and an alert insurance agent. Following an automobile accident in which he suffered injuries to his neck and arm, he was sued for $600. He countered with a $40,000 suit, including $35,000 to compensate him for his inability to practice medicine. The insurance agent, disturbed by Phillips' dirty fingernails, questioned his story, and he was exposed in court. His medical career ended when he was sentenced to fifteen to twenty years for perjury.

How are impostors exposed? Those whose medical careers last only a few months are so inept that they give themselves away. But exposure of the "experts" has proven difficult and often comes about by accident. Maturo and the Vecchiarello brothers were exposed by chance because of an investigation by the U.S. Attorney in Washington. While looking into an unrelated matter, he became suspicious of flaws in their forged Mexican credentials. Further investigation resulted in their indictments for fraud. But the matter did not end there. The three impostors were so brash that they obtained a federal court order that allowed them to continue in practice until they were finally brought to trial and convicted six months later. Needless to say, the trial caused great embarrassment to the licensing authorities of the District of Columbia and stimulated them to adopt more stringent procedures for the issuance of medical licenses.

The notorious "Dr. Frank," was responsible for at least five deaths in Chicago, A former mental patient who had taken over the practice of a vacationing doctor, Frank was exposed by a nurse of whom he became enamored. She often made house calls with him and noticed that he was unsure about the doses of drugs and mispronounced some medical terms. Frank's downfall came about because he became too ardent in wooing the nurse and tried to choke her when she resisted his charms. She investigated his credentials, found that he was not a high-ranking graduate of Northwestern University as he had claimed, and reported him to the police. When they arrested Frank, they found a gun and a large quantity of morphine in his doctor's bag. He was sentenced to three years in the penitentiary for illegal possession of drugs.

Surprisingly few impostors have credentials in the form of medical school diplomas or state medical licenses. Of the forty-seven impostors in my study, only twelve had bothered to steal or forge such credentials. This oversight is amazing because there was a well-known firm in California that specialized in producing phony documents. At least one impostor was familiar with this company. He not only ordered complete medical credentials, but also turned himself into an author. Removing the title pages from a respectable book, he had the book rebound with his name on the cover. His fatal mistake was in failing to realize that he might be asked by a colleague to discuss the book's contents!

The attitude of some impostors seems to be, "Why bother to obtain phony diplomas when they are not necessary?" I am astonished at the number of hospitals that have accepted applicants for positions without first examining their credentials. This is not confined to state hospitals. A glaring example is the case of "Dr. David William Baker," who claimed to have graduated from Temple University Medical School in 1962. From a state hospital in Idaho he went to Seattle where he worked in two hospitals for a total of three months, including two months in the emergency room of one of them. A hospital spokesman quoted in a Seattle newspaper said that Baker had been hired on the recommendation of a doctor who had known him when he worked at the blood bank. The hospital detected the impostor only when it learned that the AMA had sent out a circular declaring that a man named Baker was posing as a doctor. The administrator's justification for employing him was that Baker claimed his credentials were in transit and he was preparing to appear before the state licensing board. Hospital officials weakly contended that Baker was not a member of the staff but worked in the emergency room where he was always under the supervision of another physician.

**Attitudes toward Impostors**

As I studied case histories, I was struck by how many people were gullible enough to lend money to impostors. I was astonished by the readiness of bankers, whom I had always regarded as paragons of caution, to help impostors start their medical practice. In one instance a physician was the victim when he lent an impostor a considerable sum. Equally fair game are citizens of many small towns with desperate shortages of doctors, who will lionize any present-able individual who claims to be a physician.

Once in practice, of course, the impostor relies on the fact that most patients who do not look seriously ill will recover by themselves. This enables him to fool many people into thinking that he has given them treatment. If he is friendly, if he shows interest and compassion, and if he quickly refers to specialists those patients who do seem quite ill, the impostor is likely to develop a loyal patient following. In fact, many people will come to "swear by him." So much so that even when he is exposed as a fraud, they will defend him and be grievously hurt because the authorities have removed their "trusted family physician."

Typical is the case of the fraud who, for some six years, successfully practiced in a small town in New York State. His following of devoted patients was large; he even won the esteem of his colleagues who frequently called upon him for consultations. When he was finally exposed by the Board of Medical Examiners, the anguished cries of his devoted followers could be heard all the way across the Hudson River. They even circulated petitions to prevent him from being banished. Nevertheless he was brought to justice and convicted of fraud.

The reactions of these people and of those in Groveton, Texas, to the unmasking of Freddie Brant are by no means isolated examples. Such reactions are particularly prevalent in small towns. One can only speculate as to why these victims of hoaxes adopt such defensive attitudes. Some, like the victims of other confidence games, are embarrassed about being taken in. Some may feel a need to justify their faith in the impostor to avoid the appearance of stupidity in the eyes of their neighbors. Others may believe they have actually been helped.

Another difficulty in exposing medical impostors stems from the indifference of district attorneys. Apparently these law enforcers are not enthusiastic about pursuing people whom they regard as petty criminals, and this is how impostors are regarded in most states. Only in a few states is the practice of medicine without a license defined as a felony; in the rest it is a misdemeanor. I remember one instance in which my board of medical examiners discovered a man who was practicing without a license. On two different occasions the investigator for the board obtained receipted bills, copies of prescriptions, and samples of drugs the man had been dispensing, certainly enough evidence for the conviction of this fraud. But the district attorney showed no interest in prosecuting him. It was not until some two years later, *after the impostor had been responsible for the death of a patient,* that the state police arrested him on a charge of manslaughter for which he was convicted and sentenced to five years in prison.

The attitude of newspapers toward some impostors is interesting. While they may make every effort to report the facts accurately, their stories sometimes contain a strong underlying note of amusement. In the case just cited, after the impostor had been arrested and charged with manslaughter, the local paper printed a feature in its Sunday edition based upon an interview in the felon's jail cell. This took the form of a human interest story that depicted the impostor as an amusing eccentric and all but ignored the charge of manslaughter.

## Serious Danger

Up to a point, many of the tales of impersonation *are* amusing, provided the reader is not one of the authorities who has been duped. But the time must come when one has to be serious, particularly in light of the dangers that impostors pose to the public. Freddie Brant, alias "Dr. Brown," tried to justify his conduct by saying, "I never lost a patient." Didn't he? How could he know? Another famous impostor, M.L. Langford of Jasper, Missouri, pointed out in his defense that he performed no surgery and referred any patient who might have complications. But could he always recognize complications or foresee them? Impostors *do* kill people, albeit not always as dramatically as the notorious Dr.

Frank, who persuaded a physician to help him obtain a listing with a medical referring service.

The harm caused by make-believe doctors has not been limited to physical trauma. This was brought forcibly to my attention by a resident of an Eastern city—whom I shall call Mr. A—who sent me the following account. In 1977, he read a newspaper account of an impostor named William J. Lott, who practiced for thirty days in the Maryland Penitentiary. The story also mentioned a similar case, that of Freddie Brant, alias Dr. Reid L. Brown. This news jolted Mr. A because he was a former patient of Brant's but had no idea that he was an impostor. In 1965, when Mr. A was sixteen years old, he had been truant from school. His stepfather decided he was insane and managed to have him committed to the State Hospital in Terrell, Texas. There he was placed under the tender care of "Dr. Reid L. Brown," who prescribed a variety of drugs and subjected him to electroshock therapy. "Dr. Brown" also signed various legal documents concerning his diagnosis. Mr. A wanted desperately to have the diagnosis of insanity expunged from the record and asked for my help. All I could do was to refer him to a good lawyer.

What motivates these people to impersonate doctors? The immediate answer of the cynic is that they do it to make money. While it is true that some yearn for the imagined rich and easy life of the doctor, this is not the only answer. Some envy the physician's authority and social position. Others are deranged, many having served terms in mental hospitals. Freddie Brant simply said, "I always wanted to be a doctor." Robert Crichton, in his fascinating book *The Great Impostor* (Random House, 1959) describes the career of Fred Demara, Jr., who adopted many identities including that of Trappist monk and Surgeon Lieut. Joseph Cyr of the Royal Canadian Navy. In the latter identity, he performed heroic feats of surgery aboard a destroyer before his final exposure. According to Crichton, psychiatrists have labeled the impostor a borderline schizophrenic with a document syndrome and something like histrionic genius. Demara expressed himself this way: "I am a superior sort of liar. I don't tell any truth at all, so my story has a unity of parts, a structural integrity. It sounds more like the truth than truth itself."

**Prevention**

So far I have confined myself to the methods of medical impostors. Now let us look at how they might be controlled. As with disease, the best strategy is obviously prevention. Several agencies are responsible for the proper screening of physicians. The most important of these are the state boards of medical examiners, the medical societies, and the hospitals. The primary duty of the licensing boards is to ensure that all who are licensed are qualified. More careful screening of applicants for positions in state hospitals should be carried out, preferably by the boards. Documents must never be accepted on faith! No matter how convincing an applicant appears, his documents must be verified at their sources. The investigations should be systematic, beginning with insistence upon completion of a detailed application blank, which must include a notarized statement from the applicant that he is indeed the person whose credentials he is presenting. It is important that the physician be required to present at least two photographs, one to be affixed to the application, the other to be filed for future reference in case of a question of identity. As an added precaution, the board might insist that the photograph be affixed to the application form before it is returned to the medical school for certification or, in the case of licensure by endorsement, to the board issuing the original license. Thus the photograph can be compared with photos filed previously.

Another important method of preventing licensure of impostors is the use of the personal interview. In states that license large numbers of physicians it might be difficult for the administrative officer to interview them all. In these states the interviews could be divided among the members of the board. Although opinions differ about the value of the interview, an experienced person should be able to learn much by observing a candidate. Examiners can be alert to danger signals such as poor personal grooming, vague answers to specific questions concerning medical subjects, and failure to identify properly professors in the school from which the applicant claims to have graduated.

Still another method of detecting impostors is the requirement that all applicants for licensure be fingerprinted. Many people feel that professionals should not be subjected to such an indignity. But this is not as drastic a requirement as many think, and most applicants submit to it with good grace. After all, fingerprinting is required in applications for many jobs, particularly those associated with the federal government. Robert Sprecher, writing about licensure problems in the legal profession *(Federal Bulletin* 55:188–200, 1968), made an interesting observation. The mere requirement that applicants be fingerprinted will encourage them to admit to previous conviction of crimes. For example, bar examinations were given in Michigan and Illinois at the same time. Michigan had 281 applicants, Illinois 273. Both states asked applicants whether they had ever been charged with a crime or arrested. In Michigan, where fingerprints were required, twenty-eight people admitted to previous arrests or convictions. In Illinois, which did not require fingerprints, only two made such admissions. Obviously, fingerprinting is a deterrent to false statements.

Years ago, when the New Mexico Board of Medical Examiners began to require fingerprinting, the cards had to be sent through the local chief of police for processing by the Federal Bureau of Investigation. The chief's response to my request was one of tolerant amusement: "If the doctor wants to play detective, I suppose we must help him. But I am sure we will not turn up anything." Two weeks later, having received some forty FBI reports, he appeared at my office waving two dossiers excitedly. One applicant had a record of nine arrests in New Jersey for crimes that ranged in seriousness from petty larceny to armed robbery. The second had served five years in the penitentiary of another state for embezzlement. While this incident did not involve physician impersonators, it does show what can be accomplished by requiring fingerprints of every applicant for licensure. Impostors frequently have criminal records. Even such a smooth confidence man as Freddie Brant might have been deterred or exposed by this method.

If the practice of medicine without a license were a felony instead of a misdemeanor, as it is in most states—and if district attorneys could be persuaded to take their duties more seriously—some impostors might think twice before establishing their practices.

Though medical impostors are rare, and some regard them with amusement, we must not forget that they are con men and potential killers. Medical examining boards, hospitals, medical societies, and concerned individuals must take every precaution to keep their number to a minimum.

**Editors' Note**

This chapter is updated from the 1980 edition of *The Health Robbers*. It illustrates how individuals with little or no scientific training may convince large numbers of people that they are skilled and caring healers. Since the 1980 version was published, medical licensing procedures have become more stringent and very few cases of "successful" medical impostors have come to light. However, the number of bogus "nutritionists" and other nonscientific practitioners has increased sharply.

# 4

# Occult Health Practices

**Ray Hyman, Ph.D.**

Major C.L. Cooper-Hunt, M.A., Ps.D., Ms.D., D.D., Ph.D., M.S.F., a practitioner of "medical radiesthesia," provided the following definition in his book *Radiesthetic Analysis*:

> Radiesthesia, or the faculty of radio-perception, is a term describing the power of detecting the vibrations, or waves of force, which emanate from all manifested nature, including the four great kingdoms, or fields, of minerals, plants, animals, and human—yes, and why not the further fields of force beyond our own particular label of consciousness, i.e., the angelic, celestial and divine. . . . In order to detect and measure these inner forces various implements have been employed from the hazel-twig and the pendulum to the latest highly sensitive apparatus evolved by such enthusiastic workers as Abrams, Drown, and de la Warr.*

In his "great crusade against the inroad of disease both physical and mental," Major Cooper-Hunt accumulated a "growing pile of testimonial

---

*Albert Abrams, M.D. (1864-1924), considered the "dean of gadget quacks" by the AMA, made millions of dollars treating patients and leasing his gadgets to others. He claimed that all parts of the body emit electrical impulses of different frequencies that vary with health and disease. Illnesses (as well as age, sex, religion, and location) could be diagnosed by "tuning in" on the patient's blood or handwriting sample with one machine; and diseases could be treated by feeding proper vibrations into the body with another machine. Abrams willed his fortune to the Electronic Medical Foundation, whose subsequent president, Fred J. Hart, founded the National Health Federation (see Chapter 28). Ruth Drown, a chiropractor who followed in Abrams' footsteps until her death in 1965, claimed that she could help patients even if they were thousands of miles away. In 1943, George and Margaret de la Warr founded Delawarr Laboratories, in Oxford, England, where work based on Abrams' principles (now referred to as "radionics" or "psychotronics") was carried out for more than thirty-five years.

letters extending for over ten years of practice from the so-called 'incurables' testifying to definite alleviation and in a multitude of cases to permanent cure." One of his simpler cases was a woman with severe insomnia that had not yielded to various types of remedies. After testing her "polarity" with a pendulum, Cooper-Hunt and his wife concluded that the woman had been sleeping with her head in the wrong direction. "Radiesthetic examination indicated a different alignment and the patient [was] advised to try it out," the Cooper-Hunts reported. "Her subsequent report was complete harmony and sound sleep."

Miss F, who practiced "regression therapy," believed that most illnesses and emotional problems result from patterns and traumas experienced in "previous lives." One of her patients, she told my psychology class, had suffered from severe lower abdominal pains for which medical doctors could find neither cause nor cure. When "regressed" to a previous existence, the patient showed signs of intense pain and complained that a dagger had been thrust into his lower abdomen. At Miss F's suggestion, the patient went through the motions of "removing" the dagger. The pain was immediately relieved and never returned.

Miss F also enlightened us about a California physician who had suffered from overwhelming guilt. In six of his "previous lives," it turned out, the doctor had been the innocent victim of false accusations and punishments. This indicated to Miss F that he was still punishing himself for doing something wrong during some still earlier life. With further probing, Miss F discovered that the doctor, as "one of the major scientists on Atlantis," had made a decision that had contributed to the island's destruction. His subsequent feelings of guilt were based on the assumption that he had been completely responsible for the disaster. Miss F convinced him that he had punished himself enough and that she had another patient who, in a previous life, had also contributed to the destruction of Atlantis! These revelations, according to Miss F, lifted the burden of guilt from the doctor's shoulders and enabled him to resume living with increased effectiveness.

In *The Psychic Healing Book,* Amy Wallace and Bill Henkin reported the following case:

> Martha, a 22-year-old woman, had scarred Fallopian tubes and was supposedly sterile. Doctors told her she would never have another child. After several healings, she returned to one of these doctors, who discovered that the scar tissue had disappeared.

Using methods that the authors felt could be taught to most people, Ms. Wallace claimed to have helped, to at least "partial recovery," cases of hemophilia, multiple sclerosis, cancer, arthritis, and spinal disorders.

Mary Coddington's book *In Search of the Healing Energy* cites a dramatic case of instant healing. At a beach party, a slightly intoxicated man tripped while emerging from an automobile parked near the edge of the beach. "As he fell, there was the characteristic snapping sound of breaking bones. Inspection showed a compound fracture of the left leg just above the ankle," the book reported. An old woman, a practitioner of Hawaiian (*huna*) magic, pressed the man's bones together and recited a healing prayer. After a while, she said: "The healing is finished. Stand up. You can walk." The injured man stood up and walked. His leg was apparently completely healed.

Former NASA physicist Laura Brennan says she has been healing illness through the "human energy field" for more than fifteen years. In the October 1990 *East West* magazine, she stated that she communicates with spirit guides and that "internal viewing" enables her to see inside the human body. She also claimed that reading "auras" enables her to detect tumors, heart disease, hepatitis and many other problems, and that her own case of cervical dysplasia was diagnosed and healed by a practitioner who "balanced and cleansed" her aura. Her first book, *Hands of Light,* was said to have been published in eight languages, with about 135,000 copies distributed in English.

## Characteristics of Occult Healing

Each of the above cases involves the use of a supposed force or technique unrecognized by medical science. Such forces are the hallmark of occult healing. The word "occult" means hidden, secret, or mysterious. Some occult healers claim psychic powers; others say they use a force or energy that is natural but as yet unrecognized by science. Some healers don't specify the source of their alleged power, while others credit a Supreme Being, "spirit guides" (who may or may not be souls of the dead), a previous incarnation, beings from other "planes" or worlds, or similarly esoteric sources. Many healers are eclectic, eagerly embracing all theories and claims, even contradictory ones.

In addition to crediting mysterious forces, occult practitioners share another characteristic: They do not use measurable data to support their claims. Nor do they even try to collect such data. Instead, they offer *testimonials* from satisfied clients.

So what? Is there anything wrong with using reports from satisfied customers as evidence that a healing system works? Isn't the goal of medical treatment to make people better? If people say they have gotten better, isn't this evidence in favor of a treatment? What better way to evaluate a treatment than to try it? Is not the proof of the pudding in its eating?

Life would be simpler if medical treatments could be tested as easily as puddings. But healing is far more complicated than cooking. If a woman says she sleeps better after being advised to change her position, should we accept this as proof that a pendulum can determine "polarity"? If two patients improve after undergoing intense emotional experiences with Miss F, does this argue for the reality of "previous existences"? If scar tissue or abnormal cervical cells disappear after consultation with a psychic healer, does this prove that psychic forces did the job?

## Why Testimonials Are Undependable

For several reasons, such testimonials are worthless as evidence. The first reason should be obvious: In each case, nonoccult causes could have produced the improvement. No control comparisons are available.

Instant healing of a compound fracture, *if it took place as described above,* would provide powerful evidence in favor of *huna.* But how can we be sure that a fracture occurred? No doctor was present and no x-ray film was obtained. We are told that a man fell down while getting out of a car and that someone heard "the characteristic snapping of breaking bones." Does such a sound exist? If it does, is there reason to believe that the storyteller was experienced enough to recognize it? We also are told that "inspection" showed a compound fracture, but whether a qualified observer was present is not specified in the account. Worse yet, can we be sure that the entire story is not fabricated?

Another reason, then, why testimonials are useless as evidence is that they lack timely, objective documentation. Unaided human observation and memory are highly fallible. That's why scientists rely on carefully designed experiments rather than unaided and nonstandardized human testimony. The scientific method was created to ensure that scientists base their conclusions on data that are meaningful. Unlike investigators who follow scientific rules to measure outcome, testimonial-givers make their own rules about what counts as "improvement." If objective observations are not recorded before and after "healing" is performed, the situation is ideal for self-deception.

Dr. Louis Rose, in his book *Faith Healing,* tells how he tried for eighteen years to find evidence of healing due to a spiritual or supernatural power. Enlisting the cooperation of Harry Edwards, Britain's most famous faith healer, and other occult healers, Rose collected ninety-five cases of reported cures. In fifty-eight of these cases, he could find no medical records. In twenty-two others, available records contradicted the reported results. The remaining cases were ambiguous in other ways.

The late Dr. William A. Nolen, a surgeon from Minnesota, spent two years watching faith healers at work and examined many of their patients (see Chapter 24). He concluded that no patient with organic disease had been helped. James Randi, a prominent conjurer and paranormal investigator, reached the same conclusion in *The Faith Healers.* My own experience in tracking down cases has been similar. Adequate records of diagnosis and outcome are either unavailable or contradict the reported accounts.

## "But It Works"

Despite the lack of "scientific" evidence, it would be a mistake to dismiss occult healing as unworthy of scientific investigation. Huge numbers of people believe that occult practices work. Every system—whether based on the position of the stars, the swing of a pendulum, the fall of cards or dice, the accidents of nature, or the intuitions of a psychic—claims its quota of satisfied customers. We need to understand why so many people believe in and patronize occult healers.

It is not difficult to understand how people can be misled into thinking that an illness has been healed by an unorthodox method. For most ailments, recovery occurs without treatment. When spontaneous recovery occurs in conjunction with occult healing, patients typically credit the occultist. Some illnesses respond favorably to suggestion and other psychological factors. The positive and confident attitude of the healer may actually relieve symptoms, especially those related to tension.

An additional factor is what psychologist Daryl Bem calls "self-perception theory." People consider themselves to be rational creatures and like to believe that they do things for sensible reasons. If they patronize a healer, they are strongly motivated to believe this makes sense and will look for reasons to support this belief. Even if, by objective standards, their condition deteriorates, they may find something positive to say about the healer. They may claim, for example, that they feel better or that without the healer's intervention, their condition would have become much worse.

To scientists who insist upon objective evidence, random sampling, double-blind tests, and the like, believers respond that "people should be treated as individuals, not statistics." The abstract nature of scientific data pales when compared with emotionally charged personal experience. As psychologists have amply demonstrated, one vivid example will often take precedence over statistical data based on controlled experiments with thousands of people. But rather than question the nature of their own beliefs, those who "know" that occult practices work see science as too dogmatic.

## The Fallacy of Personal Validation

Reliance on testimonials is a form of what psychologists call "the fallacy of personal validation." In 1948, the psychologist Bertram Forer administered a personality test to the thirty-nine students in one of his courses. One week later, he gave each student a typed personality sketch with his name on it—supposedly the "results" of the tests. Unknown to the students, however, each one actually received an identical list of thirteen statements that Forer had copied from an astrology book:

- You have a great need for other people to like and admire you.

- You have a tendency to be critical of yourself.

- You have a great deal of unused capacity which you have not turned to your advantage.

- While you have some personality weaknesses, you are generally able to compensate for them.

- Your sexual adjustment has presented problems for you.

- Disciplined and self-controlled outside, you tend to be worrisome and insecure inside.

- At times you have serious doubts as to whether you have made the right decision or done the right thing.

- You prefer a certain amount of change and variety and become dissatisfied when hemmed in by restrictions and limitations.

- You pride yourself as an independent thinker and do not accept others' statements without satisfactory proof.

- You have found it unwise to be too frank in revealing yourself to others.

- At times you are extroverted, affable, sociable, while at other times you are introverted, wary, reserved.

- Some of your aspirations tend to be pretty unrealistic.

- Security is one of your major goals in life.

After reading the sketch, students were asked to rate how well it revealed their basic personality characteristics. On a scale of 0 (poor) to 5 (perfect), thirty-five out of thirty-nine rated it 4 or better; and sixteen of these rated it as perfect! Many other investigators have confirmed and added to these findings.

It turns out to be surprisingly easy to get people to accept a fake personality sketch as a unique description of themselves.

Forer remarked that psychic readers depend solely on personal validation to evaluate their practice. Because his research showed clearly that personal validation is unreliable, he called reliance on such evidence "the fallacy of personal validation." This phenomenon also plays a role in the acceptance of occult healing and other paranormal claims. It is another reason why objective measurements obtained under double-blind conditions are necessary to validate treatment methods. How people feel——or how they say they feel—is not enough.

In 1984, the Committee for the Investigation of Claims of the Paranormal (CSICOP) asked all 1,200 American newspapers that published astrology columns to carry a disclaimer saying "astrological forecasts should be read for entertainment value only. Such predictions have no reliable basis in scientific fact." More than forty papers are doing this, and a few others have reported CSICOP's request as a news item.

## Cold Reading

If a fake sketch can convince people, think how much more effective a presentation can be if actually tailored to the client. Such tailoring is the essence of "cold reading." Using this technique, the "reader" (using palms, tea leaves, a crystal ball, tarot cards, or whatever) is able to persuade a client encountered for the first time ("cold") that the reading captures the essence of the client's personality and problems.

The reading may begin with general statements like those in Forer's sketch. By carefully observing the client's reactions, the reader gradually adapts the description to fit the specific attributes and problems of the client. Much useful information can be gained by observing clothing, hair style, complexion, carriage, physique, speech, and mannerisms. As the reading progresses, the client unwittingly supplies other clues in his reactions to specific statements. Sometimes these reactions are spoken approval or denial. More often they are nonverbal cues such as pupil size, breathing rate, posture, and facial expressions.

A skilled reader can quickly tell which statements "hit the mark" and develop these further. As this happens, the client will usually be persuaded that the reader, by some uncanny means, has gained insight into the client's innermost thoughts. His guard goes down and he actually tells the reader the details of what is bothering him. After a suitable interval, the reader repackages and feeds back this information and the client is further amazed at how much the reader "knows" about him. The client never realizes that everything he has been told is based on what he revealed to the reader.

John Mulholland, a magician well known during the 1930s and 1940s, published a classic illustration of cold reading. During the Great Depression, a character reader was visited by a young lady wearing expensive jewelry, a wedding band, and a black dress of cheap material. The reader also noted that she was wearing shoes that were advertised for people with foot trouble. (Pause for a moment, imagine that you are the reader, and see what you can make of these clues.)

The reader proceeded to flabbergast the woman with his "insights." He assumed that she wanted help, as did most of his female customers, with a love or financial problem. The black dress and wedding band indicated that she had recently become widowed. The jewelry suggested financial comfort during the marriage, but the cheap dress was a sign that her husband's death had left her penniless. The orthopedic shoes suggested that she was standing on her feet more than usual. From this he deduced that the woman had to work to support herself.

The reader drew the following conclusions, which turned out to be correct: The lady had met a man who had proposed to her. Although she wanted to marry him to end her economic hardship, she felt guilty about marrying so soon after her husband's death. The reader told her what she had come to hear— that it was all right to marry without further delay.

Notice what made this a "successful" reading. The reader picked up information that the client unwittingly provided. In addition to feeding this back to the client to create the illusion of an all-knowing guru, the reader also told her what she desperately wanted to hear. Consider how these factors operate in the context of occult healing—where the client seeks hope and comforting answers.

"Psychics" and healers have another powerful force working for them: what the psychologist Sir Frederic Bartlett called "the effort after meaning." People constantly search for the meaning of what they see. We try to make sense out of what others tell us, what they do, and what we ourselves say and do. We are better than the best computers at finding patterns and meaning hidden in the complexity of the world and human behavior. But sometimes we overdo it and attribute meaning to coincidental events.

In the client's mind, correct statements confirm the power of the reader— and the more powerful the reader, the more likely the client's problems will be solved. So the client works hard to confirm the reader's power. Suppose, for example, a reader suggests that you have found it unwise to be too frank in revealing yourself to others (item #10 of Forer's fake sketch). If you trust the reader, you will try to make sense out of his statement by thinking of circumstances in your life that confirm it. Suppose you recently offended a friend by calling the friend's obsession with astrology foolish. Then you upset your parents by announcing that you just moved in with this friend. So you assume that the reader is referring to these events. The more you want the reading to succeed, the harder you will search your memory for evidence to "verify" the reader's statements.

### "Psychic Hotlines"

During the past few years, many enterprising individuals have marketed "psychic" advice by telephone. In the typical operation, callers dial a "900" number and are charged $2 to $4 per minute for the advice. In February 1993, ABC-TV's "Prime Time Live" aired the results of a three-month investigation of a lucrative "psychic hotline." One undercover investigator had no prior knowledge of occult matters. After being hired, she underwent a few days of training in tarot cards, astrology, and numerology. She then used her intuition (plus code words written on tarot cards) to formulate her responses to callers. She reported being instructed to permit suicidal callers to run up their bill before referring them to a legitimate suicide hotline. Another undercover investigator, posing as a prospective investor, interviewed a company director who said, "Most of the people's personal lives—who work for us—are just total shambles. How they could even give the stuff out is incredible."

### Self-Deception Can Be Extremely Powerful

Still another factor that helps readers succeed is what psychologists call "the power of the situation." Even if a client is skeptical or believes that psychic reading is nonsense, the very fact of participation can set up psychological forces that encourage belief. Most people underestimate how powerful these forces can be.

A reporter once checked with me before he visited a well-known psychic. After the visit, he declared it an unqualified success. The reading had lasted approximately an hour. During most of that time, the reader had made statements that were either wrong or so general that they could apply to anyone. Near the end of the interview, the reporter's mind began to wander and he thought about trouble he was having with his girlfriend. The reader then said, "I see that you are having trouble with a relationship." The impact of this remark, coming at the very moment he was concerned about his affair, was so powerful that the reporter swept aside consideration of all the other wrong statements and useless banter. Even though the reporter agreed with me that just about everyone his age was probably experiencing a problem with a relationship, he could not shake the conviction that the reader was talking about the reporter's specific relationship. He was convinced that this reader had special powers.

The client is not the only person who can be taken in by what happens during the reading. During my teens I began reading palms as a way to supplement my income as a magician and mentalist. I did not believe in palmistry, but I knew that to convince clients I had to act as though I did. After a few years, I became a firm believer in palmistry because it appeared to work. One day a friend for whom I had considerable respect suggested an interesting experiment: to deliberately give readings opposite to what the lines in the hand indicated. I tried this with a few clients. To my surprise and horror, these readings were just as successful as my previous ones! Ever since then I have been interested in the powerful forces that can convince people that something is so when it isn't. It is clear that the way people feel about a "treatment" they have experienced is very often unrelated to its effectiveness.

## Spiritualism and the "New Age"

The spiritualist movement was launched in 1848 when Margaret and Kate Fox claimed they were able to communicate with the dead. Through a series of rapping noises, the "spirits from beyond" gave advice, made predictions, and consoled loved ones. The Fox sisters performed in large arenas and charged clients for the opportunity to communicate with spirits. Soon after the Fox sisters began performing, thousands of mediums around the world claimed similar abilities. Years later, Maggie Fox admitted that she and her sister had been perpetrating a hoax. But this had no effect on committed believers.

A modern descendent of mediumship is "trance-channeling." This can be defined as the communication of information to or through a live person (the medium or channel) from a source purported to be from another dimension or reality. One well-known practitioner is J. Z. Knight, who claims that a 35,000-year-old man named Ramtha uses her body to speak words of wisdom. Another is actress Shirley MacLaine, who claims that channeling provides useful information about "past lives." Channeling differs from "classic" mediumship in that the entities speaking through the medium are not limited to people who once lived on our planet. Many are said to be from other galaxies or dimensions—which, of course, makes their existence untestable by earthly means.

Trance-channeling is one of the recent systems encompassed by the "New

Age" movement. *Time* magazine described the New Age as "a whole cornucopia of beliefs, fads, [and] rituals" to which some followers subscribe and others do not. The beliefs include crystal healing (said to help the body balance and realign its "energy fields"), therapeutic touch, healing through mental imagery, pendulum power, and dozens of others. In a recent article in *Natural Food and Farming,* a radionics advocate describes how a "black box" can be used to determine the "subtle energies" of plant nutrients and to design optimum programs for fertilizing crops and selecting vitamin and mineral supplements for animal feed.

A survey conducted by *New Age Journal* illustrates the depth of its readers' beliefs. In 1987, the magazine reported that almost 100 percent who responded to a questionnaire had used "alternative" health methods and that 97 percent would be willing to choose such methods for treatment of a potentially life-threatening illness. The respondents reported using the following methods with mostly satisfactory results: acupuncture (used by 33 percent), acupressure (42 percent), chiropractic (56 percent), crystal healing (25 percent), colonics (21 percent), energy therapy (25 percent), Feldenkrais bodywork (13 percent), aromatherapy (26 percent), herbal medicines (47 percent), homeopathy (47 percent), mental imagery (70 percent), iridology (19 percent), macrobiotic diet (26 percent), meditation (85 percent), polarity therapy (24 percent), reflexology (38 percent), rolfing (19 percent), and yoga (53 percent).

Despite the popularity of these methods, 73 percent of the respondents said that an "alternative" practice had harmed them and 57 percent felt that closer regulation was needed—preferably by "experts in various holistic therapies." The methods most often judged harmful were chiropractic, acupuncture, colonics, fasting, and various "natural" diets. Almost all of the respondents felt that "maintaining an emotional, physical, and spiritual balance" and "maintaining a positive attitude" were vital to good health, but only 57 percent thought it was important to have regular check-ups by a medical doctor.

## Unmet Needs

The apparent success of occult healers suggests that some are appealing to needs that the medical profession should be handling more effectively. And the fact that millions of clients not only consult occult practitioners but also believe in their claims implies that our educational system is failing. It is possible to go from kindergarten through graduate school without having to take a single course in the sort of logic that can protect people from quackery.

*Concerned citizens should insist that our educational system prepare better consumers.* This would entail providing the intellectual tools necessary to separate sense from nonsense. One set of tools would be for recognizing what constitutes good scientific evidence for a claim. A second set of tools would be for realizing how our own thoughts and feelings can mislead us. We need courses that teach about our own cognitive biases and how to correct for them. In addition the sciences, curricula should include courses in probability and statistics that teach how to separate cause and effect from coincidence. Our youth need to be inoculated against the ever-growing information pollution being dumped on all of us by the media.

Revamping our educational system is a long-range task. Meanwhile, it would help if more people could be induced to approach healing claims with a simple checklist:

- What claims are being made?

- Are the claims definite or hedged?

- Are the claims testable? Is there any outcome that would lead the proponents to admit that their claims are invalid?

- What evidence would be needed to truly support such claims?

- What arguments and evidence are offered?

- How good are the evidence and arguments?

- Are the claims based on anecdotes or testimonials?

- Are they based on well designed research? If so, have the findings been independently replicated?

- Have the findings undergone expert analysis and/or been published in a reputable scientific journal?

- Does the scientific community accept them?

- Is there any reason people believe the claims even though their acceptance is unwarranted?

Remember: Throughout history, millions of people have fervently believed things that are not so. Almost all healing systems can produce large numbers of testimonials from satisfied adherents. That doesn't mean their methods work.

# 5

# The Food-Fear Epidemic

## Elizabeth M. Whelan, Sc.D., M.P.H.

Millions of Americans are worried about "all those chemicals" in our diet. I can easily understand this fear. I've been there myself.

For me, it began in the fall of 1969. Prior to that time, I had been enjoying the noncaloric sweet life. I would shake a few drops of a miracle liquid into my coffee each morning, quench my thirst at lunch with a chilled bottle of calorie-free soda, and garnish my dinner salad with a thick, creamy, but non-guilt-provoking diet dressing. Then, suddenly, the Secretary of Health, Education, and Welfare informed me (and millions of other cyclamate users) that the innocent-looking white powder perking up my low-cholesterol, low-fat break-fast had brought about a cancerous tumor in the bladders of some unfortunate rats. Cyclamates soon disappeared—and so did my confidence in food additives.

If cyclamates were dangerous, what about all those other chemicals that are routinely added to food? I started to read labels compulsively. Butylated hydroxyanisole (BHA). Butylated hydroxytoluene (BHT). Sodium bisulfite. Lecithin. Xanthan gum. How did I know they were safe? The fact that I couldn't even *pronounce* some of them didn't make me feel any better.

Eventually I shifted from reading labels to reading books. Authors informed me that there were poisons in my food—mischievous chemicals lurking in my cupboards, waiting for the chance to pollute my "inner environment" and scramble the genes of the next generation. A very unappetizing evaluation indeed. And what did these writers suggest? A return to nature, the consumption of foods that were "100 percent pure, organically grown," packed with "no artificial anything." Natural foods, they said, were my key to a long

67

and happy life and, most important, a means of lowering my odds of contracting the most dreaded of all diseases—cancer.

So I gave it a try. For three months I shopped at the Mother Nature Spa around the corner. I bought the makings for cold lentil salad, organic omelets, fava bean casserole, desiccated liver stew, and cucumber yogurt soup with dill. I drank so much Tiger's Milk that I thought I detected stripes on my skin. I ate so much honey and granola that I began to feel like a sticky wheat product. I tried the natural way. It was expensive and time-consuming, and I didn't like it. But I was still worried about food additives. Although I had a graduate degree in public health, the subject of additives had barely been touched on during my training.

I did know how to investigate, however, and decided to look more deeply into the natural-versus-artificial controversy. I surveyed both popular and scientific literature on the subject. I examined food fads of the past to see if our current back-to-nature binge had historical roots. I talked with FDA officials, political representatives, independent scientific researchers, and food industry chemists. I learned how the food laws worked in general, and how the so-called Delaney anticancer clause had been applied to ban additives. My conclusion: *The back-to-nature mania, like similar movements throughout history, is a hoax orchestrated by a variety of opportunists who are taking advantage of a vulnerable public.*

I returned to "regular" food, comfortable about eating again but determined to share my hard-won insights with others.

### "All Those Chemicals"

All foods—indeed, all living things—are made of chemicals. A hot, steamy solution containing essential oils; butyl, isoamyl, phenyl, ethyl, hexyl, and benzyl alcohols; tannin; geraniol; and other chemicals isn't some artificially wicked brew but an ordinary cup of tea. If you have rejected boxed stuffing mix because its ingredients include sulfur dioxide, calcium propionate, turmeric, monosodium glutamate, BHA, propyl gallate, and a long list of other chemicals, consider that 100 percent natural potatoes, even those that are "organically grown," contain more than 150 chemicals, including solanine, oxalic acid, arsenic, tannin, and nitrates.

Some perfectly safe foods contain deadly toxins. For example, potatoes contain solanine, which, in high enough doses, can interfere with nerve impulses. The amount of solanine in 119 pounds of potatoes (the amount eaten in one year by the average person) is enough to kill a horse. However, when eaten one serving at a time, potatoes are harmless. Lima beans contain cyanide, but those sold in the United States do not contain enough to worry about. *Whether or not something is poisonous depends on the dose.*

These simple facts tell us something: *Most people who try to stir up public fear about "too many chemicals in our food" are confused, untrustworthy, or both.*

## But What about Additives?

The broadest definition of a food additive is anything added to food. The most widely used are sugar, salt, and corn syrup. These three, plus citric acid (found in oranges and lemons), baking soda, vegetable colors, mustard, and pepper, account for about 98 percent by weight of all food additives used in this country. The rest—about 2,800 in all—make up less than 1 percent of the food we eat each year. The FDA is responsible for judging the safety of these substances and has paid a great deal of attention to this matter. Food additives, particularly those introduced during the past twenty-five years, have survived testing procedures more stringent than those applied to the great majority of natural products. These tests must prove that the additive is not only safe but performs an important function.

Many additives are used to enhance food colors and flavors. Although naturophiles may not care if their favorite fruit juice is purple or green, most people want their food to look appealing. A ripe orange that loses its characteristic color as a result of a temperature variation may be perfectly edible and nutritious. But people who think it doesn't "look right" won't eat it. Food dyes are used to correct this situation.

Taste is equally important. Variety keeps our diet interesting, but there is simply not enough natural flavoring to satisfy our demanding tastebuds. For example, there is not enough natural vanilla in the whole world to flavor the ice cream we eat in this country in a year. So we synthesize vanillin, the flavoring substance found in vanilla extract.

Additives also perform vital functions in food preservation and enrichment. The World Health Organization estimates that almost a quarter of the food produced each year is lost before it gets into consumer hands as a result of infestation by insects and rodents and because of spoilage. Food additives slow down deterioration considerably and, as a result, make the food supply more plentiful. Antimicrobial preservatives prevent spoilage caused by bacteria, molds, fungi, and yeast. They also extend the shelf life and protect the natural color or flavor of food. Antioxidants delay or prevent rancidity or enzymatic browning. Fortification of foods with iodine and vitamin D has almost eliminated the scourges of goiter and rickets.

Now let's look at some additives that have been controversial.

## Sugar Myths

Books and magazine articles still proclaim that sugar is a "killer on the breakfast table" and is the underlying cause of diabetes, heart disease, overweight, hypoglycemia, and a host of other health problems. But the facts are as follows:

- Sugar is perfectly safe when used in moderation as part of a normal, balanced diet. (However, if you have diabetes, overuse of sugar may worsen it.)

- There is no evidence that sugar increases the risk of developing heart disease.

- Sugar is a factor in the tooth-decay process. However, the amount of sugar in the diet is only one factor. The frequency and length of time that any digestible carbohydrate remains in contact with the teeth and the extent of oral hygiene practiced are also important (see Chapter 22).

- Sugar is not the cause of obesity. Overweight is caused by eating more calories than are used up in body activity. Recent evidence suggests that high-fat diets are more likely than high-carbohydrate diets to produce obesity.

- Hypoglycemia ("low blood sugar"), which is rare, is not caused by sugar.

## The Concern About Nitrites

Sodium nitrite is used during the curing process of meats and fish and is responsible for the characteristic flavor, color, and texture of bacon, ham, and sausage products. Without sodium nitrite, bacon would simply be salt pork, and ham would look and taste like roast pork. Most important, sodium nitrite prevents growth of bacteria that cause deadly botulism poisoning.

Concern over nitrite is based on the observation that, under some circumstances, it combines with other dietary components to form chemical compounds known as nitrosamines. Some nitrosamines have been found to cause cancer when fed in large amounts to test animals. However, sodium nitrite is a normal component of human saliva, and some 80 percent of the nitrite in the body comes from eating celery, beets, radishes, lettuce, spinach, and other commonly consumed vegetables. So it seems a bit absurd to panic about adding small amounts of substances that prevent serious health threats while remaining unconcerned about larger amounts that are present naturally.

Although there is no evidence that nitrites in cured products actually pose a hazard to human health, they have been a target of scaremongers. Nitrites deserve further study. However, reducing or eliminating their use may increase the risk of botulism.

## Artificial Sweeteners

Cyclamates were banned in 1969 after more than eighteen years of use. This was done because in one study of 240 rats given a mixture that included cyclamate, eight of those consuming the highest levels developed bladder tumors. How could such meager evidence lead to a ban? During the fall of 1969, a few self-styled consumer advocates publicly, but without supporting facts, raised questions about the sweetener. When the results of the laboratory experiment became known, public concern peaked and the Secretary of Health, Education, and Welfare felt pressured to act. Subsequent studies throughout the world have not demonstrated any danger to human health. Today, many food scientists feel that the banning of cyclamates was a mistake.

And saccharin—with an eighty-year history of safe use by humans? In 1977, preliminary results of a Canadian study indicated that rats fed large amounts of saccharin developed bladder tumors. Although studies of diabetics who had used large amounts of this sweetener for up to twenty-five years had revealed no excess incidence of cancer, the FDA announced its intention to ban it.

In June 1977, the press carried reports that another Canadian study had found an increased incidence of bladder cancer in male saccharin users. The results of this study were not consistent with at least eight other epidemiologic studies done by prominent scientists from Harvard, Johns Hopkins, Oxford, and elsewhere. Indeed, the previous studies, which involved more than sixty thousand people, indicated no adverse effects from saccharin use. The new Canadian study showed a 60 percent increased risk of cancer for males and a 40 percent decreased risk for females. The study also noted that men who smoked fifteen or fewer cigarettes per day had no increase in cancer risk. *Lancet,* the British medical journal that published the original article, labeled the human evidence against saccharin "unimpressive."

The National Academy of Sciences (NAS), which reviewed the data, concluded that epidemiologic studies do not provide clear evidence either to support or refute an association between saccharin use and cancer in humans.

NAS also concluded that although saccharin is a low-potency carcinogen in male rats and may increase the potency of other cancer-causing agents, the relevance of this conclusion to humans is far from clear.

Faced with the prospect of losing their last artificial sweetener, irate saccharin users bombarded Congress and the FDA with protest messages and a law was quickly passed to delay the ban. (The FDA received more than eighty thousand comments—the most it has ever received regarding a proposed regulation.) The risk to humans from saccharin—if any—is exceedingly small; but the ultimate fate of this artificial sweetener is still undecided.

Aspartame entered the market during all the hullabaloo over saccharin and cyclamates. Aspartame was accidentally discovered in 1965 by a research worker who observed that a compound made of two amino acids (phenylalanine and aspartic acid) and methyl alcohol tasted very sweet. Although this particular combination doesn't appear in nature, amino acids are the building blocks of protein, and small amounts of methyl alcohol occur naturally in some foods. In 1981, aspartame was approved for use as a tabletop sweetener (now marketed as *Equal*) and in certain foods and beverages (marketed as *NutraSweet*). By 1983, aspartame was allowed in soft drinks.

Unlike cyclamates and saccharin, aspartame has not been associated with cancer in laboratory animal tests. However, the FDA and the U.S. Centers for Disease Control and Prevention (CDC) have received and investigated consumer complaints of nausea, diarrhea, headaches, mood changes, seizures, and anxiety, all of which were blamed on aspartame.

In 1985, both the CDC and the American Medical Association's Council on Scientific Affairs concluded that there was no evidence that aspartame represents a health risk to any group except people with phenylketonuria (PKU), an uncommon disease in which people cannot metabolize phenylalanine. Duke University researchers have studied people who complained of headache after ingesting aspartame and found that they were no more likely to have a headache when receiving the amount of aspartame in a gallon of diet soft drink than when they were given a placebo. At the National Institute of Mental Health, a similar study investigated claims that aspartame causes disruptive behavior in preschool children and failed to find such a link.

Acesulfame-K was invented by West German scientists of Hoechst Company in 1967. (The K stands for potassium.) This compound (marketed as Sunette) passes through the body without being changed and, unlike aspartame, is not broken down by heat. In 1988, the FDA approved acesulfame-K for use in powdered drink mixes, puddings, chewing gum, and tabletop sweeteners. Shortly before it was approved, the Center for Science in the Public Interest (CSPI) began a series of allegations that animal studies indicate risks of lung cancer, mammary tumors, and elevated cholesterol. In 1992, the FDA denied the group's request for a formal public hearing and stated that the new sweetener had been studied enough to demonstrate its safety.

## The Delaney Clause

A key factor in the banning of food additives is a forty-seven-word section of the 1958 food additives amendment to the federal Food, Drug, and Cosmetic Act. This section, known as the "Delaney Clause," states:

> No additive shall be deemed to be safe if it is found to induce cancer when ingested by man or animal, or if it is found, after tests which are appropriate for the evaluation of the safety of food additives, to induce cancer in man or animals.

The problem with this clause is its inflexibility: it calls for banning whether a risk is great or infinitesimal. Followed literally, it fails to allow regulators to weigh possible risks against known benefits. Congressman James Delaney, prime sponsor of the legislation that bears his name, had not been concerned about such subtle distinctions. An avowed antifluoridationist, he regarded carcinogens as "stealthy, sinister saboteurs of life." Passage of his controversial amendment may well have laid the groundwork for the current public fear of additives.

The requirement that animal tests be "appropriate" might appear to offer some regulatory flexibility. But the very existence of the Delaney Clause has made the FDA too vulnerable to public pressure. Despite flimsy evidence, the Delaney Clause *was* invoked in the banning of cyclamates, diethylstilbestrol (DES), and a few unlucky coloring agents.

## Do Additives Cause Cancer?

Cancer, which was the eighth leading cause of death in 1900, is now second on the list. At first glance, the parallel rise in the use of food additives might make them logical suspects. But a closer look indicates that the rise in cancer deaths in this country in the last sixty years is largely attributable to *lung* cancer due to cigarette smoking. The rates of most other forms of cancer have either stabilized or declined. This includes cancer of the stomach, an organ that has considerable contact with food chemicals—both natural and added. Ironically, use of the antioxidants BHA and BHT may be responsible for a decline in human stomach cancer. These actually decrease the incidence of stomach cancer when added to the diet of laboratory animals.

You will continue to read and hear stories about how additives are dangerous, untested, and put into our food just so food companies can make more money. The reality is, however, that we know more about additives than we do about the chemistry of food itself. *Without the intelligent use of additives, it would be far more difficult to feed all of us. Food prices would be much higher, and most women would be back in the kitchen for many long hours.*

## Do Additives Cause Hyperactivity?

In 1973, Benjamin Feingold, M.D., a pediatric allergist at the Kaiser Permanente Medical Center in San Francisco, issued a sweeping accusation against food additives. In a book called *Why Your Child is Hyperactive,* he proposed that salicylates, artificial colors, and artificial flavors caused hyperactivity in children. To treat or prevent this condition, he suggested a diet that was free of these chemicals.

Two different types of scientific investigations have been carried out to test Feingold's theory. In "diet-crossover" studies, one group of hyperactive children followed a diet based on Dr. Feingold's recommendations, while a similar group of children were given food that looked the same but actually contained salicylates, artificial colors, and artificial flavors. After a few weeks, the diets were reversed. The results of these early studies varied considerably. Some children appeared to improve, some were unchanged, and some became worse. Scientists soon realized that the crossover type of study could not indicate which change—family diet or lifestyle—was affecting the children.

Next, "specific challenge" experiments were conducted. In these trials, children whose behavior had seemed to improve on the Feingold diet were kept on the diet but given occasional "treats." Some treats contained artificial food colors; but others, which appeared identical, did not. The experiments were "double-blind"—neither the researchers nor the participants knew which treats were which during the trial periods. These experiments show that additives have little if any effect on behavior. This subject is discussed further in Chapter 29.

## The Apple Scare

Alar is a chemical that, when sprayed on apples, makes them redder and firmer, lengthens their shelf life, and enables whole crops to ripen at the same time. In 1978, it was found that this product, which had been widely used since 1967, breaks down into UDMH, a substance that can cause cancer in laboratory animals. Uncooked apples don't contain UDMH. Cooked apples may contain small amounts, but the risk to humans is extremely small.

In February 1989, the Natural Resources Defense Council (NRDC) claimed that children were developing cancer due to pesticide residues in vegetables and fruits, especially the Alar used on apples. NRDC's claims were then foisted on the American public through a media blitz led by actress Meryl Streep. CBS-TV's "60 Minutes" aired a segment called "Intolerable Risk: Pesticides in Our Children's Food," and Phil Donahue also addressed the subject with a program that began with "Don't look now, but we're poisoning our kids" and told listeners how to obtain a book critical of pesticides. Ironically, Alar is not a pesticide but a growth regulator.

Even *Consumer Reports* carried a cover story headlined "Bad Apples," which said that no risk should be tolerated when an additive provides no health benefit. Apple sales plummeted, and both consumers and sellers threw out perfectly good apples, apple juice, applesauce, and apple pies. Some school systems even banned apples and apple products from their school lunches. In response to the fuss, most apple growers stopped using Alar. In mid-1989, after the U.S. Environmental Protection Agency said it would seek a ban, Alar's major manufacturer stopped marketing it in the United States.

The apple industry, which estimates that growers lost more than $100 million due to unfair negative publicity, has sued "60 Minutes" and NRDC. The suit may provide an opportunity to bring out the truth about Alar under courtroom conditions.

**The Assault on BST**

In August 1989, *The New York Times* reported that five of the nation's largest supermarket chains had announced their intention to "make sure that dairy products that carry their stores' brands do not contain milk from cows treated with an experimental genetically engineered drug." The object of this attack was bovine somatotropin (BST), a hormone produced naturally in the anterior pituitary gland of cattle. Injections of supplemental BST can boost the milk output of cows by about 15 percent. Using recombinant DNA technology, scientists have been able to make it at a price low enough for commercial use.

Milk produced by BST-treated cows is no different from milk produced by untreated cows. Since lactating cows produce BST naturally, small amounts are found in all cows' milk. BST treatment does not increase these levels. Moreover, BST is a protein that is digested like any other protein in milk and is not biologically active when ingested.

Why, then, would anyone oppose producing the same milk at lower cost without the slightest risk to consumers? The strongest opposition has come from parties claiming to be interested in protecting the small family farm. Two of the leading milk-producing states, Minnesota and Wisconsin, have temporarily banned BST because of an unfounded fear that it will drive small farmers out of business. Some detractors claim BST can cause unwanted growth and induce breast cancer in humans, increase the prevalence of resistant bacteria, and cause AIDS-related diseases that might be transmitted from cows to humans. Others object because they oppose all types of biotechnology. Experts consider all of these fears groundless.

## The Assault on Food Irradiation

Food irradiation is accomplished by treating foods with ionizing radiation (gamma rays) from radioactive cobalt or cesium or from devices that generate electron beams (beta rays) or electrons. Irradiation can kill harmful microorganisms and insects and can extend the shelf life of fruits, vegetables, and certain other foods by retarding spoilage. Some irradiated foods have better flavor and texture than their heat-treated counterparts because, unlike heating, irradiation doesn't cook the foods. The pork industry strongly favors irradiation because it can virtually eliminate the hazard of trichinosis at a cost of less than one cent per pound of pork. Irradiation of chicken is equally important because it kills the *Salmonella* bacteria that can cause severe diarrhea.

Despite all this, opponents of food irradiation have been working hard to prevent irradiated food from becoming established in the marketplace. Irradiation's opponents have lobbied for labeling requirements (assuming that the label will frighten people) and state laws to ban or delay its implementation. They have also persuaded many food companies—under threat of a boycott—to pledge not to sell irradiated food. One group distributed bumper stickers with the message: "Don't nuke my food." The "health food" industry is telling its followers that irradiated foods are dangerous, and many of its manufacturers and retailers have pledged not to market them.

Some of the propaganda involved resembles that of opponents of fluoridation. For example, to whip up its troops, the National Health Federation's magazine *Health Freedom News* published a letter stating:

> Eventually, all edibles will be zapped with radiation. . . . When this happens, all life-giving vitamins, minerals, enzymes, amino acids, and other food nutrients necessary to health will be destroyed. Foods POISONED to death! . . . Literally millions of people will develop cancer and other degenerative diseases to suffer and die five to ten years down the road.

The magazine's editors thanked the writer for "manifesting this very real problem."

Like fluoridation, food irradiation is a valuable public health measure. It would be a terrible shame if irresponsible critics succeeded in driving it from the marketplace. The biggest safety problem with our food supply is the prevalence of food poisoning due to bacterial contamination. Irradiation could help solve this problem but is opposed by the some of the very groups clamoring for increased safety. The tragic loss of life in the recent Jack-in-the-Box hamburger incident could would not have occurred had the meat been irradiated!

## The Assault on Genetic Engineering

Next in the parade of "new stuff in our food supply to be scared about" is genetic engineering or biotechnology. Biotechnology is the use of living things to create new products or to change old ones. Contrary to what opponents of biotechnology would have you believe, it has been around for a long time. Cattle-breeding is a time-honored example of improving stock by selectively breeding two superior animals to produce offspring with certain desired characteristics. Beefalo, on the other hand, is the result of breeding cattle with buffalo to create an entirely different animal. The tangelo is the result of crossing a tangerine with a grapefruit.

Today's critics of biotechnology don't seem concerned about tangelos. They are fighting new approaches that take the guesswork out of selective breeding of plants and animals by allowing direct alteration of DNA, the material in living cells that carries inherited characteristics. In the new biotechnology, the gene carrying a desired trait is transferred from the DNA of one organism to that of another. This technology is not being applied to produce new plants and animals, however. In most cases, it is used to improve on what we already have.

Billions of dollars are spent each year for insecticides and herbicides to protect plants used for food and animal feed. Biotechnology has enabled the development of hardier plants. It can also provide foods with superior keeping qualities, appearance, flavor, and nutritional value (such as reduced-fat meat or corn with increased protein). In the long run, introducing products like these into the food supply will help lower food prices by reducing losses from insects, weeds, viral infections, droughts, freezing weather, and spoilage. The first genetically engineered food scheduled to reach the American dinner table is the *Flavr Savr* tomato, which keeps longer without getting soft.

In 1992, the government announced a policy of promoting the development of new, safe foods through biotechnology by reforming the process of regulating this industry. The policy was developed by the FDA, which has the responsibility of overseeing that foods and other products created through biotechnology pose no risk to the public. It describes the scientific basis for evaluating and ensuring the safety of new varieties of foods that are developed using any technique, including biotech. Biotechnology opponents have threatened that unless the FDA conducts a formal rule-making procedure (a lengthy process of review and public comment), they will initiate legal action to prevent genetically engineered products from being sold. They have also threatened to organize a boycott and take other steps to stop marketing of the *Flavr Savr* tomato. Their tactics are similar to those of the opponents of food irradiation.

## A Brief History of Food Fears

Food faddism is not a new phenomenon. In a 1910 book called *Stover at Yale,* a fictional character called Ricky Rickets told his friend Dink Stover how to become a millionaire within ten years:

> First, find something all the fools love and enjoy, tell them it's wrong, hammer it into them, give them a substitute, and sit back, chuckle, and shovel away the ducats. Why, in the next 20 years, all the fools will be feeding on substitutes for everything they want . . . and blessing the name of the foolmaster who fooled them.

Ricky was commenting on the patent medicine craze of his day. But his remarks also reflect what has happened in the field of nutrition. Food choices are highly susceptible to rumors, and rumors promote food faddism. At some point in history, concerns have probably been expressed about almost every item in the human diet.

Sylvester Graham (1794–1851) mixed religious fanaticism with a zeal for the natural, "uncomplicated" life. "The simpler, plainer, and more natural the food," he said, "the more healthy, vigorous, and long-lived will be the body." Among the prohibited foods were salt and other condiments (these and sexual excesses caused insanity), cooked vegetables (against God's law), and chicken pies (caused cholera). His most vigorous attacks were against "unnatural" substances such as meat, white flour products, and water consumed at mealtime. Although Graham's health petered out at the age of fifty-seven, his spirit remains with us in the cracker that bears his name.

John Harvey Kellogg (1852–1943) supposedly ate his way through medical school on a diet of apples and graham crackers. He belonged to a Seventh-day Adventist group that had founded a religious colony and health sanitarium at Battle Creek, Michigan. It has been said that he and his brother, Will, were the first men to make a million dollars from food faddism. Under Dr.

Kellogg's leadership, the Battle Creek Sanitarium attracted hordes of wealthy clients whose intestines he "detoxified" with enemas and high-fiber diets. In an effort to provide a dried bread product upon which his clients could exercise their teeth without breaking them, he hit upon the idea of a wheat flake. By 1899, the flakes had evolved into a cereal-based company that soon had many competitors. One was Charles W. Post, a former Kellogg patient, who ground up wheat and barley loaves, called his new product "grape nuts," and marketed it as a cure for appendicitis, malaria, consumption (tuberculosis), and loose teeth. Such were the humble beginnings of two of today's giant cereal producers: the Kellogg Company and the Post Division of General Foods (now part of Philip Morris).

Adolphus Hohensee (1901–1967) began training to be a nutrition expert by taking a job as a soda jerk. After dabbling in real estate (with time in jail for mail fraud) and the field of transportation (during which time he was arrested for passing bad checks), Hohensee resumed his education. In 1943, he acquired an Honorary Degree of Doctor of Medicine from a nonaccredited school and followed this with Doctor of Naturopathy degrees from two schools that he did not attend. In 1946, he acquired a chiropractic license in the state of Nevada.

A master showman, Hohensee could lecture for hours about the terrible American diet that would stagnate the blood, corrode blood vessels, erode the kidneys, and clog the intestines. He said that most people had intestinal worms, which, fortunately, could be cured by his special cleansing. He promised a long life to those who consumed his wonder products. Repeated prosecution by the FDA made him more cautious about selling his products during lectures, but his promotion of the gamut of food myths sent his audiences flocking to nearby "health food" stores whose shelves just happened to be well-stocked with his product line. In 1955, alert reporters caught Hohensee eating a meal of forbidden foods after one of his lectures. In 1962, he began serving an eighteen-month prison term for selling honey with false claims. But neither of these setbacks dampened his enthusiasm or that of his loyal followers.

Gayelord Hauser (1895–1984) promised to add years to your life with wonder foods: skim milk, brewer's yeast, wheat germ, yogurt, and blackstrap molasses. He lectured frequently and was a partner in Modern Food Products of Milwaukee, Wisconsin, a company that produces products bearing his name. Hauser wrote a syndicated newspaper column and more than a dozen books reported to have sold close to fifty million copies in the United States and abroad. One book, *Look Younger, Live Longer,* led the bestseller list in 1951. That same year, the FDA seized copies of the book, claiming they were being used to promote sales of blackstrap molasses as a cure-all.

William Howard Hay warned against eating protein and white bread and urged frequent use of laxatives. D.C. Jarvis, M.D. (1881–1966), believed that bodily alkalinity was the principal threat to American health, recommended apple cider vinegar as the antidote, and advised against eating meat, wheat foods, citrus fruits, white sugar, and maple sugar. Melvin Page, D.D.S., who warned that milk was an underlying cause of cancer, persuaded many of his followers to stop drinking it or giving it to their children. And on they went— one faddist after another—each with his own brand of food fear and magic.

Although the "health food" industry was well established by the mid-1960s, it had not yet penetrated the average consumer's mind. Most of its customers were considered cultists. Two developments changed this, however. The first was the explosive growth of mass communication—particularly television. The second was a growing public concern about pollution. Rachel Carson's *Silent Spring,* though filled with errors, increased public concern about pesticides and decreased public confidence in governmental protection. The concept of "organic farming" enabled faddists like J.I. Rodale (1898–1971) and Adelle Davis (1904–1974) to arouse the interest of many people who weren't looking for miracle foods, but just wanted to feel that their food was safe. Sales pitches like "Make sure you have enough" and "Beware of chemicals in your food" converted the majority of Americans into at least occasional "health food" customers. Rodale and Davis made millions from the sale of their publications.

Into the 1970s, promoters of faddism kept pounding away: "Our food supply is poisoned!" "Our soil is depleted!" "Buy natural!" "Don't trust the government!" Carlton Fredericks, Lendon Smith, and a host of other spokespersons dominated the airwaves and bookshelves, supported by a vocal following of health food store operators and chiropractors. Linus Pauling turned millions of people on to megadoses of vitamin C. And the cyclamate scare turned additional millions more off the FDA, paving the way for a different chorus of voices.

**"Consumer Advocates"**

In 1970, a team of "Nader's Raiders" led by attorney James Turner published *The Chemical Feast,* a blistering attack on the FDA. The book stated that the FDA would not acknowledge "the relationship between deteriorating American health and the limited supply of safe and wholesome food." During the following year, other Nader associates formed the Center for Science in the Public Interest (CSPI) to investigate and report on a variety of food and chemical issues.

CSPI said it intended to "improve the quality of the American diet through research and public education." It promised to "watchdog" federal agencies that oversee food safety, trade, and nutrition. It also launched an annual National Food Day to call public attention to food issues. What issues? A 1975 Food Day brochure claimed: "Chemical farming methods create environmental havoc." A 1976 brochure stated: "Every few months, it seems, another common food additive is found to be harmful. . . . And agricultural chemicals have polluted everything from the nation's water supply to mother's milk." In 1986, CSPI launched Americans for Safe Foods (ASF), a coalition of more than forty consumer, environmental, and rural groups. ASF charged that much of the nation's food supply was riddled with pesticides, bacteria, drugs, and other hazards. During the past several years, CSPI has campaigned vigorously for government certification of "organically grown foods" and sponsored annual conferences on this subject.

CSPI, which now has more than 400,000 members, is still led by one of its co-founders, microbiologist Michael F. Jacobson, Ph.D. Its monthly publication, *Nutrition Action,* contains many attacks on food companies that CSPI believes are "more concerned with big profits than with good nutrition."

Unlike the traditional attackers of chemicals, Jacobson and his colleagues don't stress magical ideas about foods and are not obviously outlandish. Nor do they appear to be motivated by personal financial gain. They have stimulated several valuable government actions to protect consumers against misleading claims in food and vitamin advertising. They have campaigned vigorously to strengthen FDA regulation of food supplements, which the health food industry wants to weaken. However, their unjustified attacks have undermined public confidence in the government and the food industry and lent credibility to what the faddists have been saying all along.

## Food Industry Response

Many of our country's largest and most respected food companies have jumped on the back-to-nature bandwagon. Today the words "natural" and "additive-free" are applied to almost every type of edible product. Even beer and candy bars (so-called "health bars") bear these magic words.

Two years ago, after passage of a federal law to establish "organic" food standards, Beech-Nut Nutrition Corporation introduced a line of "organic" baby food products—which cost about 40 percent more than their regular counterparts.

Companies that exploit the growing public fear of additives may make windfall profits—but they also ignore their responsibility to the American public. Promoting accurate nutrition information and exposing food faddism would be much more commendable actions.

## A Balancing Force

For many years, I have been associated with Fredrick J. Stare, M.D., who founded and was Chairman of the Nutrition Department at Harvard University School of Public Health. In 1978, we formed a scientific organization whose purpose is to investigate chemical issues in our lives. The American Council on Science and Health (ACSH), which is nonprofit and tax-exempt, now has a full-time staff of researchers and more than three hundred prominent scientific advisors.

Every few months, ACSH selects a topic for investigation and assigns a staff member to coordinate research for the project. We perform a computer search of the scientific literature, collect and analyze pertinent literature, interview experts, and review unpublished research projects. After an initial draft is written, we circulate copies to appropriate members of our advisory board and outside experts. After their comments are received, additional drafts may be circulated until differences of opinion are resolved. When each final draft is published, it is available to the news media and the public.

ACSH has added a rational voice to the discussion of chemicals in our society—a voice that represents a consensus of scientific thinking about each topic we investigate. Of course, with environmental issues, there is no such thing as "absolute safety." The benefits of each chemical used should be weighed carefully against any actual or potential hazards. ACSH's approach is in marked contrast to that of others who base their calls for government bannings on emotional appeals or political advantage.

Even before ACSH issued its first report, CSPI began suggesting that we were "biased" and a "front" for industry. There is, however, no substance to these allegations. ACSH's activities are supported by grants from foundations, government research grants, and individual and corporate contributions. While support comes from companies that have a commercial interest in the issues we investigate, such support has not stopped ACSH from criticizing several sponsors whom we felt had advertised unethically.

ACSH considers the American food supply to be the safest in the world. It isn't perfect, and we don't know all there is to know about food safety— but responsible scientists *are* working to protect us. Widespread fear that our food supply is unsafe is simply unjustified.

# 6

# "Alternative" Cancer Treatment

## Stephen Barrett, M.D.

John Miner was deeply shaken by what he saw:

> The right side of her face was that of an angel. The left half was covered with a growth so monstrous as to seem beyond nature's capacity to be cruel and grotesque. . . . When I walked out of her room, I knew two things: Linda Epping would soon die; second, when it happened, I would seek a murder indictment.

When Miner made this report, he was Assistant District Attorney for Los Angeles County. The case had started routinely in 1961 with a complaint from Linda's parents. A chiropractor named Marvin Phillips had bilked them out of $739 by falsely promising to cure their eight-year old daughter of cancer of the eye.

Linda had been scheduled for surgery that would remove her left eye and surrounding tissues. Cure was possible, her doctors thought, because the tumor did not appear to have spread. But shortly before the operation could be performed, a fateful conversation took place. In the hospital waiting room, Linda's distraught parents met a couple who said that Phillips had cured their son's brain tumor without using surgery.

Her hopes aroused, Mrs. Epping telephoned Phillips and informed him of Linda's diagnosis. Without even seeing the child, he replied, "Yes, absolutely," he could help by "chemically balancing" her body.

Elated by this promise, the Eppings removed Linda from the hospital and took her to Phillips for treatment with vitamins, food supplements, and laxatives (up to 124 pills plus 150 drops of iodine solution daily). In addition, Phillips "adjusted" Linda's spine at his office and told the Eppings to manipulate the ball of her foot each day until she cried.

Despite the new "treatment," the tumor grew quickly. Within three weeks, it was the size of tennis ball and had pushed Linda's eye out of its socket. There was no longer any hope that surgery could save her. She died within a few months. Phillips was subsequently convicted of second degree murder and sentenced to prison.

Charles "Chuckie" Peters, Jr., and his family were luckier. In 1979, eight-year-old "Chuckie" entered a University of Chicago hospital suffering from headaches, extreme sensitivity to bright lights, severe bone pain, mental confusion, and a ten-pound weight loss. Previously diagnosed as leukemic, the boy had been receiving effective doses of chemotherapy. But his mother—who was concerned about its severe side effects—had been persuaded to give him large doses of vitamin A as part of a program of "metabolic therapy."

One year later, according to Mrs. Peters' testimony to the Illinois state legislature's Commission on Cancer Quackery, Chuckie reached a point where "he couldn't walk at all and the touching of his arms and legs brought screams of pain." The cause: vitamin A poisoning.

Chuckie stayed in the hospital for about two weeks so the doctors could relieve his bone pain with narcotics and monitor the gradual return of the function of his brain. After returning home, he was unable to attend school for another two months. "Almost half the time we carted him around in a wheelchair," his mother told the Commission. "Our son was a shell of what he was a few months before. The three years on the chemotherapy program never yielded the amount of pain he experienced from vitamin A toxicity . . . which almost cost him his life!"

Fortunately, this story has a happy ending. Chuckie recovered completely from the vitamin A poisoning. Following his final course of chemotherapy, his leukemia did not recur. He is alive and well today and is considered cured. His parents sued the people who had led them astray and settled out-of-court for an undisclosed sum.

## Empty Promises

Cancer quackery is big business, with an estimated yearly income in the billions. It is also cruel business, for its customers come in desperate fear. Customers who come while also undergoing sound medical care buy only empty promises. Those like the Eppings, who delay or abandon medicine's best, will purchase death.

Promoters of quackery are often closely attuned to the emotions of their customers. They may exude warmth, interest, friendliness, enthusiasm, and compassion. They pitch their methods as safe, natural, and nontoxic. Most important, they assure their frightened patients that they will be helped.

Quacks pitch their methods as "alternatives"—*which they are not.* A method that does not work is not a true alternative to one that might. Misuse of the word "alternative" is the cruelest form of doublespeak in the propaganda arsenal of quacks.

Unfortunately, recognizing quackery is not always easy. Its promoters may present a professional appearance. They may wear white coats and use scientific-sounding words. They may use the title "Doctor" and display a variety of elaborately framed diplomas. Close investigation might reveal that their credentials come from "diploma mills" that have no recognized academic standing. It is important to realize, however, that some promoters of questionable methods are highly educated individuals who have strayed from their fields of competency.

**Proven Versus Questionable Methods**

Quacks tend to be isolated from established scientific facilities and associations. They report their results through nonmedical channels rather than scientific journals. Sometimes their cure is "secret" or bears their own name. They claim persecution by the medical profession or government agencies. Typically, they keep scanty records or no records at all. Many demand large amounts of cash in advance for methods that cost very little to administer.

Cancer quacks rely heavily on stories of people they have supposedly cured. But such evidence is not reliable. Many cancer patients have given testimonials, believing they have been cured, only to find out later that they still have the disease. Others did not have cancer to begin with, but thought they did. Some satisfied customers are patients who used unproven methods together with good medical care. Charmed by the quack, however, they believe that his treatment was what helped them.

Predicting survival time is much more difficult than most people realize. When a doctor says that a cancer patient has a year to live, the estimate usually refers to median survival time for the type and stage of the tumor. About half of the patients will outlive the "predicted" time. Every facility that treats a substantial number of cancer patients will have some who live "unusually" long. Occasionally, a patient will experience a complete spontaneous remission. Ethical physicians, however, do not use testimonials from long-term survivors to promote themselves.

To be classified as effective or proven, a treatment method must meet certain standards. Patients treated with a particular method must do better than similar patients who do not receive that treatment. Proof that the patients actually had cancer must be available in the form of specimens that can be examined by microscope. Patients must be followed for many years to measure the true outcome of their cases, and the number of patients must be large enough to rule out chance as a factor. Experiments that are valid can be repeated and thus confirmed by the scientific community. To date, all drugs shown to be effective in treating cancer in humans have also been effective against some form of animal or human cancer cells in laboratory test systems. For this reason, drugs ordinarily will not be tested in humans unless anticancer activity is demonstrated in laboratory tests.

The words "quackery," "unproven," and "questionable" are often used interchangeably although they do not have identical meanings. Medical progress requires the study of unproven methods *in a responsible manner.* Quackery, as defined by the National Council Against Health Fraud and used throughout this book, is "the promotion of a false or unproven method for profit." Questionable methods, as defined by the American Cancer Society, are "lifestyle practices, clinical tests, or therapeutic modalities that are promoted for general use for the prevention, diagnosis, or treatment of cancer and which are, on the basis of careful review by scientists and/or clinicians, not deemed to have real evidence of value."

## Questionable Methods

Cancer quackery is as old as recorded history and probably has existed since cancer was recognized as a disease. Thousands of worthless folk remedies, diets, drugs, devices, and procedures have been promoted for cancer management.

• *Corrosive agents* have been applied directly to tumors with the hope of burning them away. Turpentine is an old favorite, having been used by quacks since ancient times. In recent years, scientists have found chemicals that can destroy very superficial skin cancers. Except for that, however, corrosive agents are worthless.

• *Folk remedies* have included red clover tea, salves made from zinc chloride and blood root, plant material sun-dried in pewter, and even "live green frogs applied to external cancer till they die." Plants said to be used by Indians to shrink heads have been promoted—with the theory that if they could shrink heads, they could shrink cancer.

Beginning in 1922, a naturopath named Harry M. Hoxsey amassed a fortune treating cancer patients with dubious folk remedies. He used a combination of internal and external substances. The internal medicine, taken by mouth, was prescribed "in all cases" to "restore the body to physiological normalcy." It contained potassium iodide and such things as red clover, licorice, burdock root, Stillingia root, Berberis root, poke root, cascara, prickly ash bark, and buckthorn bark. Hoxsey's external medicines contained corrosive agents such as arsenic sulfide. He had acquired the formulas for his remedies from his father while the latter was dying of cancer.

Three times during the late 1920s, Hoxsey was convicted in Illinois of practicing medicine without a license. In 1930, he was permanently enjoined from violating the Iowa State Medical Practice Act. In 1936, after unsuccessful attempts to practice in several other states, Hoxsey moved to Texas, where he was able to practice for many years. Vigorous action by the FDA during the 1950s and early 1960s finally drove him out of business in the United States. However, the treatment is still available to patients at a clinic in Mexico run by Hoxsey's former head nurse, Mildred Nelson.

Essiac is an herbal remedy that was prescribed and promoted for about fifty years by Rene Caisse, a Canadian nurse who died in 1978. Shortly before her death, she turned over the formula and manufacturing rights to a Canadian company that can provide it to patients under a special agreement with Canadian health officials. Animal tests using samples of Essiac have shown no antitumor activity. Nor did a review of data on eighty-six patients performed by the Canadian federal health department during the early 1980s.

• *Diets* are also claimed to remedy cancer. The usual theory behind them is that cancer is caused by an "imbalance" in the body or by accumulated "poisons" or "impurities." Proper diet would then "detoxify" the body. One such regimen is promoted by Johanna Brandt, N.D., in her book *The Grape Cure*. The patient must eat one-half pound of any "good variety of grapes," starting at 8 A.M. and repeating every two hours, for seven meals a day. For one or two weeks, nothing else may be added except for water. Then sour milk, raw vegetables, salads, dried fruits, nuts, honey, olive oil, and certain fresh fruits may be eaten. Neither the Grape Cure nor any other special diet has any proven value in the prevention or treatment of cancer.

Proponents of the Gerson diet claim that detoxification is accomplished by frequent enemas and a diet consisting primarily of fresh fruit and vegetable juices. Salt, spices, sodium bicarbonate, alcohol, and tobacco are forbidden. After several weeks, milk proteins, vitamins, and various other food supplements are added. This method was developed by Max Gerson (1881–1959), a German-born physician who emigrated to the United States in 1936. Still available at a clinic near Tijuana, Mexico, Gerson therapy is actively promoted by his daughter, Charlotte Gerson, who believes that "by healing the body, you can heal cancer and almost any other chronic disease and it doesn't matter what the cause. . . . All chronic diseases are deficiency diseases."

In 1947, the National Cancer Institute reviewed ten cases selected by Dr. Gerson and found his report unconvincing. That same year, a committee appointed by the New York County Medical Society reviewed records of eighty-six patients, examined ten patients, and found no scientific evidence that the Gerson method had value in the treatment of cancer.

Charlotte Gerson claims that treatment at the Tijuana clinic has produced high cure rates for many cancers. A few years ago, however, investigators learned that patients were not monitored after they left the facility. Although clinic personnel later said they would follow their patients systematically, there is no published evidence that they have done so.

Even a simple follow-up study may yield meaningful data. In 1983, a naturopath named Steve Austin visited the Gerson Clinic and asked about thirty cancer patients to permit him to follow their progress. He was able to track twenty-one of them over a five-year period (or until death) through annual letters or phone calls. At the five-year mark, only one was still alive (but not cancer-free); the rest had succumbed to their cancer. The study is remarkable because Austin had been favorably predisposed toward Gerson therapy.

Proponents of the macrobiotic diet (see Chapter 16) contend that cancers arise from imbalances in the body and build-ups of poisons or impurities, and that "detoxification" can be accomplished through dietary means. However, no published evidence meeting accepted scientific criteria supports these views. Claims that the macrobiotic diet can cure cancer are based on anecdotes and personal testimony rather than controlled studies of the diet versus other treatments or a placebo. Critics also warn that the diet can be nutritionally inadequate for cancer patients and lead to undesirable weight loss.

Revici Cancer Control (also called lipid therapy) is based on the idea that cancer is caused by an imbalance between two types of lipids (fats), acid and alkaline. Its proponent, Emanuel Revici, M.D., was born in Rumania in 1896. To treat patients, he prescribes lipid alcohols, zinc, iron, and caffeine, which he says are "anabolic," and fatty acids, sulfur, selenium, and magnesium, which he classifies as "catabolic." His formulations are based on his interpretation of the specific gravity, pH (acidity), and surface tension of single samples of the patient's urine. Revici also claims success against AIDS.

Scientists who have offered to evaluate Revici's methods have never been able to reach an agreement with him on procedures to ensure a valid test. However, his method of urinary interpretation is obviously not valid. The specific gravity of urine reflects the concentration of dissolved substances and depends largely on the amount of fluid a person consumes. The acidity depends mainly on diet, but varies considerably throughout the day. Thus, even when these values are useful for a metabolic determination, information from a single urine sample would be meaningless. The surface tension of urine has no medically recognized diagnostic value.

In 1988, after reviewing charges that he had inappropriately managed three patients with cancer, New York State licensing authorities placed Revici on five years' probation. One patient was a forty-nine-year-old woman who had consulted Revici after several other doctors had advised her to have a marble-sized lump removed from her left breast. Revici persuaded her to undergo treatment with him. After fourteen months, the tumor had filled one breast and spread to the opposite breast and to many lymph nodes—requiring removal of both breasts and treatment with radiation and chemotherapy.

Proponents of dietary therapy typically claim that cancer is caused by immune deficiency and can be cured by "strengthening the immune system"— which their methods supposedly do. The fact that AIDS patients—who are immunosuppressed—are prone to develop cancer may seem to support this theory but actually proves it wrong. AIDS patients contract a rare form of cancer called Kaposi's sarcoma. If immune suppression caused the common forms of cancer (breast, lung, colon, stomach, prostate, etc.), then AIDS patients would get them. But they don't.

• Useless *biological products* used to treat cancer include vaccines and preparations derived from the patient's own blood and/or urine or from animal blood and/or urine. One such vaccine was the "Radio-Sulpho Cancer Cure" which originated in Denver, Colorado. Philip Schuch, Jr., President of the Radio-Sulpho Company, claimed he could "culture cancer germs direct from the cancer vaccine" he discovered. Although he was not a physician, he called himself a "cancer specialist." Schuch's treatment consisted of washing the cancer with Radio-Sulfo Brew, applying a Limburger cheese "poultice," and repeating every twelve hours. However, "to stand the powerful drawing power of the cheese," Schuch warned, "a person must be strong and healthy."

Virginia Livingston, M.D., who died in 1990, postulated that cancer is caused by a bacterium that invades the body when resistance is lowered. To combat this, she claimed to strengthen the body's immune system with various vaccines (including one made from the patient's urine); a vegetarian diet that avoided chicken, eggs, and sugar; vitamin and mineral supplements; visualization; and stress reduction. She claimed to have a very high recovery rate but published no clinical data to support this. Attempts by scientists to isolate the organism Livingston postulated were not successful. Researchers at the University of Pennsylvania Cancer Center compared seventy-eight patients treated at the center with seventy-eight similar patients given various vaccines, a vegetarian diet, and coffee enemas at the Livingston-Wheeler Clinic. All of the patients had advanced cancers for which no proven treatment was known. As expected, the study found no difference between average survival time of the two groups. However, patients in the Livingston-Wheeler program reported more problems with appetite difficulties and pain.

Immuno-augmentative therapy (IAT) was developed by Lawrence Burton, Ph.D., a zoologist who claimed to have discovered a way to treat cancer patients by manipulating an immune defense system that he postulated. He claimed to accomplish this by injecting protein extracts isolated with processes he had patented. However, experts believe that the substances Burton claimed to use cannot be produced by these procedures and have not been demonstrated to exist in the human body. Moreover, he did not publish detailed clinical reports, divulge to the scientific community the details of his methods, publish meaningful statistics, conduct a controlled trial, or provide independent investigators with specimens of his treatment materials for analysis. During the mid-1980s, it was reported that several of Burton's patients developed serious infections following IAT.

In 1979, Burton's efforts received an enormous boost when the CBS-TV's "60 Minutes" gave them favorable publicity. A prominent physician stated that one of his patients treated by Burton appeared to have undergone a miraculous recovery. The patient died within two weeks after the program was shown; but despite prodding from several people (including me), "60 Minutes" never informed viewers of this fact. In 1982, William A. Nolen, M.D., visited Burton's clinic, reviewed many records, and had follow-up conversations with at least ten patients and some of their doctors. Dr. Nolen concluded that most of the patients had never had cancer or else had tumors that typically grow slowly, while some had undergone conventional treatment that was probably responsible for any positive results.

Burton's clinic has published a booklet summarizing the experiences of thirty-five IAT patients and their status as of February 1988. However, cancer specialist Wallace I. Sampson, M.D., has concluded:

> The sampling of cases is not meaningful. To estimate prognosis accurately, the stage and grade of a tumor are needed. Only a few of these vignettes provide both of these. Any facility that treats large numbers of cancer patients will have some patients who survive a long time—with or without treatment. It would not be possible to determine IAT's effectiveness without knowing how these outcomes compare with the rest of Burton's patients who had similar cancers. Moreover, thirty of the thirty-five received standard or near-standard treatment

before undergoing IAT. All of these had a significant probability of living as long as was recorded in the booklet.

In 1986, the Congressional Office of Technology Assessment (OTA) appointed a group of technical experts and representatives of Burton to design a clinical trial to evaluate IAT. However, the OTA report states that communication between Burton and U.S. government authorities broke down after he insisted that a "pre-test" be conducted at his clinic. The report also concluded that "no reliable data are available on which to base a determination of IAT's efficacy." Burton died in March 1993, but the clinic is still operating

Stanislaw R. Burzynski, M.D., has given the name "antineoplastons" to substances that he claims can "normalize" cancer cells that are constantly being produced within the body. He has published many papers in which he claims that antineoplastons extracted from urine or synthesized in his laboratory have proven effective against cancer in laboratory experiments. He also claims to have helped many people with cancer get well. Saul Green, Ph.D., a biochemist who worked for many years at Memorial Sloan-Kettering Hospital doing research into the mechanisms and treatment of cancer, has written a detailed analysis of Burzynski's claims. Green does not believe that any of the substances Burzynski calls "antineoplastons" has been proven to "normalize" tumor cells.

In 1988, Burzynski got a tremendous boost when talk-show hostess Sally Jesse Raphael featured four "miracles," patients of Burzynski, who, she said, were "cancer-free." The patients stated that Burzynski had cured them when conventional methods had failed. In 1992, "Inside Edition" reported that two of the four patients had died and a third was having a recurrence of her cancer. (The fourth patient had bladder cancer treated by conventional means before he saw Burzynski. Bladder cancer has a good prognosis.) The widow of one of Raphael's guests stated that her husband and five others from the same city had sought treatment after learning about Burzynski from a television broadcast— and that far from being helped, all had died.

• *Diagnostic testing* is another fertile field for quackery. One worthless test was developed by Dr. H.H. Beard, a biochemist. Beard claimed that by measuring a sex hormone in the urine, he could detect cancer in the body within two or three weeks after it started. His book, *A New Approach to Conquering Cancer, Rheumatic Fever and Heart Disease,* contained a chapter on preventing malignancy by using his "Beard Anthrone Test." Advertisements for the book included instructions for collecting specimens that could be mailed to Beard in Fort Worth, Texas.

In 1965 the California Cancer Advisory Council and the Department of Public Health studied the Beard Anthrone Test and found it useless in the detection of cancer in humans. In 1967, Beard was indicted by a Federal Grand Jury for mail fraud. Pleading "no contest," he received a six-month suspended sentence and one year probation. But before the court had halted his activities, Beard had conducted an estimated fifteen thousand tests for which he had received approximately $150,000.

The Arthur (or Automated) Immunostatus Differential (AID) test, according to its proponents, "can lead to a diagnosis and early treatment several months to several years prior to the crisis we usually call cancer.... The test also helps to detect general immune reserve deficiencies before a serious challenge occurs to destroy health and well being." To carry out the test, a few drops of blood are taken from an earlobe by pricking it with a pin. The blood is then smeared on a slide, stained, and examined by a computerized microscope. One practitioner in Ohio claimed that the test is 98.67 percent reliable.

Two tests were used by William Donald Kelley, D.D.S., as guides to his dietary program to treat cancer. His Protein Metabolism Evaluation Index was based on the premise that cancer is a foreign protein. His Kelley Malignancy Index was claimed to be "the most accurate and extensive cancer detection system ever developed." It was claimed capable of detecting "the presence or absence of cancer, the growth rate of the tumor, the location of the tumor mass, prognosis of the treatment, age of the tumor and the regulation of medication for treatment." A booklet by Kelley claimed that "at least 86 percent of all cancer conditions could be adequately treated and/or prevented by diet alone" and that "cancer is nothing more than a pancreatic enzyme deficiency" caused by eating too much of the wrong kind of protein. "If people would not eat protein after 1:00 P.M.," the booklet stated, "83 percent of cancer in the United States could be eliminated."

According to a report in the newspaper of the American Dental Association, Kelley was convicted in 1970 of practicing medicine without a license after witnesses testified that he had diagnosed lung cancer on the basis of blood from a patient's finger and prescribed supplements and a diet as treatment. In 1973, Kelley was brought before the Texas State Board of Dental Examiners on charges of unprofessional conduct. The complaint contended that he had obtained a fee by fraud or misrepresentation by offering diagnosis and treatment of cancer in his dental office. The board's decision to suspend Kelley's license for five years was later upheld in court and went into effect in 1976. However, he continued to promote his methods for several more years through his Dallas-based International Health Institute. Kelley's last moment of notoriety came when he treated well-known actor Steve McQueen for lung cancer at a Mexican clinic. McQueen died under Kelley's care shortly after broadcasting a raspy testimonial that he was getting better.

Methods claimed to be similar to Kelley's are still used today by Dr. Nicholas Gonzales, a physician in New York City who claims to have performed an extensive analysis of Kelley's former patients and drafted a book about his findings. As far as I know, the manuscript was never published, but conventional physicians who evaluated its chapter on fifty cases found no evidence of benefit.

Hariton Alivizatos, a Greek physician who died in 1991, claimed to have a blood test that could determine the type, location, and severity of any cancer. He also asserted that his "serum" enabled the patient's immune system to destroy cancer cells, and helped the body rejuvenate parts destroyed by cancer. Knowledgeable observers believe that the principal ingredient of the so-called Greek Cancer Cure was niacin.

• *Psychic surgery* is claimed to remove tumors without leaving a skin wound. Actually, its practitioners use sleight-of-hand to create the illusion that surgery is being performed. A false finger or thumb may be used to store a red dye that appears as "blood" when the skin is "cut." Animal parts or cotton wads soaked in the dye are palmed and then exhibited as "diseased organs" supposedly removed from the patient's body. Most "psychic surgeons" practice in the Philippines or Brazil, but some have made tours within the United States. A few have been prosecuted for theft and/or practicing medicine without a license.

• Many worthless *drugs* have been promoted for cancer prevention or cure. During the early 1940s, William Koch, M.D., Ph.D., acquired a large following of believers in a remedy that he claimed was 1.32 parts of glyoxylide per trillion parts of water! More than three thousand assorted practitioners bought it for $25 per ampule and charged patients up to $300 per injection. Analysis of the product could find only distilled water.

Iscador is an extract of mistletoe first proposed for the treatment of cancer in 1920 by Dr. Rudolph Steiner, a Swiss physician who had strong beliefs in the occult. Steiner founded the Society for Cancer Research to promote mistletoe extracts and occult-based practices he called Anthroposophical medicine. A 1962 report by the society typifies his thinking. "In order to make an efficacious remedy," the report states, "it is necessary to pay attention to the time of picking ... [since the plants] not only react to the influences of the Sun and Moon, but also to those of the planets." Various mistletoe juice preparations have been studied with the hope of finding an effective anticancer agent. In 1984, however, the Swiss Society for Oncology (a scientific organization) warned patients not to use Iscador because its expert working group found no evidence that Iscador was effective against human cancers.

Cancell, originally called Entelev, is a liquid purported to cure cancer by reducing the voltage of cancer cells until they become "primitive" and self-destruct. It has also been promoted for the treatment of AIDS and many other diseases. In 1989, the FDA reported that Cancell contained inositol, nitric acid, sodium sulfite, potassium hydroxide, sulfuric acid, and catechol. Subsequently, its promoters claimed to be modifying the formulation to make it more effective. Laboratory tests conducted between 1978 and 1991 by the National Cancer Institute found no evidence that Cancell was effective against cancer. The FDA has obtained an injunction forbidding its distribution to patients.

"Hyperoxygenation therapy" is based on the erroneous concept that cancer is caused by oxygen deficiency and can be cured by exposing the cancer to more oxygen than it can tolerate. The most commonly used modalities are hydrogen peroxide, germanium sesquioxide, and ozone. Although these compounds have been the subject of legitimate research, there is little or no evidence that they are effective for the treatment of any serious disease, and each has demonstrated potential for harm.

Laetrile heads the all-time list of quack cancer remedies. It contains the chemical amygdalin, a substance abundant in the kernels of peaches, apricots, bitter almonds, and apple seeds. Such seeds are dangerous to eat because amygdalin breaks down into a toxic cyanide. Although laetrile is sometimes referred to as "vitamin B-17," it is not a vitamin.

Although laetrile has been used for many years, there is no evidence that it is safe or effective. In 1953, the Cancer Commission of the California Medical Society published information on forty-four cancer patients who had been treated with laetrile during the previous year. Nineteen had died of their disease, and there was no evidence that laetrile had helped any of the others.

Claims for laetrile's efficacy have varied considerably. First it was claimed to prevent and cure cancer. Then it was claimed not to cure, but to "control" cancer while giving patients an increased feeling of well being. More recently, laetrile has been claimed to be effective, not by itself, but as one component of "metabolic therapy," a program (with inconstant components) which may include enzymes, enemas, megadoses of vitamins, "pangamic acid" (also referred to as "vitamin B-15"), and a diet that excludes protein from animal sources.

In response to political pressure, a clinical trial was begun in 1982 by the Mayo Clinic and three other U.S. cancer centers under the sponsorship of the National Cancer Institute. Laetrile and "metabolic therapy" were administered as recommended by their promoters. The patients had advanced cancer for which no proven treatment was known. Of 178 patients, not one was cured or even stabilized, and none had any lessening of any cancer-related symptoms. The median survival rate was about five months from the start of therapy. In those still alive after seven months of treatment, tumor size had increased.

Several patients experienced symptoms of cyanide toxicity or had blood levels of cyanide approaching the lethal range.

In 1975, a cancer patient named Glenn Rutherford filed a class action suit to stop the FDA from interfering with the sale and distribution of laetrile. Early in the case, a federal district court judge in Oklahoma issued orders allowing cancer patients to import a six-month supply of laetrile for personal use if they could obtain a physician's affidavit that they were "terminal." A higher court partially upheld this ruling, but in 1979 the U.S. Supreme Court disagreed, stating that drugs offered to "terminal" patients should not be exempted from FDA authority. The court reasoned that it is not possible to determine with certainty who is terminal and that even if it were possible, both terminally ill patients and the general public deserve protection from fraudulent cures. In 1987, after further appeals were denied, the district judge (a strong proponent of laetrile) finally yielded to the higher courts and terminated the affidavit system. Today, few sources of laetrile are available within the United States, but it still is utilized at a few Mexican clinics.

In a more recent case involving FDA attempts to restrict the sale of antineoplastons, an appeals court judge concluded:

> The patients who appear in this suit are in a critical plight. They seek any treatment that offers them the slightest hope, for they think it better to exhaust any possibility than to resign themselves to a fate that seems otherwise certain. The FDA has been assigned the duty of protecting such desperate persons from deception, abuse, and exploitation and of assuring that the treatment they are given is safe and effective. It cannot perform these tasks if those professing to offer new cures can refuse to work with the system and obey the law, whether their motives be noble or ill. The court, therefore, must not allow sympathy for the plight of persons suffering from cancer to cause us to interfere hastily with the mission of the FDA or to distract us from our duty to uphold the law.

• Various *psychological methods* are being promoted to cancer patients as cures or adjuncts to other treatment. The techniques proposed for this purpose include imagery, visualization, meditation, and various forms of psychotherapy. A positive attitude may increase a patient's chance of surviving cancer by increasing compliance with proven treatment. However, there does not appear to be any evidence that emotions directly influence the course of the disease.

Bernie Siegel, M.D., author of *Love, Medicine & Miracles* and *Peace, Love & Healing* is a surgeon who espouses meditation, support-group meetings, and other psychological approaches for cancer patients. He claims that "happy people generally don't get sick" and that "one's attitude toward oneself is the single most important factor in healing or staying well." Siegel also states that "a vigorous immune system can overcome cancer if it is not interfered with, and emotional growth toward greater self-acceptance and fulfillment helps keep the immune system strong." However, he has published no scientific studies to support these claims.

O. Carl Simonton, M.D., medical director of the Simonton Cancer Center, Pacific Palisades, California, believes that cancers may be affected by relaxation and visualization techniques. He claims that this approach can lessen fears and tension, strengthen the patient's will to live, increase optimism, and alter the course of a malignancy by strengthening the immune system. However, he has not published the results of any well-designed study to test his ideas. Simonton theorizes that the brain can stimulate endocrine glands to inspire the immune system to attack cancer cells. In line with this theory, Simonton and his wife Stephanie (a psychotherapist) taught cancer patients to imagine their cancer being destroyed by their white blood cells. However, Edward R. Friedlander, M.D., a pathologist at the University of Missouri, has noted:

> When the Simontons developed this technique, many people thought that the white blood cells of the immune system were the body's major defense against cancer. Cancerous cells supposedly are produced on a steady basis but destroyed by the body's white cells; and malignancies that become evident are the ones that "got away." Unfortunately for the "immune surveillance" theory, we now know that people who are given immunosuppressant drugs . . . or who are immunodeficient because of hereditary disease or AIDS, are not prone to develop any of the common cancers. . . . Nevertheless, imagers still meditate about white cells making their cancers go away.

Simonton's book *Getting Well Again* included reports on patients who got better after using his methods. However, Friedlander, who analyzed five of the reports he thought might impress laypersons the most, noted that two of the patients had undergone standard treatment, one had a slow-growing tumor, and one probably did not have cancer. The fifth patient's tumor was treatable by standard means.

Some people suggest that programs like those of Siegel or Simonton may have positive psychologic effects that help people to relax and to feel that they are "doing something" positive. Although their method are physically harmless, they may waste people's time and money and encourage some patients to abandon effective care.

A British study has disclosed how evangelical zeal can lead people to misjudge the effectiveness of psychological approaches to cancer. In 1986, the staff and patients at Bristol Cancer Help Center "felt a need to validate scientifically the results they felt had been achieved" with counseling, "healing," a vegetarian diet, homeopathy, acupuncture, and various other therapies said to enhance the quality of life and to help develop a positive attitude toward cancer. They invited a research team, which compared the course of 334 of the center's breast cancer patients and 461 similar patients treated at conventional hospitals during a sixteen-month period. Survival times and metastasis-free periods were significantly shorter among the center's patients. The study demonstrated how people who believe in a treatment can overestimate its effectiveness.

**Promoters of Questionable Methods**

Many individuals and groups are involved in the promotion of questionable methods. Some emphasize methods related to cancer, while others have a broader scope.

The International Association of Cancer Victors and Friends (IACVF) was formed in 1963 to "restore the cancer victim's life and free choice of treatment and doctor." The Association's founder, Cecile Pollack Hoffman, was a San Diego schoolteacher who underwent a radical mastectomy for breast cancer in 1959. In 1962, she had further surgery due to the spread of the cancer. Her husband, while sitting in an airport waiting room, happened to pick up a paperback book entitled *Laetrile: Control for Cancer* by Glenn D. Kittler. After reading the book, Mrs. Hoffman sought further information. Not long afterward, she became a staunch supporter of laetrile and developed a belief that it had saved her life. Although she died of metastatic cancer in July 1969, IACVF has continued to sponsor conventions and distribute literature promoting questionable methods.

The Cancer Control Society was formed in 1973 in Los Angeles by dissident IACVF members after disputes arose over major policy and the distribution of the proceeds of book sales. Both groups have similar activities today.

The National Health Federation (NHF) promotes the gamut of questionable health theories and practices (see Chapter 28). Since its founding in 1955, it has fought vigorously against government regulation of unproven methods. NHF's main impact has been its ability to generate huge amounts of mail to Congress and other agencies. In 1957, for example, an NHF campaign resulted in 200,000 communications to the FDA to protest its interference with the Hoxsey cancer treatment.

The Foundation for Alternative Cancer Therapy (FACT) publishes a newsletter, holds public meetings, and engages in letter-writing campaigns.

The Committee for Freedom of Choice in Medicine (CFCM) was founded in 1972 by Robert Bradford, a Stanford University technician (see Chapter 28). It publishes a newsletter and campaigns against government regulation of "alternative" methods.

People for Cancer evolved from a previous group formed to promote Lawrence Burton's immuno-augmentative therapy. It publishes a newsletter, recruits patients for Burton, and promotes other "alternatives" as well.

Project Cure distributes literature and campaigns for the gamut of "alternative" methods.

Several individuals and organizations offer lengthy reports said to provide detailed, individualized reports on both proven and "alternative" forms of cancer treatment. The best-publicized are Health Resource, the World Research Foundation, and CANHELP. No evaluation of the quality of their information has been published in the scientific literature. However, the operator of CANHELP (Pat McGrady, Jr.) has been severely criticized by investigative reporter David Zimmerman. In the November 1991 issue of his newsletter *Probe,* Zimmerman described how a man with virulent lung cancer had been advised to use a restrictive diet, coffee enemas, and 100 to 150 supplement pills per day—and that report had overlooked a promising new treatment whose results had not yet been published in a scientific journal, but which were readily available to physicians and the public from the National Cancer Institute's information services. In plain words, the $400 CANHELP report had suggested worthless treatment and failed to mention the one treatment that might save the patient's life.

## Promotion through the Media

Freedom of speech and of the press are important factors in the promotion of unproven cancer remedies. Books, especially if they are on so-called "controversial" medical problems, are quite appealing to the public. Many books on "alternative" methods are cleverly written so that readers may think they are getting valuable information when they are not. Some books deal with one method, sometimes reporting a personal experience, while others deal with the gamut of such methods.

*Laetrile Case Histories,* by John Richardson, M.D., and Patricia Griffin, R.N., illustrates how survival statistics can be deceptively packaged. (Richardson, a prominent laetrile promoter, had his medical license revoked in 1976 and was convicted in 1977 of conspiring to smuggle laetrile.) Although the book's cover promises ninety case histories, it actually contains only sixty-two, more than half of whom received some conventional treatment in addition to treatment by Richardson. Dr. William Jarvis has found that only fifty-one of the sixty-two histories contain enough information to enable comparison with published statistics of similar patients treated by conventional means. He concluded:

> These fifty-one hand-picked patients constitute 1.3 percent of the four thousand cases treated at the Richardson Clinic between 1971 and 1976. They survived an average of 29.9 months against odds which suggest that 70 percent of similar cases would normally be alive that long without metabolic therapy. Statistically speaking, this is quite unimpressive.

The writings of Anthony Sattilaro, M.D., provide misleading testimonials about his struggle with prostate cancer. In *Recalled By Life* (1982), he credited macrobiotics with helping him even though he had undergone conventional treatment. In *Living Well Naturally* (1984), Sattilaro stated that his doctors had pronounced him in a state of permanent remission. He died of his disease in 1989, but readers of these books may not learn of this fact.

Entertainers, politicians, and other socially prominent persons are often called upon to promote unproven methods. These individuals, while presumably sincere, seldom have the scientific background to judge the value of what they are promoting. Cancer quackery gets additional support from sensational mass circulation newspapers and magazines and from radio and television talk shows. Several "health" magazines and newsletters are especially interested in unproven treatment regimens and publish information on the latest "theories" and "advances" in cancer management. Examples of these are CFCM's *The Choice*, NHF's *Health Freedom News*, People for Cancer's *Cancer Chronicles*, the *Health Victory Bulletin*, and *Let's Live*.

**Reliable Information Banks**

In 1954, the American Cancer Society began a program to help fight cancer quackery. At that time, there was little factual information concerning this problem and no state laws to combat it. The society formed a Committee on Unproven Methods of Cancer Management to serve as a central coordinating force in this field. The committee (recently renamed the Committee on Questionable Methods of Cancer Management) is concerned with public and professional education as well as legal matters. Its membership includes experts in these fields. The Committee has issued many reports on individual unproven cancer remedies and tests.

The national office of the American Cancer Society has established an information clearinghouse that contains one of the country's largest collections of information about cancer quackery. Material from its files is used to answer thousands of inquiries from health professionals, writers, and the general public. Information about unproven methods is also published in *CA—A Cancer Journal for Clinicians* which is distributed free of charge to about 350,000 physicians and other health professionals in the United States. Close communication is also maintained with the FDA, the National Cancer Institute, the U.S. Postal Service, the U.S. Customs Service, and other interested parties—both government and private. Information about cancer treatment—both proven and questionable—can be obtained from local chapters or by dialing the national office at 1-800-227-2345.

The National Cancer Institute also has an active information program. Its Cancer Information Service can answer questions and may provide literature about the latest cancer treatments, clinical trials, early cancer detection, reducing cancer risk, and community services for patients and their families. Physicians can obtain additional information on treatment protocols, results, and clinical trials through Physician Data Query (PDQ), a computerized database maintained and updated monthly by the National Cancer Institute.

These services enable most cancer patients to benefit from the latest scientific knowledge without having to travel far. By dialing 1-800-4-CANCER, callers from most parts of the United States will be connected with the Cancer Information Service office serving their area. The only areas not tied into the toll-free number are Washington, DC (1-202-636-5700), Alaska (1-800-638-6070), and Hawaii (1-800-524-6070).

**The Bottom Line**

Most cancer patients can be cured if treated properly and in time. Several million Americans are alive today because their cancers were cured by prompt use of *proven* methods of surgery, radiation, or chemotherapy.

You might think that as medical treatment has become more effective, quackery would diminish in proportion. That has not happened, however. Modern communication and our free press have enabled questionable methods to get enormous publicity—luring many unsuspecting Americans to try them.

Many people who promote questionable methods of cancer management are well-meaning individuals who are sincere in their beliefs. The rest are profiteers. Regardless of their motivation, however, one thing is clear. Incurable cancer patients who waste their life's savings on false hopes, and potentially curable patients who die from delay of proper treatment, are victims of quackery at its cruelest.

# 7

# The Misery Merchants

### Diana Benzaia
### Stephen Barrett, M.D.

*"Do you ache all over when you wake up in the morning? Are your joints stiff and swollen during the day? Do you fall asleep in pain? Then you don't need a doctor to tell you have arthritis. And a doctor can't cure you either. But our out-of-this-world treatment can cure you!*

*Government scientists have never revealed the fantastic medical benefits of soil samples brought back from the moon. But now the secret is out! This amazing moondust will cure you of arthritis—as it has cured others—and you can have it right now, without a doctor's prescription! The cure is quick and the price is cheap when you think of the happy life ahead of you—without arthritis!"*

Would you believe the above sales pitch—that a single salesman has obtained closely guarded samples, that an arthritis cure is being kept secret, that a layman can cure what a doctor cannot?

Millions of people have believed such yarns in the past and continue to fall for modern-day versions. Gadgets used to be the mainstay of phony arthritis "cures." Today nutritional approaches are emphasized and the pitches tend to be more subtle, but most still follow the above pattern. Let's examine it closely.

*"You don't need a doctor to tell you have arthritis."* False! There are close to a hundred different kinds of rheumatic disease. Arthritis can strike at any age, even in infancy, and can last a lifetime. Proper treatment requires proper diagnosis. Symptoms similar to those of arthritis may even be caused by other types of disease. Only a qualified physician can properly diagnose and treat arthritis.

*"Government scientists have never revealed the fantastic medical benefits of soil samples brought back from the moon."* False! No scientist would

have reason to keep an arthritis cure secret. Sharing a "secret cure" is a favorite sales trick of quack promoters. It is also a way to sell newspapers, as the sensational tabloids have discovered. Their headlines promise "cures" while referring to the promises of quacks or the unconfirmed, preliminary findings of researchers.

*"This amazing moondust will cure you."* False! Except for a few infectious types, there is *no* cure for arthritis. It is common, however, for the disease to have ups and downs. Some people, after having been troubled by pain for months, may suddenly feel free of all symptoms. The absence of pain may last for days, weeks or even months. If, by pure coincidence, someone has used a quack product just before this period of temporary improvement, he will be tempted to believe that the product has cured him.

*"The cure is quick and the price is cheap."* False! Arthritis sufferers waste close to a *billion* dollars a year on remedies that range from useless to dangerous. They can also waste valuable time. Although the medical profession can't promise quick results, doctors can plan programs of medication, surgery, physical therapy, exercise, and self-help devices that can minimize pain, deformity, and disability. Early diagnosis and treatment offer the best results. People who walk away from their doctor when they learn that proper treatment may be slow and limited will delay treatment that might make a crucial difference in the outcome of their disease. If inflammation is not controlled, for example, their joints may be permanently damaged. Yet their chronic pain can make them desperate enough to try anything that sounds good.

Arthritis hucksters, who can do nothing but exploit their victims, are truly "merchants of misery." Now let's look at some of the "treatments" they have offered.

### Gadgets and Devices

The supposed curative powers of various metals have been glorified by quacks for years. You may have seen arthritis sufferers sporting copper bracelets. For best results, promoters recommend wearing one on each wrist to set up a so-called "curative circuit." Pure hokum, of course, but that doesn't stop the salesman from selling or the desperate from buying.

"Magnetic induction" to cure arthritis was claimed for the "Inductoscope." This strange device consisted of metal rings that were to be placed over afflicted parts of the body. The rings were connected by wires to an electric wall outlet. The Inducto-scope provided no medical benefit and also exposed its users to dangerous electric shocks. For these reasons, the FDA stopped its sale. The

"Solarama Board" is another gadget that was based on mixed-up electronic theory. Also known as the "Earth Board" or "Vitalator," it was to be placed under the victim's mattress at night. The board supposedly emitted "free electrons" to rejuvenate the body.

Radioactive healing powers, which sound good to many laymen, were claimed for the "Vrilium Tube," a brass tube about two inches long that contained barium chloride. It cost a few cents to manufacture, yet was sold to arthritis victims for hundreds of dollars. The "Oxydonor" was claimed to "reverse the death process into the life process" as well as cure arthritis. Buyers were told to clip metal disks to their ankles and immerse an attached cylinder in water—the colder the water the better. Victims of this fraud soon discovered that all they got for their money was cold toes.

Quacks keep up with the times by developing "new models" of their devices just as other businesspeople do. The "Polorator," an electric heatshocking machine, first appeared as a large, bulky item to be applied to areas of pain. Later it was issued as an attractive, slim metal wand with a small metal roller at one end. Needless to say, it "polarized" nothing.

Vibrators of all sorts are immensely popular with arthritis quacks. While these may offer some relief of minor muscle pain caused by overexertion or fatigue and relax some muscular tension, their effect is merely temporary. Vibrators cure nothing and can sometimes do serious harm by increasing joint inflammation. This is a far cry from the "miraculous" relief promised in some advertisements. Whirlpool baths are also sometimes promoted in misleading fashion. The moist heat of a whirlpool device may temporarily soothe an aching body, but many are no more effective than a plain hot bath. In addition, those that fail to maintain constant temperatures may stress the patient's cardiovascular system.

Lotions, oils, creams, and liniments are similarly overrated by some promoters. These products may exert a temporary soothing effect, but advertising which suggests that they hold greater potential is a cruel deception. Such items applied to the outside of the body can have no effect on the internal course of the disease. Magnets applied with band-aids are also popular for arthritis.

### Dietary Methods

So the food faddists claim to work inside your body. Although medical researchers continue to explore the role that diet may play in certain types of arthritis, so far it seems that only a tiny percentage of individuals with arthritis have indiosyncratic reactions to food. Only carefully controlled experiments can determine whether dietary manipulation actually works for a given person. So far, no compelling evidence exists that any diet is consistently helpful for arthritic conditions. Yet myths persist that dietary factors can cause or cure them.

There is hardly a food item that has not been promoted at one time or another as a "cure" for arthritis. One widely publicized food product was "immune milk." This was said to be derived from antibodies produced by cows that had been injected with streptococcus and staphylococcus vaccines. Scientific studies showed that this milk had no effect on arthritis, yet gullible buyers paid premium prices. Other foods touted for arthritis have more or less appeal, depending on your point of view. How does cod liver oil and orange juice sound? Not too good? Then the "healer" down the street will suggest honey and vinegar, or molasses, or megadoses of vitamins.

The idea of "natural" approaches as beneficial to health is getting a lot of publicity these days. Diets based on raw foods, foods without chemical additives, and other supposedly "natural" items are being hustled by health food stores and a variety of offbeat practitioners. So are misleading books that, unfortunately, have been best-sellers. Many of these approaches are based on the notion that arthritis and other "degenerative diseases" are caused by a build-up of (unspecified) toxins that can be corrected by whatever method they happen to advocate.

"Natural" faddists overlook the fact that prehistoric humans—who certainly ate no additives—also suffered from arthritis. This fact has been documented by studies of fossilized bones. But the "health" and "natural" food peddlers go on offering alfalfa tea, sea brine, citrus concoctions, green-lipped mussel, vitamin concoctions, and a wide variety of other nostrums that are absolutely useless to arthritis sufferers. In fact, promoters of nutrition nonsense sometimes harm their followers. Fad diets that omit essential nutrients or encourage avoidance of proper medical care will endanger the arthritis sufferer as they will anyone else.

## Folklore

Dietary myths derive from our past. Before the advent of modern medicine, people looked to their environment for "cures." Knowing little about the real nature of disease, they relied on methods used by their ancestors. The Indian medicine man, grandma, and others may have had no impact on disease; but if someone, somewhere, went into spontaneous remission while following their advice, that advice might become part of folklore. That is why some people with arthritis carry buckeyes, horse chestnuts, or potatoes with them to "draw out" the disease. And why others wrap themselves in the skins of snakes, wolves, or wildcats.

"Burial" in horse manure is another remnant of folk medicine. Although the moist heat of manure may have a temporary soothing effect, there are certainly more pleasant ways to reach such a goal. However, people don't always expect treatment to be pleasant; they may be prepared to suffer a bit. Maybe that's why so many submit to another old technique—rubbing turpentine over the affected areas. This also provides warmth, but offers burning pain as well, not to mention an unpleasant odor.

Of course, not all folk remedies are painful. Some of grandpa's elixirs can be quite delightful. Their high alcohol content doesn't stop pain, but may make sufferers less aware of it. But if that's your approach to dealing with pain, why not take it straight?

### From "Radioactivity" to Real Estate Promotions

Nothing is ever "straight" about the quack's promises. Merchandisers of the "Radon-pad" claimed it contained a mixture of radioactive materials from Swiss uranium mines that could reverse the arthritic process when applied to afflicted areas. It was nothing but a costly and useless device that emitted less radiation than a wristwatch. Owners of an inactive uranium mine have promoted radon gas as beneficial for arthritis. Victims pay to sit in the dank caverns, supposedly soaking up helpful rays. The radiation level in the mine is so low that it can have no effect on the body at all—which is fortunate, because high radiation levels can increase peoples' chances of developing cancer. Even though there is no scientific evidence that radiation helps arthritis, some sufferers still travel long distances to visit this mine.

In fact, traveling around for a cure is still common for arthritis victims. Some seek cures from clinics and spas that offer special diets, mineral baths, and even such unpleasant treatments as daily colonic enemas. Others search for a climate that will cure their arthritis, and real estate promoters capitalize on the hope that a warm climate will be the answer to their problem. (Never mind that Eskimos and Laplanders, who live in cold, damp climates, have fewer cases of rheumatoid arthritis than people who live in warmer, drier ones. Or that rheumatologists in states like Arizona have thriving practices.) The "weather myth" of arthritis seems to come from evidence that some people feel worse when barometric pressure drops. While a more stable climate may make them feel better, it will not influence the course of their disease.

## Painkiller Promotions

Even effective drugs can be promoted in misleading ways. People with arthritis are bombarded with television ads suggesting that many different nonprescription products can help relieve their pain. The ads seldom reveal, however, that many competing products contain the same ingredients. Nor—despite claims to the contrary—does one product work significantly faster than another.

Most nonprescription pain-relievers contain either aspirin, acetaminophen, or ibuprofen. Small doses of any of these may be effective against the aches and pains of mild forms of arthritis. In high doses, aspirin or ibuprofen (but not acetaminophen) can be effective against the *inflammation* of arthritis, but these doses should not be used without medical guidance. Consumers who self-treat without first seeking medical attention may be risking irreversible damage to joints (as well as serious side effects)—damage that might be prevented with appropriate treatment.

## Medical Mismanagement

Some doctors harm their arthritis patients because they don't know any better. At present, there are about 3,200 physicians in the United States who specialize in treating arthritis—nowhere near enough to supervise those among the 37 million arthritics who might benefit from their expertise. So most people rely on their family doctor for arthritis treatment. Some family doctors provide good care; others are sincere in their wish to help but are not up-to-date in their knowledge of arthritis treatment. An example of this would be a doctor who recommends removal of teeth or tonsils on the theory that they might harbor infections. (The theory that hidden tooth or tonsil infections can cause arthritis has long been disproven.)

A more common response of the untrained doctor is to sympathize with the patient, shrug his shoulders, indicate that "nothing much can be done," and recommend aspirin to alleviate pain. (Although aspirin can be useful for relieving pain, it must be taken on a regular schedule to reduce inflammation—and not just when pain arises.) You can't call this approach quackery, but it often drives sufferers to quacks. People who are discouraged, and have more pain than they think they should, are often willing to try anything that offers hope.

## Dangerous Drugs

Shoulder-shruggers are nothing compared to the doctors who falsely promise "miracles" to arthritis victims. A prime example was Dr. Robert Liefmann, a

Canadian physician who claimed a drug he made would cure arthritis. Called *Liefcort,* the drug contained steroids and other potentially dangerous hormones. Because side effects from steroids can be dangerous, and even fatal, they have limited value in the treatment of arthritis. Patients who take them should have close medical supervision. After paying high prices at Dr. Liefmann's Montreal clinic, patients returned home with a several-month supply of medication — typically taken without medical supervision. As a result, many experienced infections, cataracts, adrenal shock, thinning of the bones, compression fractures, stomach ulcers, and even death.

In 1969, Dr. Liefmann was convicted on sixteen counts of violating Canada's Food and Drugs Act and was fined $2,400. He died in 1972 with the case still under appeal. *Liefcort* has never been approved by the FDA for distribution in the United States, but formulas like the one he concocted are still dispensed under various names at clinics in Canada and Mexico.

Since the late 1970s, Oriental arthritis remedies said to be "all-natural" herbal products have been illegally marketed in the United States under the names *Chuifong Toukuwan, Black Pearls,* and *Miracle Herb.* Government agencies have found that in addition to herbs, these products contain various potent drugs not listed on their label. The drugs have included antianxiety agents (diazepam [*Valium*], chlordiazepoxide [*Librium*]), anti-inflammatory drugs, (indomethacin, phenylbutazone, prednisone, dexamethasone), pain-relievers (mefenamic acid, acetaminophen, aminopyrine), and the male sex hormone methyltestosterone. Aminopyrine was banned in the United States in 1938 because it can cause agranulocytosis, a life-threatening condition in which the body stops producing white blood cells. Prednisone and dexamethasone are steroids. Some batches of *Chuifong Toukuwan* have contained amounts of diazepam high enough to cause addiction. In 1975, four users of *Chuifong Toukuwan* were hospitalized with agranulocytosis and one died. The FDA has banned importation of the product and helped Texas authorities obtain criminal convictions against several marketers. However, it is still illegally imported and marketed through clandestine channels.

## Quackery in Print

How do arthritis victims in Maine hear about clinics in Mexico? By word-of-mouth and the power of the printed word. Freedom of the press allows anyone to plug a remedy for arthritis, and quacks take full advantage of the media.

Many books—including some from supposedly reputable publishers—promote false theories about the cause and treatment of arthritis. Some push special diets; others make overblown claims for good techniques. For example, promotional ads for *Pain-Free Arthritis,* by Dvera Berson with Sander Roy, said, "It's not just a book. It's a promise." The ads also quoted a physician, supposedly an Arthritis Foundation member, as calling the book "the first truly helpful innovation in the physical therapy of arthritis in the past hundred years." Angered by the book's bogus claims, the Arthritis Foundation fired off a strong protest to its publisher, Simon and Schuster. Noting that the physician was not a Foundation member, the organization said: "It is Dvera Berson's thesis that exercise under water helps arthritis. That's true. It does. It's called hydrotherapy. . . . It has been around for years. But it is not a panacea."

Another popular title has been Dale Alexander's *Arthritis and Common Sense,* which, according to its publisher, has sold more than a million copies. Alexander, who died in 1990, was endearingly referred to as "the Codfather." The book states that Alexander was inspired by treating his mother's crippling arthritis. He concluded that the basic cause of arthritis is "poorly lubricated joints" and that dietary oils (particularly cod liver oil) relieve arthritis by lubricating the joints. This theory is ludicrous. The lubricating fluid within the joints is not oil but a fluid that resembles blood plasma and is secreted by the tissue lining the joints. Moreover, dietary oils can't reach the joints intact because they are broken down into simple substances by the digestive process. Alexander also stated that arthritics should allow at least six months to assess the results of taking cod liver oil because "it could take that long for the whole body to lubricate itself." That, of course, would be sufficient time for many arthritics to undergo spontaneous improvement.

Authors and book publishers are not the only ones who profiteer in print at the expense of arthritis victims; media that accept ads for misleading books are equally to blame. And so are the health-food industry's publications, which abound with claims that food supplements can help virtually every health problem. In 1990, Alexander's theories appeared in a two-page interview in Swanson's *Health Shopper* together with an ad for Twin Laboratories, Inc.'s *Emulsified Norwegian Cod Liver Oil,* whose label bore Alexander's signature.

Tabloid newspapers seem to "specialize" in reporting so-called arthritis cures—often with front-page headlines. Articles of this type tend to fall into three categories: (1) sensationalized presentations of useful methods already known to the arthritis community, (2) preliminary reports of research findings that have no practical significance, and (3) one-sided reports touting quack nonsense. For example:

- In a *Sun* article headlined "Miracle Caves Cure Thousands of Arthritis," the "miracle caves" were tunnels in the mines described earlier in this chapter.

- In another *Sun* article, "Bible Cures for Arthritis and High Blood Pressure," "powwow doctors" in Pennsylvania are said to "restore people to perfect health" by reciting Biblical verses and laying hands on them.

- "Nature's Miracle Cures for Arthritis and High Blood Pressure, according to the *National Examiner*," were fruits that supposedly rid the body of toxins that cause arthritis.

- The *National Examiner's* "New Diet to Ease Pain of Arthritis" was a standard low-fat, high-fiber diet plus vitamin supplements. Its "How to Wash Away Arthritis Pain Instantly" was simply a hot bath.

- *Weekly World News* has touted "Bottled Love Water," a bottled spring water said to contain lithium and be effective not only against arthritis but also against alcoholism, heart ailments, colon cancer, and a dozen other problems.

Many arthritis "cures" are characterized by unscientific theory, lack of controlled tests, and refusal to permit other physicians to examine patient records. When any such "breakthrough" is reported in the press before review by medical colleagues, the arthritis patient should be suspicious. Some "breakthroughs" may merit further investigation, but those with no scientific basis will merely raise false hopes.

## Acupuncture

Promotion before the facts are all in may not be as unethical as promotion of the definitely phony; but it can still be harmful. Acupuncture is another illustration of this problem. When this ancient Chinese technique arrived on the American medical scene, it was hailed as a surgical anesthetic. Then it was promoted as a cure for various ailments (see Chapter 18). Massive publicity led many arthritis hopefuls to join the long lines at acupuncture clinics, hoping for a cure. Research to date seems to indicate that acupuncture may provide temporary relief of pain for some arthritis patients—but has no long-range effect on the course of the disease. At this point, it seems unlikely that acupuncture will find a place in the list of legitimate treatments for arthritis.

Another example of irresponsible publicity for a supposed cure garbed in a medical aura is that which surrounded the antifungal drug, clotrimazole. This drug was hailed by a British physician as a cure for rheumatoid arthritis, which he said was a protozoal infection. His claims received front-page coverage in many newspapers. Few newspapers gave much space to the follow-up, however, which revealed that: the physician involved was neither an arthritis specialist nor then licensed to practice medicine in Britain; the manufacturers of the drug he recommended reported no knowledge that it had antiprotozoal activity, even if rheumatoid arthritis were a protozoal infection, which it is not; the physician had not conducted a controlled trial and did not even have any clotrimazole to dispense. Pity the poor people who wasted thousands of dollars traveling to England for a "cure" after the first newspaper reports.

## Other Quasi-Medical Approaches

Dimethyl sulfoxide (DMSO) has been touted as a possible treatment for various ailments, including musculoskeletal injuries and some arthritic diseases. In 1978, the FDA approved its use for interstitial cystitis, a rare bladder disorder. However, DMSO has not been demonstrated to have any long-term benefit for any form of rheumatic disease, and most reputable physicians don't prescribe it. Several clinics in Mexico claim to treat arthritis patients with DMSO, although some drugs brought back to the United States from some of these clinics have contained potent (and sometimes dangerous) ingredients other than DMSO.

Capsules of omega-3 fatty acids—commonly referred to as "fish oils"— have been marketed with claims that they are effective against several types of arthritis. A few experiments in both animals and humans have had positive results, but it is not known whether there is a dose that is both practical and safe. Fish oil supplements can interfere with blood clotting and increase the risk of stroke, especially when taken with aspirin or other nonsteroidal anti-inflammatory drugs. Fish oils can also cause diarrhea and upset stomach. Responsible medical authorities believe that including oily fish (mackerel, salmon, sardines, or lake trout) to the diet is preferable to taking fish oil supplements.

Homeopathic products, discussed in Chapter 13, are also promoted for arthritis. In a recent issue of *Let's Live,* a leading homeopath stated that there may be 150 remedies available for different types of arthritis and that they work by stimulating the body to heal itself. He claimed that, "Mild or relatively recent cases can be cured completely. Cases of many years' duration can usually be greatly relieved, sometimes cured, and, at the very least, the degenerative process can be halted." There is no scientific evidence to support these claims.

## The Reality of Arthritis

Arthritis victims who are disappointed by one "miracle" after another may develop a sense of hopelessness. When told that rheumatologists really *can* help, they may react like the townspeople did to the boy who cried "wolf" once too often. They may disbelieve.

The reality of arthritis is that it is a chronic disease. When it comes, it usually stays and lasts a lifetime. It is the nation's number one crippling disease, but much of its pain and disability can be alleviated through early diagnosis and proper treatment. Most arthritis patients can be helped with a well-designed program of medication, special exercises, rest, and other measures—prescribed by a well-trained physician.

What's also very real is the research now being conducted to find the causes of arthritis. What a "miracle" it would be if the money wasted on arthritis quackery could be used for research instead.

# 8

# Weight Control:
# Facts, Fads, and Frauds

## Stephen Barrett, M.D.

Year after year, "new" diet books are published amid claims of "quick, safe, and painless weight reduction—without hunger." Newspapers and magazines abound with ads for diet plans, reducing pills, and gadgets for slimming of selected body parts. Weight-loss clinics are everywhere. With all this hoopla, you might think that Americans overall are getting thinner, but such is not the case. The prevalence of obesity has actually increased during the past two decades. Approximately one quarter to one third of adults are now classified as overweight, depending on the criteria used.

Health and insurance statistics show clearly the penalties of being 20 percent or more overweight. One serious problem associated with obesity is high blood pressure. There is also considerably increased risk of sickness and/or death from diabetes; liver, kidney, heart, blood vessel, and gallbladder diseases; and other health problems.

Many promoters of dietary schemes would have us believe that a special substance or combination of foods will automatically result in weight reduction. But you can't fool Mother Nature! To lose weight, you must eat less, or exercise more, or do both.

There are about 3,500 calories in a pound of body weight. To lose one pound a week, you must consume about five hundred fewer calories per day than you metabolize. Most fad diets, if followed closely, will result in weight loss—as a result of caloric restriction. But they are invariably too monotonous and are often too dangerous for long-term use. Moreover, dieters who fail to adopt better exercise and eating habits will regain the lost weight—and possibly more.

**Fasting**

The most drastic way to reduce caloric intake is to stop eating completely. Indeed, fasting has been used for weight reduction since ancient times. Fasting can produce dramatic weight loss, particularly in its early stages. Losses will be greatest in the heaviest subjects and least in those who weight the least. Loss of body water is partially responsible for the weight lost during the initial stages of fasting. In the short run, this may trick some dieters into thinking that they have found a magical way to lose weight. In the long run, however, losing water is not the same as losing true body fat. Body water will be restored quickly when eating is resumed.

Prolonged fasting will throw the body into a state of ketosis. Under ordinary circumstances, the preferred fuel for every tissue is the simple sugar, glucose, which can be obtained easily from carbohydrates, less easily from proteins, but not at all from fats. After a few days of total fasting, body fats and proteins are metabolized to produce energy. The fats are broken down into fatty acids that can be used as fuel. In the absence of adequate carbohydrate, the fatty acids may be incompletely metabolized, yielding ketone bodies and thus ketosis. But proteins must also be broken down to produce glucose. In ketosis, these are taken from lean body mass—muscles and major organs such as the heart and kidneys. A prolonged fast may also lead to anemia, impairment of liver function, kidney stones, postural hypotension, mineral imbalances, and other undesirable side effects. Deaths due to prolonged fasting have occurred, usually in people who believed this would "purify" their body or cure them of some disease.

**Supplemented Fasting**

Although most body tissues can adapt to using ketone bodies for fuel, the brain requires at least 20 percent of its fuel in the form of glucose. This must be supplied from somewhere—dietary carbohydrates, dietary proteins, or one's own tissues. It might seem that the simplest way to prevent loss of protein from vital tissues during a fast would be to give just enough food to supply the central nervous system with its daily glucose requirement and thus "spare" the protein in the body. But researchers have found that carbohydrate is unsuitable for this purpose. Even a small amount will stimulate insulin secretion that leads to hunger attacks that don't occur when the body is running on ketone bodies. Dietary protein works better because it breaks down more slowly to glucose without triggering an insulin response.

It was this rationale that inspired a method called the "protein-sparing modified fast" or very-low-calorie (VLC) diet. The original program, developed by George Blackburn, M.D., Ph.D., in the early 1970s, was intended for people who were markedly overweight and for use under strict medical supervision. Within a few years, however, the concept was popularized by a book called *The Last Chance Diet.* Although the book warned readers to seek medical supervision, it also told them how to administer their own program with a liquid protein product. "Do-it-yourself" products soon flooded the marketplace. Unlike the high-quality protein used by Dr. Blackburn, the protein in many of these products was of poor quality. This resulted in more than fifty deaths, many from sudden disturbances of heart rhythm.

Nowadays, properly supervised VLC programs take precautions to minimize complications. These programs typically use 400 to 800 calories per day, most of them from high-quality proteins, plus vitamins and minerals, particularly potassium. Some use liquid formulas, while others utilize food sources (poultry, fish, and lean meats). Programs this drastic should be restricted to individuals who are at least 30 percent overweight and should be administered only under close medical supervision as part of a comprehensive program. A well-run program includes a weekly examination by a physician familiar with the metabolic effects of VLC diets, blood tests to detect potentially dangerous metabolic abnormalities, and behavior modification. Weight gain is still common after the eating of food is resumed, but it is more likely to occur with do-it-yourself plans than with medically supervised ones. Fewer than half of the people who sign up for a VLC program actually reach their goal weight.

**Low-Carbohydrate Diets**

Weight-reduction diets can be divided into two broad groups, those that restrict calories *per se,* and those that restrict intake of one or more of the macronutrients (carbohydrates, proteins, and fats) that are the main sources of calories. Carbohydrates in particular have been singled out as villains in the battle of the bulge for more than a century, especially during the past two decades. Examples of low-carbohydrate diets are the Air Force Diet, the Calories Don't Count Diet, the Drinking Man's Diet, the Doctor's Quick Weight Loss Diet, Dr. Atkins' Diet Revolution (old and new versions), the Mayo Clinic Diet (which, by the way, has no connection with the Mayo Clinic), and the Loma Linda or T-3 Diet (which has no connection with Loma Linda Medical Center). Diets like these have been extremely popular. Many people have actually lost weight on them—often temporarily—but not necessarily for the reasons suggested by their promoters.

Most low-carbohydrate diets do not limit the intake of proteins, fats, or total calories. Promoters claim that unbalancing the diet will lead to increased metabolism of unwanted fat whether or not calories are restricted. What actually happens, however, is that obese individuals who drastically reduce their carbohydrate intake are apparently unable to make up the ensuing deficit by increasing their intake of protein and fat. It is very difficult to unbalance a diet to this extent and consume the same number of calories as before. Weight loss on such diets is due mainly to reduced intake of calories—as a result of the restrictive diet's monotony—rather than some special metabolic response to the contents of the diet.

A diet that is low in both carbohydrates and calories will produce ketosis. As with fasting, hunger may be suppressed and weight loss may be rapid during the first few weeks (due primarily to water loss). Medical complications are similar to those of the fasting state.

### Nonsensical Diets

If a contest were held for the most ridiculous diet book ever written, the result might be a tie between *The Beverly Hills Diet* (1981) and *Fit for Life* (1986).

*The Beverly Hills Diet* was based on the notion that fully digested food passes through the body without causing weight gain, but undigested food gets "stuck" in the body and becomes fat. The book also alleged that if foods are not eaten one at a time, the enzymes they contain will cancel each other out and interfere with digestion. Fruits are ideal, the book claimed, because their enzymes can make hard-to-digest foods less fattening. During the first ten days, the dieter was supposed to eat nothing but fruit—with at least two hours between types.

The author, Judy Mazel, had studied dramatics in college and had no academic training in medicine or nutrition. At first, the media treated her as a novelty. But the book's popularity waned sharply after the *Journal of the American Medical Association* published a devastating analysis by Gabe Mirkin, M.D., and Ronald N. Shore, M.D., two physicians practicing in Silver Spring, Maryland. First they explained in detail why Ms. Mazel's basic theory was nonsensical. (Among other things, the only enzymes involved in the digestive process are those made within the body.) Then they selected eighteen statements from the book and explained why they were wrong. Then they described how three of their patients had developed severe diarrhea, muscle weakness, and dizziness during their first week on the diet—which is not surprising because large amounts of fruit usually will cause diarrhea. Finally, they indicated why more serious complications might well occur.

*Fit for Life* was written by "Dr." Harvey Diamond and his wife Marilyn, neither of whom had any scientific training in nutrition (see Chapter 16). The book states that when certain foods are combined in the body, they "rot" and "putrefy," creating digestive cesspools that somehow poison the system and make a person fat. To avoid this, the authors recommend that fats, carbohydrates, and protein foods be eaten at separate meals, concentrating on fruits in the morning and vegetables in the afternoon. They favor fruits and vegetables because foods high in water content can "wash the toxic waste from the inside of the body" instead of "clogging" the body. Actually, digestion is a process of controlled disintegration in which digestive juices break down the foods into smaller chemical components so they can pass through the intestinal wall. Contrary to the Diamonds' assertion, the process is completed within a few hours.

Katherine Musgrave, Ph.D., a professor of nutrition at the University of Maine, used a computer to analyze seven days of menus printed in *Fit for Life*. She found that the diet was marginal in iron and deficient in zinc, calcium, vitamin D, and vitamin $B_{12}$. Over a period of several weeks, these shortages are unlikely to cause trouble. But as a life-long program (which the authors recommend), significant deficiencies could result. The book's recommendation to avoid milk and most dairy products is an invitation to calcium shortage and osteoporosis.

Despite its nonsense, the book was a great commercial success. Appearances on the Merv Griffin and Donahue shows helped generate sales of well over a million copies. Commenting on this, Dr. William Jarvis, president of the National Council Against Health Fraud, stated:

> *Fit for Life* seems unprecedented in the amount of misinformation contained. It is appalling that such a book can become a best seller in the latter half of the twentieth century. Its only socially redeeming feature is that its popularity may alert American educators to their failure to impart the most fundamental knowledge about health and nutrition to the students entrusted to their care.

Another nonsensical approach that is equally imaginative, but not as well known, is the "body type" system described by Elliot D. Abravanel, M.D., and his wife Elizabeth A. King in *Dr. Abravanel's Body Type Diet & Lifetime Nutrition Plan* (1983) and *Dr. Abravanel's Anti-Craving Weight-loss Diet* (1991). These books maintain that there is a "dominant gland" at the root of every weight problem and that weight can be controlled by soothing the errant gland and moderating its cravings. The book advises that the corrective plan be tailored to the individual's "body type," which is determined by examining the person's shape, body fat distribution, food cravings, sleep patterns, and various other characteristics. Women can be classified as a "thyroid," "pituitary," "adrenal," or "gonadal" type, while men can be classified as "thyroid," "pituitary," or "adrenal." The personality traits described for each type resemble those of a typical horoscope.

Nature's Sunshine Products (NSP), a multilevel company discussed in Chapter 17, markets this approach as the GlanDiet Program, which is intended "to bring balance to out-of-balance systems." The program includes two types of meal-replacement powders whose protein-to-carbohydrate ratios are said to be formulated to stimulate either the thyroid and pituitary glands or the adrenals and gonads. To help distributors design the correct program, NSP provides a "body type" questionnaire said to be based on the person's shape and build. For each type there also are "foods to eat or avoid" and various herbal teas and supplement products. All dieters are advised to begin with a "two-to-three-day cleanse," engage in aerobic exercise, and aim for an overall calorie count of 1,200/day for women or 1,400/day for men. Of course, virtually everyone who can achieve such exercise and calorie-restriction levels will lose weight whether or not they use NSP products.

## Diet Aids

Nonprescription diet aids sold in pharmacies and "health food" stores enjoy popularity despite their questionable effectiveness. Ads for many of them make dieting sound like more fun than eating. These products, sometimes accompanied by a printed diet, generally fall into six classes: (1) candies alleged to curb appetite; (2) anti-appetite agents, such as phenylpropanolamine; (3) local anesthetics; (4) diuretics; (5) bulking agents; and (6) secret cures—which usually turn out to contain such ingredients as kelp, fructose, caffeine, or protein. Most of these products are discussed in the quick-reference guide at the end of this chapter.

Diet plans that substitute a protein-containing preparation for one or more meals are sold person-to-person and at retail stores. There has been little clinical testing of these programs, but it seems likely that they will prove too monotonous for long-term use.

Non-nutritive sweeteners are also very popular because they enable people to enjoy sweet drinks that contain almost no calories. Many people hope that use of artificial sweeteners will result in lowering of total caloric intake. This would be true if the rest of one's diet remained rigidly fixed. However, most people eat to a given caloric satisfaction and are likely to replace the "saved" sugar calories with others.

Mail-order products are typically marketed with claims that they can cause weight loss of several pounds a week without exercise or calorie restriction. Some of these products are claimed to suppress appetite through hormonal manipulation ("growth-hormone releasers"). Others are supposed to block the absorption of fats, carbohydrates, sugar, or calories in general. I have never seen a product advertised in this manner that was not a complete fake. Not only that, but countless people have complained to government agencies and Better Business Bureaus that money-back "guarantees" for such products were not honored.

## Behavioral Modification

The purpose of behavior modification therapy is to help people gain control over their eating behavior. This may be accomplished by understanding the factors that produce the "abnormalities" and retraining toward a more favorable behavior pattern. But there is more to it than mere suppression of the cues to eat or overeat.

A number of books outline detailed steps such as removing from sight all suggestions of food, eating at only one place at designated times, eating slowly while chewing thoroughly, and keeping a diary of food eaten. These ideas may be helpful to some individuals, but are not a substitute for more individual analysis and retraining under professional supervision. Most reliable medical clinics include behavioral modification in their programs.

Preventing overweight during childhood may lower the chance of obesity in adult life. Obesity is related to both the number of fat cells and the amount of fat they contain; the more fat cells a person has, the more likely he or she will become and remain obese. Excessive caloric intake tends to increase the number of fat cells in the body, particularly during childhood. When people lose weight they decrease the fat content of their cells but not their number. Thus the more excess weight gained early in life, the more difficult it will be to lose or maintain weight.

## What Should You Do?

Any diet that contains fewer calories than you expend will cause you to lose weight. A deficit of five hundred calories per day will yield a weight loss of one pound a week. This may not seem like much, but it will add up to fifty-two pounds in a year. While crash diets can provide faster initial weight loss, they may also lack important nutrients, may injure health, and will not help people learn to readjust their long-range eating habits. Most nutritionists recommend a low-calorie, low-fat, balanced diet plan that aims for a weight loss of one to one and a half pounds a week. For most people, successful weight-control requires a lifelong commitment to a change in lifestyle, eating habits, and dietary practices. No matter how much weight one wants to lose, modest goals and a slow course will maximize the possibility of both losing the weight and keeping it off.

A thirty-two-year study of more than three thousand men and women has shown that regardless of initial weight, people whose weight repeatedly goes up and down (referred to as "weight cycling" or "yo-yo dieting") have a higher overall death rate and as much as twice the normal risk of dying of heart disease. The researchers found that people who dieted tended to vary their weight more than people who did not. They also concluded that many women who are not overweight create trouble for themselves by dieting.

An adult whose weight is just right should eat the amount of food that permits maintaining that weight. (Most people who lead a moderately active life need about fifteen calories per pound.) If weight begins to rise, or is too high to begin with, total caloric intake (and probably fat intake) should be cut down. This can be done either by counting calories or by intuitively reducing portion sizes and eating lower-calorie foods until the desired rate of weight loss is achieved.

Although it takes a considerable amount of exercise to match the effect of calorie restriction, exercise on a regular basis is also important. The idea that exercise is self-defeating is a myth. In most cases, physical activity does not unduly increase food intake. Even if a regular exercise program does not result in the desired amount of slimming, it may increase one's quality of life by increasing physical fitness. The 1992 National Institutes of Health Technology Assessment Conference on Methods for Voluntary Weight Loss and Control concluded:

> Methods whose primary goal is short-term rapid or unsupervised weight loss, or that rely on diet aids such as drinks, prepackaged foods, or pharmacologic agents but do not include education in and eventual transition to a lasting pattern of healthful eating and activity, have never been shown to lead to long-term success. . . . A focus on approaches that can produce health benefits independently of weight loss may be the best way to improve the physical and psychological health of Americans seeking to lose weight.

Remember: Losing weight is trouble enough without wasting money and risking one's health in the pursuit of false hopes.

**Quick-Reference Guide to Weight-Reduction Methods**

*"Amazing diets"* of one kind or another produce amazing profits for their promoters. They are all based on the fantasy that a magic combination of ingredients can cause you to lose weight no matter how much you eat. Use one and you are more likely to shed dollars than pounds. Here are some clues to help you recognize an unreliable book or diet promotion:

- It suggests that a nutrient or food group is either the "key" to weight reduction or the primary "villain" that keeps people overweight.

- It offers "effortless" weight loss, with neither calorie restriction nor exercise.

- It claims to be a revolutionary or miraculous new idea.

- It reports testimonials rather than documented research.

- It refers to the author's own case histories, but does not describe them in detail.

- It claims 100 percent success.

- It claims persecution by the medical profession.

*Amphetamines* (e.g., Dexedrine) are sometimes used to suppress appetite at the beginning of treatment. Their effect is temporary, and they can have unpleasant side effects.

*Artificial bulk-producing agents* frequently are sold with the claim that they will curb appetite by tricking the stomach into thinking it is full. Your stomach won't be tricked, so don't you be tricked either.

*Artificial sweeteners,* used in place of sugar, provide another means of reducing calorie intake.

*"Cellulite"* spot-reduction plans are supposed to get rid of "unsightly, unevenly distributed pads and lumps of fat which dieting and exercise will not dissolve." The plans consist of diet plus exercise and massage. Exercise and the recommended diet are good for general weight-reduction, but the "cellulite" concept is mere window dressing.

*Counting calories.* Safe and effective, the low-calorie balanced diet is ranked highest by professional nutritionists.

*"Diet candies"* to be taken before meals, are supposed to reduce appetite by raising blood sugar. They typically contain about twenty-five calories per candy. When taken as recommended, they have little effect on blood sugar and no effect upon appetite.

*Diuretics* can make you lose weight by causing your body to shed water.

This effect is short-lived; the weight will come back when you stop the pills. Diuretics can also have bad side effects. If you want to lose fat, not water, stay away from diuretics as a "weight-reducing" pill.

*Exercise machines* tend to be overpriced, and most people find their use monotonous. Good exercise programs can help you burn up calories and improve your body tone.

*"Fat blockers"* are usually "bulking agents (such as guar gum) claimed to form an indigestible gel that carries fat out of the body as it is excreted. Although small amounts of dietary fat may be absorbed in this manner, there is no evidence that this helps people to lose weight.

*Formula diets* (usually liquid) containing specified numbers of calories offer a simple regimen that does not require much knowledge of nutrition. They may substitute usefully for one meal a day, but most people find them too monotonous to use more often.

*"Growth-hormone releasers"* usually contain one or more of the amino acids arginine, ornithine, and tryptophan. Claims that they cause "weight loss while you sleep" are false because: (1) swallowing amino acids does not cause the body to release growth hormone; (2) even if it could, growth-hormone release would be unlikely to cause weight loss; and (3) if significant amounts of growth hormone were released in the body, they could cause acromegaly, a disease in which the hands, feet, and face become abnormally large and deformed. The FDA has banned the marketing of products claimed to cause weight loss by releasing growth hormone.

*Gymnema sylvestre* is claimed to block absorption of sugar into the body. Although chewing the plant's leaves can prevent the taste sensation of sweetness, there is no reliable evidence that the chemicals they contain can block the absorption of sugar into the body or produce weight loss.

*HCG (human chorionic gonadotropin)*, a hormone derived from the urine of pregnant women, is not effective. The 500-calorie diet that typically accompanies injections is a semi-starvation one that is likely to result in protein loss.

*Herbal remedies.* Many types of herbs are touted as effective for controlling weight control. No herbal product has been approved by the FDA as safe and effective for weight control. In fact, many contain laxatives or other ingredients that cause adverse effects.

*Homeopathic products*, such as drops placed on the tongue or adhesive dots applied to "acupuncture points" on the wrist, are said to suppress appetite. Such products are total frauds.

*Kelp, lecithin, cider vinegar, and B₆*—accompanied by a 1,000-or-so-calorie diet will cause weight loss—as a result of the diet alone. The kelp and other supplements are of no benefit in a weight reduction program.

*Low-calorie foods* can give you a bit more food with fewer calories. Non-caloric sweeteners and low-calorie dressings may make food more interesting, but choosing foods by calories alone is seldom a useful approach.

*Obesity specialists* should be approached with caution. Some are excellent, but many are overpriced and follow questionable nutritional theories.

*Protein supplements* are a waste of money. You can and should get all the protein you need from ordinary foods.

*Reducing clubs* may offer moral support and nutritional information. If you join a weight-reducing club, make sure it has a consulting nutritionist.

*Reducing pills* (nonprescription type) are often promoted with exaggerated claims that you can eat all you want and still lose weight. This type of false claim has made millions for some of its promoters. (*Regimen* tablets, claimed to shed pounds without dieting, sold for an estimated $16 million between 1956 and 1962. In the court case that ended in conviction of the manufacturer and the advertising agency, it was shown that TV models who reduced during an advertising campaign had done so by *dieting.*) Diet pills sold in pharmacies typically contain phenylpropanolamine, a decongestant drug that can produce some temporary lessening of appetite. This drug, which is also a mild stimulant, can be dangerous to persons with heart disease, high blood pressure, diabetes, or hyperthyroidism.

*Reducing salons* may give you moral support in keeping to your program of exercising, but if you can't afford one, don't use one.

*Registered dietitians* and many *home economists* are trained in dietary counseling.

*"Slimming teas,"* Oriental or otherwise, have no proven value for appetite suppression or any type of "automatic" weight loss.

*Sole diets*—such as a fruit diet or any diet restricted to one food—are unhealthy because they do not provide adequate nutrition.

*Spas* vary their practices all the way from total starvation at fancy prices to well-run retreats that feature proper diet and exercise instruction. Thus people considering such facilities should investigate them beforehand with great care.

*Spot-reducers,* such as creams, sauna belts, and electric shock devices, may *appear* to work by causing water loss or muscle contraction. These are temporary effects. Spot-reducers do *not* roll it off, rock it off, or bake it off!

*Starch blockers* were claimed to contain an enzyme, extracted from beans, which could block digestion of significant amounts of dietary starch. The enzyme works in the test tube, but the body produces more starch-digesting enzymes than starch-blocker pills could possibly block. If undigested starch does reach the large intestine, it is fermented by bacteria, causing gas production and digestive disturbances. In 1982, the FDA ordered these products off the market after it received many reports of adverse reactions, including thirty cases requiring hospitalization and one death from pancreatitis.

*Starvation diets* cause protein breakdown and are potentially dangerous.

*Surgical procedures* that constrict the stomach or bypass part of the small intestine can have severe side effects and rarely produce satisfactory results.

*Thyroid hormones* in large amounts can cause you to burn calories faster, lose weight, and *strain your heart.* If your thyroid is normal, small amounts of prescribed thyroid will simply cause your body to produce less of its own. Thyroid preparations must carry a label statement that they are not for use in weight reduction. If you suspect "hypothyroidism" (underactive thyroid gland) as the cause of your overweight problem (a very rare disease, by the way), get checked by a physician who does not rely on the basal metabolism test (BMR) or armpit temperature to make the diagnosis.

*Vitamin supplements* are not necessary on a balanced diet unless it is prolonged and contains fewer than 1,200 calories per day.

*Weight-control clinics and health clubs* vary widely in their reliability. Claims that a center is medically supervised or has a physician on the premises may or may not be true. Some facilities have qualified paramedical profession-als, while others use inadequately trained laypersons. Some programs reflect the latest diet fads and promote quack notions. Few have conducted long-term studies of their program's effectiveness. In 1991, an investigation of fourteen weight-loss centers by the New York City Department of Consumer Affairs found that some even attempted to sell services to people who were normal or underweight. The Federal Trade Commission recently secured agreements in which several marketers of very-low-calorie programs pledged to stop making unsubstantiated claims about their success rates.

*"Wrapping"* the body so that a concentrated salt solution can take the water out of the outer layers of the skin can produce only temporary shrinkage at best. At worst, if enough of you is wrapped, you can get seriously ill from dehydration.

*Your doctor* may be able to help you plan a proper diet or refer you to someone else for that purpose.

# 9

# Avoiding the "Marginal" Medic

### Philip R. Alper, M.D.

Fortunately, very few physicians nowadays are quacks. This wasn't always the case, however. Before 1910, there were more than three hundred "medical schools" in the United States. But most were "diploma mills," from which an M.D. degree could be obtained by little more than attending a few lectures and paying a fee. Then the landmark *Flexner Report* was issued, which boldly outlined the deficiencies of American medical education. The report, together with Abraham Flexner's vigorous personal efforts for reform, resulted in the closing of 80 percent of the then-existent medical schools. High standards for medical training were developed, and so was an accreditation system to ensure that medical schools follow these standards.

Counting premedical education, medical training now takes from nine to fifteen years. Both the length and the intensity of this training tend to minimize the number of budding quacks that graduate. But some still enter the health marketplace each year.

Once in practice, most physicians are subject to "peer review" by their colleagues. This process is most significant for physicians who practice in accredited hospitals, where utilization committees review the management of patients to determine whether their treatment was necessary and proper. Pathologists carefully examine tissues removed during surgical operations to see whether they were diseased. In a properly run hospital, practitioners who are not up to standard will hear from their colleagues and have their hospital privileges curtailed if they fail to mend their ways.

Outside of hospitals, medical societies can examine complaints—primarily involving unethical conduct—that are brought to their attention. Doctors who violate the ethical standards required by their societies can be expelled.

Unfortunately, however, neither hospitals nor medical societies can ensure that all practicing physicians are competent and ethical. For one thing, physicians tend to have a sympathy for each other that sometimes interferes with the forcefulness of self-policing. For another, it is possible to practice medicine without belonging to a medical society or to the staff of an accredited hospital. If a doctor you consult belongs to neither, ask for an explanation. If the doctor was expelled, watch out! If the doctor never joined, make sure the reason makes sense to you.

State boards of medical licensure have the ultimate power to stop errant physicians from practicing altogether. But most state boards do not have adequate funding or tough enough laws to do this job properly.

Though I have pointed out some of the problems that the medical profession and the government have in protecting you from marginal practitioners, I would not like to leave you feeling alarmed. Very few practicing physicians are marginal, and fewer yet are outright quacks.

### Avoiding the Outright Quack

Quacks, who often are charming and project a feeling of greater-than-usual concern, are the despair of "straight" physicians. A charismatic quack can produce a legion of adoring clients to testify on his behalf. But certain behavior should make you suspect that a doctor has abandoned medical science:

- Claiming to have a special machine or formula

- Making blanket statements that surgery, x-rays, or drugs do more harm than good

- Claiming that other doctors are persecuting him or are afraid of his competition

- Using testimonials from patients or flamboyant advertising to build his practice.

If you encounter any of these traits, you should not merely seek another doctor but also report your experience to your local medical society and your state board of medical licensure. What you observed may not merely be poor medical practice—it may be illegal.

## The "Marginal" Medic

The above list should help steer you clear of the small percentage of doctors whose involvement with unproven methods is extreme. It is important to realize, however, that quackery is not an "all-or-none" phenomenon. A doctor who is otherwise competent may have a misguided belief in a particular medication or procedure. For this reason, it may be unwise to judge a physician's competence solely on the basis of any one action.

Nor is it possible to construct a list of what would be "proper" treatment for each and every illness. Doctors are alarmed at what has been termed the "tyranny of uniform standards"—the idea of a chart or "cookbook" to follow in treating each ailment. For under such a system, physicians could not use their judgment to tailor treatment to the individual patient. Moreover, some areas of medicine are *genuinely* controversial.

Despite these difficulties, is it possible to detect when a doctor practices a generally sloppy or unscientific brand of medicine? Or that he is a fuzzy thinker in whose hands you would be taking an unnecessary gamble? I think so—to some extent. Your doctor's management of certain common clinical situations can tell you a lot about his or her thinking.

## Infections and Their Management

Infections can be caused by many different kinds of germs. Some germs can be killed or weakened by antibiotics and some cannot. Generally, bacterial infections will respond to antibiotics. "Strep throat" is a common example. Viral infections will usually not be susceptible to antibiotics, though there are exceptions. The common cold is an example of a viral infection that will not respond to antibiotics.

The "ideal" way to treat an infection is to identify the germ that is causing it and prescribe an antibiotic that is specific for that particular germ. A doctor can often tell which germ is infecting you by the pattern of your illness. The diagnosis can be more certain, however, if the doctor obtains a *culture*—whereby your germs are grown so that they can be positively identified. "Sensitivity" tests can then help to determine which antibiotic is likely to be most effective.

The medical school professor, speaking as a pure scientist, may want all infections cultured. But a doctor who treats many patients should be concerned with the costs involved, not only to individual patients but also to society's total health care budget. Where clinical judgment can be accurate most of the time, clinicians should consider how much extra cost is justified for a slight increase in accuracy.

The wise physician must be prepared to use whatever tests are necessary for conditions that require greater diagnostic precision. Bladder infections in women illustrate this point. It is usually not necessary to obtain a culture with the first such infection—particularly if the patient is a young woman who has just begun sexual activity. If the infection keeps coming back, however, cultures should be obtained to ensure precise use of antibiotics. It may also be wise to obtain a kidney x-ray series (intravenous pyelogram) to rule out possible underlying causes of the infections.

Thus, in the overall management of infections, the important consideration may not be whether a doctor takes a culture or uses an antibiotic in a particular case. Rather, it is whether he or she follows a carefully thought-out approach. The wise physician will use cultures to advantage and will prescribe antibiotics *selectively*. Complete avoidance of cultures and routine use of antibiotics for treating ordinary colds are signs of fuzzy thinking.

## The Use of Tranquilizers

Articles in the medical literature point to a worrisome level of tranquilizer use. Some reports, however, suggest that most patients who receive tranquilizers have serious and sometimes disabling symptoms.

Many patients have strong feelings on this subject. Some think it is wrong to depend upon medications; others want quick relief. People who simply swallow pills may be missing the chance to learn about what makes them nervous and what other ways they can use to help themselves. Similarly, doctors who prescribe tranquilizers too readily—without trying to understand the nature of their patients' tensions—may be doing them a disservice.

## The Use of Placebos

Placebos, sometimes referred to as "sugar pills," are substances that have no real effect on the body. Any benefits they confer are through the power of suggestion—a response to the idea that something is being done. Today it is rare for physicians to prescribe totally inactive drugs as placebos. The public is too sophisticated for this form of "psychotherapy." Instead, vitamins or low doses of regular medications are likely to be used.

Many situations exist where *scientific* treatment does not call for the use of medication. However, some patients cannot accept such treatment. Unless they get a shot or a pill, they feel that the doctor "isn't doing anything." Faced with such patients, ethical doctors may find themselves in a quandary. Should they give in to the patient's wishes and become unscientific physicians themselves? Or should they flatly refuse and worry that the patient will shop around and wind up in the hands of a marginal physician or even a quack? Meaningful discussion may be impossible unless the doctor and patient have gotten to know one another and have developed a relationship of trust.

To illustrate the issues involved, consider the case of a married man who developed sexual impotence. This man was convinced that something serious must be wrong with his "glands." So he went to Dr. Z and pressed for a hormone shot. Dr. Z could simply have given the shot, but he did not. Instead, he performed a thorough physical examination and took a careful history.

It turned out that during a period of stress at work, the patient's potency had diminished to the point where he could barely have intercourse. Both he and his wife were modest people who found it difficult to discuss the subject of sex. The patient was ashamed of himself and afraid of "failing" again. His wife didn't want to seem forward by complaining. So they had stopped having intercourse for several months.

The physical exam revealed nothing to suggest a glandular disorder. Here, then, was a problem that was purely psychological. But when Dr. Z suggested that the patient discuss his doubts and fears with his wife, the man was crestfallen. So intense was his lack of confidence that he could barely imagine doing it. Eventually, Dr. Z and his patient struck a compromise. The doctor explained that no glandular deficiency existed, but if the patient still insisted, he would give him a hormone shot anyway. In turn, the patient promised to talk things over with his wife.

With the injection to bolster his confidence, the patient did speak with his wife. A month later, when he returned to the doctor's office, all was well. No more hormone shots were given or requested.

Some doctors might criticize the handling of this case for not being "100 percent scientific." But the patient was not deceived. Nor was the injection used as a substitute for confronting the real issues. *The placebo was used merely to gain the patient's cooperation.* Suppose, however, that the doctor had put the patient on a series of injections after only a brief discussion. This would have reinforced the patient's fears and probably would have made him become dependent upon medication he didn't need.

There are purists who feel that the use of *any* placebo is quackery. But the better view is to look not only at *whether* a doctor uses placebos but *why, how,* and *how often*. Doctors who use them judiciously, but who stress their limited value; who try to deal with the real problems of their patients; and who try to wean their patients, are still practicing the art of good medicine. But doctors who give placebos frequently when they are not requested, who make extravagant claims for them, or who make patients dependent upon them, should be suspect. Such practices are unethical because they *create* a demand for placebos.

Throughout this book it is stressed that patients are usually in a poor position to judge whether a given treatment has helped them—or whether they got better with time or experienced a placebo effect. Quacks capitalize on this difficulty by crediting *all* improvement to their healing powers. Although physicians rarely *try* to mislead patients in this way, they occasionally do so inadvertently. Sometimes medications are marketed that are later shown to be ineffective. But some doctors who have seen patients improve while taking these medications may mistakenly conclude that they were effective. Confidence in a drug that does not work may thus result in its unknowing use as a placebo. So there is another aspect of placebo evaluation: Does the doctor who prescribes a placebo know that he is using one?

Guarding against the use of outmoded treatment is one part of what physicians accomplish by undergoing "continuing education." This means reading current journals, attending conferences, and doing whatever else is necessary to keep up with medical advances. *The Medical Letter is* one publication that provides an excellent discussion of the effectiveness of treatment methods. Whether your doctor reads it is one indicator of an interest in keeping up-to-date.

### "Fad" Diagnoses

Years ago, many nervous or tired people were said to have "adrenal insufficiency." The vast majority of these people were not only misdiagnosed but were also treated with adrenal gland extract, a substance they did not need and that is potentially harmful. "Low thyroid" was likewise unjustifiably diagnosed in many cases of fatigue. Today's "fad" diagnoses—each used to explain neurotic nervousness, fatigue, and many other common symptoms—are chronic fatigue syndrome, "hypoglycemia," "candidiasis hypersensitivity," and "environmental illness."

Chronic fatigue syndrome originally was thought to be related to infectious mononucleosis—the "kissing disease" of adolescents and young adults. Other viruses are now suspected, but some physicians feel the condition doesn't exist. Assuming it does exist, only a small percentage of chronically tired people have it. Either way, doctors who diagnose it in most of their patients should be regarded with suspicion.

Real cases of adrenal insufficiency, hypothyroidism, and hypoglycemia definitely exist, *but they are rare* and should be carefully checked by laboratory testing before the diagnosis is made.

The diagnosis of hypoglycemia, for example, should be reserved for patients who get symptoms two to four hours after eating, develop blood glucose levels below 45 mg per 100 ml whenever symptoms occur, and are immediately relieved of symptoms when blood sugar is raised. The glucose tolerance test is not reliable for evaluating most cases of suspected hypoglycemia. Low blood sugar levels without symptoms have no diagnostic significance because they occur commonly in normal individuals fed large amounts of sugar. The only way to reliably diagnose hypoglycemia is to prove that blood sugar is low whenever symptoms occur during the patient's usual living pattern. The most practical way to do this is probably with a home testing device.

Doctors who overdiagnose hypothyroidism often base their diagnosis on "low" temperature readings determined by placing the thermometer under the armpit. This is not a valid test of thyroid function.

"Candidiasis hypersensitivity" and "environmental illness" are a slightly different story: they are based on concepts that the vast majority of doctors consider invalid. *Candida albicans* is a common yeast that can cause vaginal infections (moniliasis) and various other problems. "Candidiasis hypersensitivity" is based on the notion that "allergy" to this yeast can cause a multitude of symptoms that require treatment with vitamins, antifungal drugs, and special diets that "starve" the yeast. The American Academy of Allergy and Immunology regards the concept of "candidiasis hypersensitivity" as "speculative and unproven"—which is a polite way of saying it is bunkum.

"Environmental illness"—sometimes referred to as "allergy to everything"—is based on the notion that when the total load of physical and psychological stresses exceeds what a person can tolerate, the immune system goes haywire, and hypersensitivity to tiny amounts of common foods and chemicals can trigger a wide range of symptoms. Doctors who advocate this notion call themselves "clinical ecologists" or specialists in "environmental medicine." Their treatment approach involves elimination of exposure to foods and environmental substances to which they consider the patient hypersensitive. Extreme restrictions can involve staying at home for months or living in a trailer designed to prevent exposure to airborne pollutants and synthetic substances. In many cases, the patient's life becomes centered around the treatment. Chapter 10 discusses "candidiasis hypersensitivity" and "environmental illness" in detail.

"True believers" in "candidiasis hypersensitivity" and "environmental illness" are diagnosing and treating them in most or even all of the people who consult them. Some of these doctors are also diagnosing "hypoglycemia" and/or "chronic fatigue syndrome" excessively. Critics believe that state licensing boards should scrutinize these practices and consider revoking the licenses of the doctors involved.

### Thyroid for Weight Reduction

Thyroid hormone is sometimes used as part of a weight-reduction program. Evaluation of this practice should consider why and how it is prescribed. Does the patient really have hypothyroidism as a cause of overweight? (It is possible but uncommon.) Is the hormone being used as a placebo? Or is a fad diagnosis involved?

Some overweight patients insist upon "diet pills." They simply cannot accept the idea that the best way to lose weight is to develop sensible eating habits. For these patients, half a grain or one grain a day of thyroid hormone can be used as a placebo to gain their cooperation with the rest of the weight control program. Used in this way, it is a safe and inexpensive placebo—in marked contrast to the human chorionic gonadotropin (HCG) injections used at weight reduction clinics that exploit their clients.

A few doctors, however, prescribe *large* doses of thyroid to patients whose thyroid function is normal. This treatment is designed to "burn off fat" by raising metabolism *above the normal level.* But this practice is dangerous because it can strain the heart and other organs. Any doctor who suggests it should be dismissed.

### The "Shot Doctor"

Most medications are just as effective by mouth as by injection. Shots are less comfortable and cost more. So the *general* use of injections rather than oral medication should be questioned. Doctors who inject *most* of their patients should be suspected of poor medical practice. But note that I say *suspected* rather than rejected out-of-hand. For it is conceivable that some doctors who prescribe many injections have valid reasons for doing so.

The rules for judging injection use are not black-and-white. Take penicillin, for example. This drug will usually do its job quite well when taken orally, and routine use of shots will run an unnecessary risk—if the patient is allergic, a shot will produce a more troublesome reaction. But there are times when penicillin shots are appropriate. Shots start to work faster and may be indicated when the doctor wants the treatment to take effect as soon as possible. Shots can produce a higher blood level and are the route of choice for syphilis. Strep throats require ten days of treatment, and where patients cannot be relied upon to complete the treatment, a single shot of long-acting penicillin will do it for them.

These are just some of the many factors which a doctor should take into consideration when using penicillin—one drug among the thousands in use today. Complicated? Yes, it can be—but let me give you my personal guidelines for evaluating a suspected "shot doctor."

The first thing to consider is whether the medications being injected would be just as effective by mouth. If so, the next consideration is what stimulates the use of shots. Is it patient demand or is it the doctor's own idea? If patients demand, does the doctor resist? Some patients have such confidence in shots that refusing to give them might only result in driving them into the hands of a marginal practitioner. The better practice is to give in at first but work toward making patients less dependent upon them. If shots cannot be stopped altogether, at least they can be given infrequently.

So far I am talking about effective medications. The same principles apply to placebo shots—but there is far less excuse for frequent use. Vitamin $B_{12}$ shots are frequently used as placebos. $B_{12}$ does have a lifesaving medical use—the treatment of pernicious anemia, *a rare* disorder that affects the blood and nervous system—but other uses of $B_{12}$ are unscientific. The doctor who tells you that $B_{12}$ or "liver" shots "will really fix you up" when you feel "run down" is using them as placebos. The use of $B_{12}$ to treat iron-deficiency anemia is fuzzy thinking. Surveys of doctors' practices have shown that frequent use of $B_{12}$ injections is often associated with poor standards of care in other areas.

I don't want to give you the impression that I am totally "against placebos," or that you should look down on all doctors who use them. The practice of medicine is very complex, and there are situations where placebos have real value. I can recall one woman whose severe problem with itching baffled both me and a topnotch skin specialist. After standard treatment failed, in desperation, we tried a $B_{12}$ shot—which worked. To this day, I don't understand why. Nor do I understand why some injections (like female hormones for menopausal symptoms) sometimes seem to be more effective than the same medicine in pill form. We doctors don't have a scientific explanation for everything we see.

The point here is that some doctors *may* have valid reasons for giving more shots than average. On the other hand, shots should not be used as a substitute for taking enough time with patients to reach an adequate understanding of their individual cases.

Sometimes I encounter people whose doctors have given them vitamin or hormone shots two or three times weekly for many months or years. Such treatment angers me. It may not be immediately clear whether such doctors are motivated more by fuzzy thinking or by greed. Either way, however, their patients have a lot to lose.

## "Magic" Treatments

Gerovital H3 (GH3), developed by a Rumanian physician, has been promoted by the Rumanian National Tourist Office and a few American physicians as an anti-aging substance—"the secret of eternal vigor and youth." Claims have been made that GH3 can prevent or relieve a wide variety of disorders, including arthritis, arteriosclerosis, angina pectoris and other heart conditions, neuritis, deafness, Parkinson's disease, depression, senile psychosis, and impotence. It is also reported to stimulate hair growth, repigment gray hair, and tighten and smooth the skin. (The very length of this list should make you suspicious of the claims!) The principal ingredient of GH3 is procaine, a local anesthetic. Although many uncontrolled studies describe great benefits from the use of GH3, controlled trials have failed to demonstrate any improvement in elderly patients.

Another treatment promoted with miraculous claims is "chelation therapy." This involves intravenous injection of a synthetic amino acid (EDTA) into the blood stream where it is supposed to remove unwanted mineral deposits or "toxic metals" from various parts of the body before exiting via the kidneys. Vitamins, minerals, and other substances are used also. A course of treatment may consist of twenty to fifty infusions and cost thousands of dollars.

According to its promoters, chelation therapy can reverse or prevent the accumulation of fatty deposits (atherosclerosis) in the coronary arteries and elsewhere in the body. Some promoters refer to it as a "chemical roto-rooter" and "a way of producing a powerful rejuvenation of cell functions." Other promoters claim that it works by decreasing the body's production of "free radicals." None of these claims is valid.

Chelation therapy is used most often in cases of heart disease but is also claimed to be effective against kidney disease, arthritis, Parkinson's disease, emphysema, multiple sclerosis, gangrene, psoriasis, and other serious conditions. However, no controlled trial has shown that chelation can help any of these conditions. In 1985, the American Heart Association concluded that chelation therapy is unproven for heart disease and can be dangerous as well.

If I were you, I would steer clear of anyone who does chelation therapy or even recommends it.

Early in 1993, an investigator from ABC-TV's "Nightline" used a hidden camera to record what happened when a man complaining of fatigue consulted a "holistic" medical doctor in Virginia. The man had been undergoing appropriate treatment for high blood pressure and a heart-rhythm disturbance. Although the doctor correctly identified the heart problem that was readily apparent on an electrocardiogram, she did not consider that a medication he had been taking might be the source of his fatigue. Nor did she ask about the pattern of his fatigue, his sleeping habits, or other standard questions that belong in any proper evaluation of fatigue. Her recommendations included chelation therapy (at least thirty treatments at $105 each), vitamin and mineral supplements, and homeopathic remedies. The vitamins included huge doses of vitamin C daily, beginning with 3 grams per day (fifty times the Recommended Dietary Allowance) and increasing by 1 gram daily until a dosage of 20 grams per day was reached. These levels can cause severe diarrhea. The charge for the first visit was $415.

To reduce their time spent on paperwork, many physicians use preprinted billing forms on which frequently used diagnoses can be checked off. When Dr. Stephen Barrett examined the patient's bill, he noted that the form included chronic fatigue syndrome, candidiasis, reactive hypoglycemia, hypothyroidism, and multiple allergies (a term some doctors use for "environmental illness") among its list of about fifty diagnoses. After viewing the videotape, he made this comment about the doctor:

> She appears to have five favorite diagnoses and . . . three favorite treatments. I suspect that she gives most of her patients several of the diagnoses and maybe even all of the treatments.

## Questioning Surgery

For many years there has been considerable discussion of "unnecessary" surgery. The most commonly questioned operations have been appendectomies, tonsillectomies, hysterectomies, and procedures on the back for chronic pain. It is often pointed out that more of these operations are done in the United States than abroad. Arguments rage about whether too many operations are done here or not enough are done elsewhere. The answer is quite likely a bit of both.

Some studies have shown that when insurance companies require a second opinion by a specialist before they will pay for elective (nonemergency) surgery, fewer operations are done. So it is probably wise to have two opinions before agreeing to elective surgery. This does not necessarily mean that two surgeons must be consulted. Capable personal physicians who are familiar with the surgeon's work will not let their patients be stampeded into an unnecessary operation. They will ask the surgeon to justify the procedure to themselves as well as to the patient.

## The Skillful Patient

Licensing laws, accreditation, and peer-review procedures play a major role in protecting patients from marginal physicians. But no system is perfect. To get the most out of our health care system, you must become a skillful patient. Choose doctors carefully and get into the habit of having them explain what they are doing for you—in language you can understand. And be wary of the fringe practices described in this chapter.

# 10

# Unproven "Allergies": An Epidemic of Nonsense

## Stephen Barrett, M.D.

During recent years, several hundred physicians have promoted concepts of allergy and immune dysfunction not recognized by the scientific community. Instead of testing these concepts with scientifically acceptable protocols, they have been marketing them to the public through books, magazine articles, radio and television talk shows, and other channels. They have also supported lawsuits and worker's compensation claims by individuals claiming to have "multiple chemical sensitivity" caused by exposure to environmental chemicals. The health-food industry has joined the fray by marketing supplement concoctions for treating the supposed conditions.

### "Clinical Ecology"

"Clinical ecology," which is not a recognized medical specialty, is based on the notion that multiple symptoms are triggered by hypersensitivity to tiny amounts of common foods and chemicals. Advocates of this belief describe themselves as "ecologically oriented" and consider their patients to be suffering from "environmental or ecological illness," "cerebral allergy," "total allergy syndrome," "20th-century disease," or "multiple chemical sensitivity (MCS)," which supposedly can mimic almost any other illness.

The signs and symptoms of this condition are said to include depression, irritability, mood swings, inability to concentrate or think clearly, poor memory, fatigue, drowsiness, diarrhea, constipation, sneezing, running or stuffy nose, wheezing, itching eyes and nose, skin rashes, headache, muscle and joint pain, urinary frequency, pounding heart, muscle incoordination, swelling of various parts of the body, and even schizophrenia. Proponents state that virtually any part of the body can have "elusive symptoms for which no organic cause can be found."

Clinical ecologists speculate that: (1) although one substance may not have an effect, low doses of different substances can add to or multiply each other's effects; (2) hypersensitivity develops when the total load of physical and psychologic stresses exceeds what a person can tolerate; (3) patients often crave and become addicted to foods that make them ill; (4) changes in the degree of exposure can affect the degree of sensitivity to offending substances; and (5) hypersensitivities may be related to "immune system dysregulation" or "immunotoxicity" that can be difficult to diagnose and treat. Some proponents inform patients that they have "an AIDS-like illness."

Clinical ecologists suggest that the immune system is like a barrel that continually fills with chemicals until it overflows, signaling the presence of disease. However, some also say that "immune system dysregulation" can be triggered by a single serious episode of infection, stress, or chemical exposure. Potential stressors include practically everything that modern humans encounter, such as urban air, diesel exhaust, tobacco smoke, fresh paint or tar, organic solvents and pesticides, certain plastics, newsprint, perfumes and colognes, medications, gas used for cooking and heating, building materials, permanent press and synthetic fabrics, household cleaners, rubbing alcohol, felt-tip pens, cedar closets, tap water, and electromagnetic forces.

To diagnose "ecologically related" disease, practitioners take a history that emphasizes dietary habits and exposure to environmental chemicals they consider harmful. A physical examination and certain standard laboratory tests may be performed, mainly to rule out other causes of disease. Standard allergy test results are usually normal.

Various nonstandard tests are also used, the main one being "provocation and neutralization." In this test, the patient reports symptoms that develop within ten minutes after various concentrations of suspected substances are administered under the tongue or injected into the skin. If any symptoms occur, the test is considered positive and lower concentrations are given until a dose is found that "neutralizes" the symptoms. Elimination and rotation diets are used with the hope of identifying foods that cause problems.

In severe cases, patients may spend several weeks in an environmental control unit designed to remove them from exposure to airborne pollutants and synthetic substances that might cause adverse reactions. After fasting for several days, the patients are given "organically grown" foods and gradually exposed to environmental substances to see which ones cause symptoms to recur.

Treatment requires avoidance of suspected substances and involves lifestyle changes that can range from minor to extensive. Generally, patients are instructed to modify their diet and to avoid such substances as scented shampoos; after-shave products; deodorants; cigarette smoke; automobile exhaust fumes; and clothing, furniture, and carpets that contain synthetic fibers. Extreme restrictions can involve staying at home for months or avoiding physical contact with family members. "Ecologically ill" patients may think of themselves as immunological cripples in a hostile world of dangerous foods and chemicals and as victims of an uncaring medical community. In many cases, their life becomes centered around their illness.

Several franchised laboratories associated with chemical decontamination programs claim to detect "toxins" in the blood with an accuracy in parts per billion. Vitamin therapy costing thousands of dollars is then recommended for any value above the "normal" level of zero. This approach is not part of "traditional" clinical ecology, but some clinical ecologists are involved.

A few practitioners who consider themselves clinical ecologists use computerized galvanometers to diagnose "energy imbalances" and select homeopathic remedies or other products to correct these imbalances (see Chapter 13). The FDA considers such devices "a significant risk" to the public and has begun efforts to stop their use.

## Critical Scientific Reports

Over the past eight years, five prominent scientific panels have concluded that clinical ecology is speculative and unproven:

- The California Medical Association Scientific Board Task Force on Clinical Ecology conducted an extensive literature review and held a hearing at which proponents testified. The task force stated that "clinical ecology does not constitute a valid medical discipline" and should be considered "experimental" only when its practitioners begin to use scientifically sound experimental methods. The task force also expressed concern that unproven diagnostic tests can lead to misdiagnosis that results in patients becoming psychologically dependent, believing themselves to be seriously and chronically impaired.

- The Ad Hoc Committee on Environmental Hypersensitivity Disorders established by the Minister of Health of Ontario, Canada, received submissions, heard testimony from a large number of professionals and laypersons, observed practitioners at work, and issued a five hundred-page report describing the concepts of clinical ecology and the evidence, if any, supporting them. An expert panel then reviewed this report and concluded that "scientific support for the mechanisms that have been proposed to underlay the wide variety of dysfunctions are at best hypothetical. Moreover the majority of techniques for evaluating the patients and the treatments espoused are unproven."

• The American Academy of Allergy and Immunology, which is the nation's largest professional organization of allergists, published a position statement based on an extensive literature review and comments by its members. The statement said, "The idea that the environment is responsible for a multitude of human health problems is most appealing. However, to present such ideas as facts, conclusions or even likely mechanisms without adequate support is poor medical practice" and that "advocates of this dogma should provide adequate studies . . . which meet the usually accepted standards for scientific investigation."

• The American College of Physicians has issued a position paper concluding that "there is no body of evidence that clinical ecology treatment measures are effective." An accompanying editorial in the same journal notes that its promotion has many characteristics of a cult and that its treatment approach should not be considered harmless.

• The American Medical Association Council on Scientific Affairs concluded in 1991 that "until . . . accurate, reproducible, and well-controlled studies are available . . . multiple chemical sensitivity should not be considered a recognized clinical syndrome. Based on reports in the peer-reviewed scientific literature . . . (1) there are no well-controlled studies establishing a clear mechanism or cause for [MCS]; and (2) there are no well-controlled studies providing confirmation of the efficacy of the diagnostic and therapeutic modalities relied on by those who practice clinical ecology."

In 1991, a National Research Council subcommittee concluded that hypersensitivity has an immunologic basis, but "multiple chemical sensitivity (MCS) syndrome" does not. (In other words, although some people are sensitive to small doses of one or a few specific chemicals, the idea that people become *generally* hypersensitive to chemicals has no scientific foundation.) The subcommittee also noted that the controversy surrounding the diagnosis of MCS cannot be resolved until MCS is clearly (and measurably) defined and then explored with well-designed studies. Following a workshop at which proponents began discussing possible research protocols, the National Research Council (NRC) summarized the deliberations and warned again that meaningful research on "multiple chemical sensitivity" cannot be conducted until clear criteria for such a diagnosis can be defined. Nonetheless, "MCS" proponents tout NRC's involvement as evidence that their beliefs and practices are legitimate.

## Case Studies

Critics of clinical ecology have suggested that "environmental illness" is psychosomatic even though its symptoms don't fit clearly into any disease category. Patients in this situation are often relieved to get a "physical" diagnosis that encourages them to play an active role in their care. However, several studies suggest that many of them give up much more than they get.

In 1986, Abba I. Terr, M.D., an allergist affiliated with Stanford University Medical Center, reported on fifty patients who had been treated by clinical ecologists for an average of two years. He evaluated most of these patients because they had made worker's compensation claims for industrial illness. Although all had been diagnosed as "environmentally ill," Dr. Terr could find no unifying pattern of symptoms, physical findings, or laboratory abnormalities. Eight of the patients had not developed their symptoms until after they had consulted the clinical ecologist because of worry over exposure to a chemical. Eleven had symptoms caused by preexisting problems unrelated to environmental factors, and thirty-one had multiple symptoms. Their various treatments included dietary alterations (74 percent), food or chemical extracts (62 percent), an antifungal drug (24 percent), and oxygen given with a portable apparatus (14 percent). Fourteen of the patients had been advised to move to a rural area, and a few were given vitamin and mineral supplements, gamma globulin, interferon, female hormones, and/or oral urine. Despite treatment, twenty-six patients reported no lessening of symptoms, twenty-two were clearly worse, and only two improved.

In 1989, Dr. Terr published similar observations on ninety patients, including forty in the previous report. Although one or more of over fifty sources of chemicals at their workplace had been blamed for the patients' problems, he noted that the testing process did not usually include extracts of the workplace materials that were presumed to be responsible. He also noted that thirty-two of the ninety patients had been diagnosed as suffering from "candidiasis (yeast) hypersensitivity"—a fad diagnosis considered "speculative and unproven" by the American Academy of Allergy and Immunology.

Since provocation-neutralization tests had played a major role in the misdiagnosis of most of the patients he examined, Dr. Terr pointed out that scientific studies have shown it is unreliable. He stated that although exposure to chemicals can cause disease, it is unlikely that the diagnostic and treatment methods of clinical ecology are effective. He also believes that its methods and theories appear to cause unnecessary fears and lifestyle restrictions.

Carroll M. Brodsky, M.D., Ph.D., professor of psychiatry at the University of California (San Francisco) School of Medicine, made similar observations after studying eight people who, following diagnosis by a clinical ecologist, had filed claims for injury primarily by airborne substances. He concluded that they became "adherents of physicians who believed that symptoms attributed by orthodox physicians to psychiatric causes are in fact due to common substances in air, food, and water." He also stated that clinical ecologists "neither promise nor give hope of eliminating the offending condition, and the patients do not seem to expect it.... [They] seem content with their condition and with the reassurance that their symptoms have a physical cause.... Yet we must also recognize that these patients have had symptoms for many years, and whether seen as neurasthenic, hypochondriacal, or phobic, they are among the most resistant and difficult to treat.... These patients search for healers who will provide them with an explanation of their experiences and symptoms that makes sense to them and fulfills a number of psychological needs."

Donna E. Stewart. M.D., associate professor of psychiatry and of obstetrics and gynecology at the University of Toronto, assessed eighteen "20th-century disease" patients referred to the university's psychiatric consultation service. She concluded:

> Virtually all had a long history of visits to physicians, and their symptoms were characteristic of several well-known psychiatric disorders.... It is important that patients with a wide range of diagnosable and treatable psychiatric conditions not receive a misdiagnosis of 20th-century disease and thereby embark on a prolonged, socially isolating, expensive, and often harmful course of ecologic treatment that reinforces their invalidism.

John C. Selner, M.D., and Herman Staudenmayer, Ph.D., operate an environmental unit in Denver, Colorado. In a lengthy report, which is probably the best scientific analysis of the subject ever published, they trace the origins of clinical ecology and illuminate the flaws in its theories and practices. They note that: (1) people do exist who are very sensitive to various micro-organisms, noxious chemicals, and common foods; (2) the key question is whether multisystem disease can be caused by generalized allergy to environmental substances; (3) when a physician is confronted by a patient claiming to be "allergic to everything," the diagnosis can usually be traced to the influence of a proponent of clinical ecology; (4) there is no scientific evidence that an immunologic basis exists for such a symptom pattern; (5) clinical ecologists assume that if even a trace of any chemical is found in the patient's environment, that chemical can be held responsible for any symptom; (6) clinical ecologists appear to lack the motivation or intellectual capacity to test their theories scientifically; (7) clinical ecologists offer a philosophy of certainty, often reassuring patients during an initial phone contact that their diagnosis is obviously ecologic disease; (8) patients with genuine allergies to noxious chemicals do not have multi-system complaints without associated physical or laboratory findings; (9) many patients with symptoms of "environmental illness" find "healers" who tell them they are "universal reactors" to environmental substances; (10) this explanation of their experience and symptoms makes sense to them and enables them to avoid facing their real problem—which is psychiatric in nature; (11) using well designed double-blind tests with more than a hundred patients, the authors were able to demonstrate that most people said to be "universal reactors" develop multiple symptoms in response to the testing process without being allergic to any of the individual substances administered; and (12) once patients understand that this can happen, psychotherapy may cure them. Drs. Selner and Staudenmayer also note that "ecologists claim a unique identity with victims of the environment by declaring themselves, or members of their families, similarly affected. . . . This is a powerful bonding tool which snares patients into a . . . cult interdependence in which facts are irrelevant."

Researchers at the University of Iowa College of Medicine have reported that the prevalence of major psychiatric disorders among twenty-six "environmental illness" patients was more than twice as high as that of a control group.

Researchers at the University of California have demonstrated that provocation and neutralization—the principal diagnostic tests used by clinical ecologists—are not valid. The determination was made with a double-blind study of eighteen patients, each of whom received three injections of suspected food extracts and nine of normal saline (dilute salt water) over a three-hour period. The experimental protocol was developed in consultation with proponents and critics who agreed that it was a fair and appropriate test. Proponent organizations also provided financial support.

The tests were carried out in the offices of seven proponents who had been treating the patients. In unblinded tests, these patients had consistently reported symptoms when exposed to food extracts and no symptoms when given saline injections. But during the experiment, the patients reported as many symptoms following salt-water injections as they did after food extract injections, indicating that their symptoms were nothing more than placebo reactions. The symptoms included itching of the nose, watery or burning eyes, plugged ears, a feeling of fullness in the ears, ringing ears, dry mouth, scratchy throat, an odd taste in the mouth, fatigue, headache, nausea, dizziness, abdominal discomfort, tingling of the face or scalp, tightness or pressure in the head, disorientation, difficulty breathing, depression, chills, coughing, nervousness, intestinal gas or rumbling, and aching legs. Clinical ecologists also claim that "neutralizing" doses of offending allergens can relieve the patient's symptoms. However, the seven patients who were treated during the experiment had equivalent responses to extracts and saline.

In 1989, a reporter from the syndicated television program "Inside Edition" visited the Dallas clinic of William J. Rea, M.D., past president of the American Academy of Environmental Medicine (formerly called the Society for Clinical Ecology). The reporter truthfully told Rea that he had been feeling more tired than usual, that he was having headaches that could be relieved by aspirin, that his eyes had been getting red more often than usual, and that his shoulder still hurt from an accident several months ago. Rea said that all the symptoms could be due to allergies and ordered a lengthy series of skin tests.

Before going to Rea's facility, the reporter had been checked by Raymond G. Slavin, M.D., past president of the American Academy of Allergy and Immunology, who had found no evidence of allergy. After the reporter returned from his visit to Rea, Slavin said that Rea's testing was a waste of money because the reporter's story did not provide a legitimate basis to suspect that his symptoms were due to allergies. Slavin also said that the skin reactions produced by the testing were caused by irritation from the injected chemicals rather than by allergies. "Inside Edition" reported that treatment at Rea's facility costs thousands of dollars and that he referred many of his patients to a trailer court near Dallas where "environmentally safe" cottages and trailers could be rented for $500 per week. Rea also has operated an inpatient unit at a hospital in Dallas. Rea's patient manual—about seventy-five pages long—contains detailed instructions about food choice and avoiding environmental chemicals. Rae's recent book, *Chemical Sensitivity: Principles and Mechanisms,* devotes more than one hundred pages to "nonimmune mechanisms" of MCS.

**Political Activities**

Rejection by the scientific community has not dampened the enthusiasm of clinical ecologists, about four hundred of whom belong to the American

Academy of Environmental Medicine. This group, which holds meetings and publishes a quarterly journal, is composed mainly of medical and osteopathic physicians. A few years ago the journal announced that the paper on which it is printed had been changed because several readers had complained that the old paper had made them ill. In the same issue, the editor complained that he was not receiving enough acceptable manuscripts to maintain a four-times-a-year schedule. Despite their questionable content, courses sponsored by the academy are accepted for continuing education credits by the American Medical Association and the American Academy of Family Physicians.

Clinical ecologists also play a significant role in the American Academy of Otolaryngic Allergy (AAOA), which was founded in 1941 by Theron Randolph, M.D., and others who espoused diagnostic and treatment procedures that mainstream allergists regarded as invalid. AAOA has about two thousand members, most of whom are board-certified otolaryngologists. The percentage who espouse the practices of clinical ecology is unknown, but some AAOA seminars are taught by leading clinical ecologists. AAOA has endorsed the use of provocation and neutralization testing.

The Human Ecology Action League (HEAL), formed in 1976, is composed mainly of laypersons and has chapters and support groups in about one hundred cities. It distributes physician referral lists and publishes *The Human Ecologist,* a quarterly magazine of news and advice for patients and their families. One area of great concern to proponents is whether insurance companies will pay for their treatment, which can be quite expensive. Advice on how to press for such payment is available from HEAL. In eighteen cases reported to the Canadian ad hoc committee, patients bore an average annual cost of $4,463, with a range from $400 to $12,378, most of which was not covered by insurance companies or government programs.

The National Center for Environmental Health Strategies (NCEHS), of Voorhees, New Jersey, is a membership organization that was started in 1986 and now has more than two thousand members. NCEHS operates a clearinghouse for information on MCS and publishes a newsletter called *The Delicate Balance.* Its founder and president, Marie Lamielle, says that she started the group following an exposure to toxic chemicals, when she "found that no public agency or private organization could answer my questions or advocate for me." In October 1992, she announced that Congress had appropriated $250,000 to develop MCS research protocols and an MCS patient registry that NCEHS will maintain.

During 1992, the U.S. Department of Housing and Urban Development (HUD) concluded that multiple chemical sensitivity and environmental illness are handicaps within the meaning of the Federal Fair Housing Act. HUD memoranda have stated that individuals so handicapped are entitled to "reasonable accommodations" to be determined on a case-by-case basis. NCEHS is lobbying, "pursuant to the Americans with Disabilities Act," to persuade employers and government agencies to adopt policies that "accommodate employees and members of the public disabled by chemical barriers." Its lengthy list of recommendations includes: (1) better ventilation systems; (2) no use of air fresheners; (3) no indoor use of pesticides except in emergencies; (4) no use of synthetic lawn chemicals near the workplace; (5) no smoking in or near the workplace; (6) purchase of the "least toxic/allergenic" building materials, office furnishings, equipment, and supplies; and (7) employee prenotification for "construction and remodeling activities and toxic cleaning activities such as the use of paints, adhesives, and solvents, carpet shampoos and floor waxes."

Caroline Richmond, a medical historian at London University who became concerned about unfounded attacks on food additives, wrote a spoof manifesto for the Dye Research Allergies Bureau (DRAB), a spin-off of a larger group which she called the Food Additives Research Team (FART). According to the manifesto, the public was being put at risk by unscrupulous manufacturers who made clothes stuffed with unnecessary dyes solely to boost their profits. After sending a copy to the leading organization campaigning for allergy sufferers in England, Ms. Richmond was surprised that the group's newsletter reported on DRAB and people wrote to her that dye fabrics had caused them all sorts of problems. After the hoax was revealed, the allergy group maintained that dyes did cause allergies and that Ms. Richmond had unwittingly performed a public service by highlighting this problem.

**Legal Action**

Many doctors who treat "environmental illness" believe that they themselves have it. In 1977, a federal tax court ruled that the extra cost of "organically grown" foods could be deducted as a medical expense by Theron Randolph, M.D., and his wife, Janet. The Randolphs claimed that when Janet inhaled or ingested contaminants, she experienced mental confusion, crossed eyes, and difficulty walking; and that Theron had suffered from sluggishness, malaise, headaches, nausea, and anorexia due to contaminated foods.

Many suits have been filed by "ecologically ill" patients seeking reimbursement from insurance companies for their treatment. These suits can be expensive to defend and may trigger an award for punitive damages if a jury concludes that an insurance company has acted in "bad faith" in refusing to pay for clinical ecology treatment. In 1987, the Association of Trial Lawyers of America voted to establish a clearinghouse on ecological illness and its legal aspects. The proposal's author was Earon S. Davis, J.D., M.P.H., a former executive director of HEAL who also published the bimonthly *Ecological Illness Law Report* and operated a referral service for two hundred interested attorneys.

Claims and lawsuits are also being filed to collect worker's compensation and Social Security Disability. Although damage awards are limited, individual cases can still be expensive to defend. Some cases involve a large number of workers who claim they were made ill by low-dose exposure to chemicals in the workplace. Others involve people who are not physically ill but are afraid that low-dose exposure to environmental chemicals has affected their immune system and may make them susceptible to cancer or other diseases in the future.

Legitimate cases exist where exposure to large or cumulative amounts of toxic chemicals has injured people. But in many of the cases described above, serious immune disorders are being alleged merely because laboratory testing has detected traces of a chemical in the body or has found a minor deviation from "normal" in some measure of immune function. Although no clinical injury is apparent, these plaintiffs are often described as suffering from "chemical AIDS." Where large numbers of plaintiffs are involved, it is prohibitively expensive for a defendant to examine all of them in order to provide evidence to rebut the claims. Such "toxic tort" suits also carry a threat of punitive damages if the defendant loses.

Some lawyers foresee a wave of lawsuits sweeping the nation, based on an approach that links many kinds of illness to immune-system injury and ties immune injury to exposure to chemicals. There appears to be a growing network among the "traditional" clinical ecologists, plaintiffs' attorneys, and physicians who use questionable interpretations of laboratory data to support claims that virtually any symptom can be caused by exposure to almost anything. These doctors testify that the immune system can become overactive (leading to numerous symptoms) or suppressed (leaving the individual at risk for infection, cancer, rheumatoid arthritis, and other diseases). This latter mechanism is referred to as "multiple chemical sensitivity" or "chemical AIDS." In 1985, based on testimony by two clinical ecologists, a jury awarded $6.2 million in compensatory damages and $43 million in punitive damages to thirty-two people who lived near a chemical plant in Sedalia, Missouri.

This case and several others involving alleged illness due to chemical exposure have been analyzed by Peter W. Huber, an expert in liability law. In *Galileo's Revenge: Junk Science in the Courtroom,* Huber concluded that clinical ecologists are "perfectly adapted to modern-day testifying" because they are "adept at prevaricating, playing on credulity, scoring verbal points, forgetting inconvenient data, and dredging up convenient anecdotes."

In 1991, a jury in New York City awarded $489,000 in actual damages and $411,000 in punitive damages to the estate of a man who committed suicide at age twenty-nine after several years of treatment by Warren M. Levin, M.D., a clinical ecologist. Testimony at the trial indicated that although the patient was a paranoid schizophrenic who thought "foods were out to get him," Levin had diagnosed him as a "universal reactor" and advised that, to remain alive, he must live in a "pure" environment, follow a restrictive diet, and take supplements. Levin admitted that since 1974, when he began practicing clinical ecology, he had diagnosed every patient he saw as suffering from environmental illness. In 1992, after a lengthy investigation involving the care of thirteen patients, the New York State Department of Health Board for Professional Medical Conduct stated that Levin "has a litany of unproven and medically unnecessary tests that he runs on virtually all patients. He uses these tests—whatever their results may be—to convince his patients that his unconventional kinds of treatment are necessary." The Board found him guilty of "gross negligence," "fraudulent practice," and "moral unfitness" and recommended that his license be revoked.

### "Candidiasis Hypersensitivity"

Closely aligned with clinical ecology is the concept of "candidiasis hypersensitivity." *Candida albicans* (sometimes referred to as Monilia) is a fungus normally present in the mouth, intestinal tract, and vagina. Under certain conditions, it can multiply and infect the surface of the skin or mucous membranes. Such infections are usually minor, but serious and deeper infections can occur in patients whose resistance has been weakened by other illnesses. Promoters of "candidiasis hypersensitivity" claim that even when infection is absent, the yeast can cause or trigger multiple symptoms such as fatigue, irritability, constipation, diarrhea, abdominal bloating, mood swings, depression, anxiety, dizziness, unexpected weight gain, difficulty in concentrating, muscle and joint pain, cravings for sugar or alcoholic beverages, psoriasis, hives, respiratory and ear problems, menstrual problems, infertility, impotence, bladder infections, and prostatitis.

According to its promoters, 30 percent of Americans suffer from "candidiasis hypersensitivity." Many clinical ecologists view it as an underlying cause of the "environmental illness" that they postulate. It is also touted as an important factor in AIDS, rheumatoid arthritis, multiple sclerosis, and schizophrenia, as well as "hypoglycemia," "mercury-amalgam toxicity," and other fad diagnoses.

The main promoters of "candidiasis hypersensitivity" have been

C. Orian Truss, M.D., of Birmingham, Alabama, author/publisher of *The Missing Diagnosis,* and William G. Crook, M.D., of Jackson, Tennessee, who wrote and published *The Yeast Connection.* Crook says his book was produced after a 1983 television talk show appearance drew 7,300 requests for further information.

According to Crook, "If a careful check-up doesn't reveal the cause for your symptoms, and your medical history [as described in his book] is typical, it's possible or even probable that your health problems are yeast-connected." He also claims that lab tests, such as culturing to determine the presence of the yeast, don't help much in diagnosis because "Candida germs live in every person's body. . . . Therefore the diagnosis is suspected from the patient's history and confirmed by his response to treatment."

Crook claims that the problem arises because "antibiotics kill 'friendly germs' while they're killing enemies, and when friendly germs are knocked out, yeast germs multiply. Diets rich in carbohydrates and yeasts, birth control pills, cortisone, and other drugs also stimulate yeast growth." He also claims that large numbers of yeasts weaken the immune system, which is also adversely affected by nutritional deficiencies, sugar consumption, and exposure to environmental molds and chemicals. To correct these alleged problems, he prescribes allergenic extracts, antifungal drugs, vitamin and mineral supplements, and diets that avoid refined carbohydrates, processed foods, and (initially) fruits and milk.

Crook's book contains a seventy-item questionnaire and score sheet to determine how likely it is that health problems are yeast-connected. Shorter versions of this questionnaire have appeared in magazine articles and in ads for products sold through health food stores.

In 1986, for example, an article in *Redbook* magazine asked readers whether they: (1) have ever taken antibiotics on a frequent basis; (2) have ever been troubled by premenstrual tension, abdominal pain, or loss of sexual interest; (4) crave sugar, breads, or alcoholic beverages; (3) have recurrent digestive problems; (5) get moderate to severe symptoms when exposed to tobacco smoke; (6) experience fatigue, depression, poor memory, or nervous tension; (7) are bothered by hives, psoriasis, or other chronic skin rashes; (8) have ever taken birth control pills; (9) are bothered by headaches; or (10) feel bad all over without any apparent cause. According to the article, "If you have three or four 'yes' answers, yeast possibly plays a role in causing your symptoms. If you have five or six 'yes' answers, yeast probably plays a role in causing your symptoms. If you have seven or more 'yes' answers, your symptoms are almost certainly yeast-connected." The article's author was said to be "on her way to recovery" from a debilitating case of "the yeast syndrome."

Proponents of "candidiasis hypersensitivity" refer to this alleged problem with several terms. Dr. Crook prefers "Candida-Related Complex." Others use the terms "Candida" and "yeast problem." (The less specific the concept, the more difficult it would be to test the proponents' theories.) During the past year, proponents have been suggesting that chronic fatigue syndrome and Candida infections are closely related. Dr. Truss has said he believes that "chronic fatigue syndrome is Candida under a different name."

## Severe Criticism

The American Academy of Allergy and Immunology has issued position statements strongly criticizing the concept of "candidiasis hypersensitivity syndrome" and the diagnostic and treatment approaches used by its proponents. These statements conclude: (1) the concept of candidiasis hypersensitivity is speculative and unproven; (2) its basic elements would apply to almost all sick patients at some time because its supposed symptoms are essentially universal; (3) overuse of oral antifungal agents could lead to the development of resistant germs that could menace others; (4) adverse effects of oral antifungal agents are rare, but some inevitably will occur; and (5) neither patients nor doctors can determine effectiveness (as opposed to coincidence) without controlled trials. Because allergic symptoms can be influenced by many factors, including emotions, experiments must be designed to separate the effects of the procedure being tested from the effects of other factors. Several years ago, Dr. Crook told me he had no intention of conducting a controlled test because he was "a clinician, not a researcher."

The antifungal drug most often prescribed by proponents of "candidiasis hypersensitivity" is nystatin (*Mycostatin, Nilstat*), which seldom has significant side effects. However, they also prescribe ketoconazole (*Nizoral*), which has an incidence of liver toxicity (hepatitis) of about one in 10,000. The liver injury usually reverses when the drug is discontinued, but ketoconazole has been responsible for several deaths. For this reason it should be prescribed only for serious infections. Both of these drugs are expensive. In a recent double-blind trial, the antifungal drug nystatin did no better than a placebo in relieving systemic or psychological symptoms of "candidiasis hypersensitivity syndrome."

## Problems Reported

In 1986, two doctors from Loyola University's Stritch School of Medicine reported seeing four young women whose nonspecific complaints included chronic fatigue, anxiety, and depression. All four mistakenly believed they had disseminated candidiasis and were taking nystatin or ketoconazole, which had been prescribed by their family physicians. All had read *The Yeast Connection* and had carried the book into the office during their visits. One patient on ketoconazole had hepatitis, which resolved when the drug was stopped.

Worse yet, a case has been reported of a child with a severe case of disseminated candidiasis who had been seen by a "Candida doctor" and given inadequate treatment. The report concluded that "the advice of yeast connection advocates may be inappropriate even for illnesses in which Candida is implicated."

Perhaps the saddest report was a letter in a health-food magazine from a woman appealing for help and encouragement. She said that a clinical ecologist had been treating her for allergies and Candida for four years, that initial tests showed she "was allergic to all foods" as well as to numerous chemicals and inhalants, and that so far nothing had helped.

In 1990, "Inside Edition" aired two segments vilifying Stuart Berger, M.D., a Park Avenue "diet doctor" who is author of *Dr. Berger's Immune Power Diet* and *What Your Doctor Didn't Learn in Medical School*. During the first program, a reporter described what happened when she visited Berger complaining of fatigue. So did a prominent New York allergist who consulted Berger with a similar complaint. Both noted that their contact with him lasted about two minutes, included no physical examination, and culminated with a diagnosis of chronic fatigue syndrome and allergy to yeast (*Candida albicans*). The reporter's cost was $845 for the first visit, with an estimated total of about $1,500 through the third visit. A former patient described a similar experience which had cost over $1,000. And a former employee said that Berger ordered his employees to indicate on blood test reports that every patient was allergic to wheat, dairy products, eggs, and yeast. The reporter's visit had been filmed with a hidden camera. Berger obtained a court order stopping "Inside Edition" from showing the tape during the initial program. But two weeks later, after the U.S. Supreme Court sided with the producers, the tape was shown. During the interim, complaints were received from more than a hundred former patients and employees.

In 1985, *Dr. Berger's Immune Power Diet* became an overnight best seller following Berger's appearance on the "Donahue" show. The book claims that overweight and numerous other health problems are the result of an "immune hypersensitivity response" to common foods, and that "detoxification" and weight loss followed by food supplements can tune and strengthen the immune system. There is no scientific evidence to support these claims. The *Harvard Medical School Health Letter* said the book "should have been listed in the fiction category" and was "selling a collection of quack ideas about food allergies that have been around for decades."

## Government Actions

Due largely to Crook's promotion, public interest in "candidiasis hypersensitivity" has grown rapidly. Several other books have been published, and many manufacturers have marketed "yeast-free" supplements that presumably are "safer" than ordinary ones. Health-food industry manufacturers, including several that market through chiropractors, offered such products as *Candi-Care, Candida-Guard, Candida Cleanse, Candistat, Cantrol, Yeast Fighters, Yeast Guard, Yeastop, Yeasterol,* and *Yeast•Trol.* Before the *Redbook* article was published, Cantrol's manufacturer notified retailers that an ad in the same issue would "specifically instruct the consumer to go to their local health food store to purchase Cantrol." The ad contained a toll-free number for ordering the product or obtaining further information. According to a company official, more than 100,000 people responded.

Under federal law, any product intended for the prevention or treatment of disease is a drug, and it is illegal to market new drugs that do not have FDA approval. "Candida" products were claimed to be "dietary supplements," not medical treatment. However, it was clear that these products were being marketed illegally. In 1989, the FDA Health Fraud Branch issued instructions and a sample regulatory letter indicating that it is illegal to market "supplement" products intended for the treatment of yeast infections.

During 1988, the FDA had initiated a seizure of *Yeastop,* a vitamin concoction claimed to be effective against yeast microorganisms that have become "overgrown" or "out of control." The manufacturer, Nature's Herbs, of Orem, Utah, claimed that the product was a "dietary supplement." But the FDA charged that the therapeutic claims on its label made it an illegal drug. In 1990, a federal judge ruled that *Yeastop* was a drug and ordered Nature's Herbs to pay for its destruction and for other court costs and fees. The FDA also seized a supply of *Cantrol* from its manufacturer, Nature's Way, of Springville, Utah.

In 1989, Great Earth International, the nation's second largest health food store chain, agreed to pay $100,000 in penalties plus $9,520 in costs to settle charges filed in 1987 by the Orange County (California) District Attorney. The case involved advertising claims for *Yeasterol* ("to control ... Candida albicans, a troublesome yeast") and several other products. Without admitting wrongdoing, the company signed a consent agreement pledging to refrain from marketing products that are misbranded or are unapproved new drugs.

In 1990, Nature's Way and its president, Kenneth Murdock, settled an FTC complaint by signing a consent agreement to stop making unsubstantiated claims that *Cantrol* is helpful against yeast infections caused by *Candida albicans*. The product is a conglomeration of capsules containing acidophilus, evening primrose oil, vitamin E, linseed oil, caprylic acid, pau d'arco, and several other substances. *Cantrol* was promoted with a self-test based on common symptoms the manufacturer claimed were associated with yeast problems. The FTC charged that the test was not valid for this purpose. The company also agreed to pay $30,000 to the National Institutes of Health to support research on yeast infections.

In 1990, the New Jersey State Attorney General secured consent agreements barring Linda Choi, M.D., and Pruyakant Doshi, M.D., from diagnosing and treating "Candida albicans overgrowth syndrome." Both were assessed $3,000 for investigative costs and had their medical license placed on probation for one year. Among other things, investigation by the State medical board had concluded that "Candida albicans overgrowth" was not generally recognized as a clinical entity and had not been established as the cause of the conditions the doctors treated.

## Overview

Clinical ecology is practiced by several hundred medical and osteopathic physicians who diagnose "environmental illness" in large numbers of patients who consult them. Many of these physicians and an unknown number of chiropractors are also treating "candidiasis hypersensitivity," while the health food industry is still marketing do-it-yourself "anti-Candida" products that lack FDA approval for their intended purposes. Instead of testing their claims with well-designed research, proponents of these concepts are selling them to the public through books, magazine articles, and radio and television talk shows. Many are also part of a network of legal actions alleging injuries by environmental chemicals.

The number of people caught up in this hoopla is unknown. Nor can it be determined what percentage of them are being helped or harmed as a result. But if "environmental illness" and "candidiasis hypersensitivity" are figments of their proponents' imagination—which I believe they are—patients who rely on these concepts run the risks of misdiagnosis, mistreatment, financial exploitation, and/or delay of proper medical care. In addition, insurance companies, employers, other taxpayers, and ultimately all citizens are being burdened by dubious claims for disability and damages. Although government regulatory actions have forced several companies to stop making illegal therapeutic claims for "anti-yeast" products, such products continue to be marketed with claims made by word-of-mouth and through the media.

Many people diagnosed with "environmental illness" or "candidiasis hypersensitivity" suffer greatly and are very difficult to treat. The work of Drs. Selner and Staudenmayer suggests that most of them have psychosomatic disorders in which they react to stress by developing multiple symptoms. Knowledgeable critics believe that the theories of clinical ecology are too vague to be defined and tested, and that proponents will cite calls for additional research as evidence that their work raises legitimate scientific issues—which it does not.

The problems described in this report will not be simple to correct. But one thing that might help would be for state licensing boards to examine the activities of the physicians involved and determine whether the overall quality of their care is sufficient for them to remain in medical practice. I believe that most of them are practicing unscientifically and should be delicensed.

# 11

# Immunoquackery

### Stephen Barrett, M.D.

Acquired immune deficiency syndrome (AIDS) is a fatal disease caused by the human immunodeficiency virus (HIV). The virus eventually disrupts the body's immune system, making the infected individual susceptible to organisms that normally would be harmless.

Most people with HIV infection are young adults, but it can occur at any age. The initial stage of the disease typically incudes fever, sore throat, skin rash, swollen lymph glands, headache, and malaise. This phase usually lasts one to two weeks and is followed by a prolonged symptom-free period. The median length of the symptom-free period in untreated individuals is about ten years, but the disease progresses much faster in some individuals and may remain quiescent indefinitely in a small percentage of others. Thus, at any given time, most people who carry the AIDS virus exhibit no symptoms. Regardless of the stage of their disease, however, infected individuals can transmit the virus to others.

Once clinical symptoms appear, the course of the disease can vary considerably, depending in part on extent of immune damage and the treatment received by the patient. Eventually, most AIDS patients become thin, easily fatigued, and prone to diarrhea, swollen lymph glands, and multiple infections. *Pneumocystis carinii* pneumonia and a skin cancer called Kaposi's sarcoma are life-threatening complications. In addition, some patients suffer from dementia.

Finding a cure for AIDS is considered very difficult because the HIV is able to copy itself into the genetic material (DNA) of certain cells, which "tricks" them into treating the virus's genes as their own. The virus is then safe from attack by the body's immune system and is reproduced whenever the host cells reproduce. AIDS develops when something triggers rapid reproduction and spillage of the virus into the bloodstream, where it destroys certain lymphocytes and weakens the patient's immune system. Although no cure has been found, a few drugs have been proven effective for helping infected individuals to live longer and have fewer complications, and many other drugs are at various stages of development in the laboratory or in human clinical trials.

## Exploiting Vulnerability

The fact that AIDS causes great suffering and is deadly has encouraged the marketing of hundreds of unproven remedies to AIDS victims. As noted by Susan Miller, M.D., an AIDS specialist at Baylor College of Medicine:

> When people find out that they are HIV-infected, their initial response is one of overriding fear and horror. They may sense that death is imminent and that their life is over. In this state of panic, they are extraordinarily vulnerable to quackery. Since scientific medicine cannot cure AIDS, these individuals may seek alternative approaches to remedy their situation.

John H. Renner, M.D., president of the Consumer Health Information Research Institute, adds that "many people with AIDS are anti-establishment to begin with and are encouraged by AIDS activist groups to seek alternatives." Dr. Renner, who has attended many expositions at which unorthodox methods were promoted, has observed that "many of the expert quacks in arthritis, cancer, and heart disease have now shifted into AIDS" and that "every quack remedy seems to have been converted into an AIDS treatment." The "cures" he has noted have included processed blue-green algae (pond scum), hydrogen peroxide, BHT (a food preservative), pills derived from mice given the AIDS virus, herbal capsules, bottles of "T-cells," and thumping on the thymus gland. Some firms have even offered to freeze and store bone marrow, claiming that it could be used to restore an AIDS victim's marrow when AIDS began to deplete the body's supply of bone marrow (which manufactures blood cells).

Several studies have shown that significant percentages of AIDS patients use one or more unproven treatments. A study of seventy-nine patients attending the St. Louis AIDS Clinical Trials Unit found that forty-four (56 percent) had tried an "alternative" remedy. The most commonly used were vitamins (46 percent of patients), herbal therapy (16 percent), imagery or meditation (14 percent ), and nonapproved drugs (14 percent). The majority of patients using these methods thought they had improved their general well-being, but readily admitted that the benefit was largely psychological. The average yearly cost was $356, but fourteen of the patients spent between $500 and $2,700, and two patients spent more than $9,000 each.

Interviews with 114 patients attending the AIDS Clinic of the University of California San Francisco Medical Center, indicated that twenty-five (22 percent) had taken one or more herbal products during the three months prior to the survey. The study's authors expressed concern that herbal extracts can produce diarrhea, liver toxicity, and other symptoms common in AIDS itself.

Many Mexican cancer clinics offer unproven treatments to AIDS victims, and a black market has developed in drugs that have shown promise but lack FDA approval here because the agency is not convinced they are safe and effective. Several drugs available without a prescription in Mexico are being smuggled into the United States. Drugs are also imported through "buyer's clubs," which obtain them from other countries where they are legally prescribed or are used in clinical trials. "Legitimate" buyers' clubs require a prescription written by an American physician who supervises the patient's care. However, some buyers' clubs will obtain drugs for people who are not under medical care. Some also supply drugs to victims of cancer, Alzheimer's disease, chronic fatigue syndrome, and other diseases.

Some AIDS support organizations advocate or engage in consumer-protection efforts because they recognize that unproven "alternatives" can cause adverse effects or shorten survival time. But others make indiscriminate referrals to promoters of these methods. Cable News Network recently called attention to a Mexican clinic that charged $2,500 for an "AIDS cure" served in cranberry juice. The investigators described how a supposedly reputable community information agency had referred patients to this clinic, even though its counterpart agencies near the Mexican border knew that the treatment was a scam.

Some AIDS activists have expressed considerable animosity toward government agencies and consumer groups that are interested in protecting the public from being exploited by quack methods. About fifty members of the AIDS Coalition to Unleash Power (ACT-UP) staged a protest at the 1990 National Health Fraud Conference in Kansas City, Missouri. The demonstrators picketed the hotel and distributed flyers stating:

> The goal of this conference is to directly challenge any type of treatment that does not currently meet AMA guidelines or FDA approval! . . . It is not to eliminate any real health fraud that is out there! It represents the efforts of the AMA and the big drug companies to suppress their competition, and the insurance industry to reduce their coverage!

Several protesters were arrested when they stormed into the meeting room blowing loud whistles and shouting their views. Seventeen others were arrested outside of the hotel and charged with trespassing.

ACT-UP's protest was misdirected. Antiquackery groups do not oppose making experimental medicines available to AIDS patients before they have been completely studied. Rather, we want them tested under scientific conditions so that knowledge can be gained about their usefulness. ACT-UP's leaders appear so alienated that they cannot distinguish between people who wish to help them and those who wish to exploit them.

Financial exploitation has also occurred in connection with normally legitimate treatment. The New York City Department of Consumer Affairs has concluded that many private home-care suppliers have been engaging in "bedside robbery." The biggest problem was the provision of total parenteral nutrition (TPN), a liquid protein and fat supplement fed intravenously through a surgically implanted catheter to AIDS patients whose digestive system no longer functions normally. The department's 1991 report, "Making a Killing on AIDS," cites instances where insurance companies and government agencies have been billed more than $15,000 a month for treatment that costs much less to deliver. Only three out of twelve companies responded to the Department's questionnaire about prices for their services. Several patients reported that buying supplies through a pharmacy and administering TPN themselves could more than halve their home-care costs.

Fear of AIDS has also spawned inappropriate promotions related to the detection or prevention of AIDS. Several companies have offered unreliable or fraudulent AIDS tests by mail. Covers for public toilets and telephone receivers have been marketed with claims that they will prevent transmission of the AIDS virus, even though the virus is not transmitted in this manner.

Some dating services require AIDS testing for prospective clients. While a negative test would make it less likely, it does not guarantee that the person is not infected with the AIDS virus. Antibodies to the virus are not present during the first few months of infection. In addition, a negative test cannot ensure that an individual will not acquire HIV infection in the future.

In 1993, postal inspectors arrested a California couple for conducting a phony charity scheme using the name American Society for AIDS Prevention (ASAP). Documents in the case charged that brochures mailed to potential donors contained numerous misrepresentations about ASAP's track record in helping AIDS victims as well as about the manner in which solicited funds would be used. Many of the services that had been claimed had not been performed, and money collected had been used to perpetrate the scheme even further.

**The Expanding Market**

Public focus on AIDS has spawned a host of products and procedures claimed to work by influencing the immune system. In recent years, many "alternative" practitioners have adopted the "immune system" as a focus of their treatment. Cancer quacks claim that cancer occurs because the immune defenses fail to destroy cancer cells before they multiply out of hand. Acupuncturists, naturopaths, chiropractors, homeopaths, Natural Hygienists, and other types of so-called vitalistic healers (see Chapter 16) equate their various forms of "life force" with immune mechanisms. Clinical ecologists claim that millions of people have become ill because their immune system has become overloaded (see Chapter 10). And the health-food industry has promoted countless nutrient combinations claimed to "strengthen" the immune system.

In 1986, the trade magazine *Health Foods Retailing* reported that vitamin sales had increased sharply in response to *Dr. Berger's Immune Power Diet,* by Stuart M. Berger, M.D., which claimed that weight control can be achieved by "rebuilding" one's immune system with dietary change and food supplements (see Chapter 10). According to the magazine's editor, the problem of AIDS had stimulated public concern about the immune system. This, plus the discovery that President Ronald Reagan had developed cancer, had forced the population as a whole "to admit the possibility that large numbers of Americans are being stripped of their ability to resist infections and, even more psychologically damaging, that no one, including the President, was beyond the reach of many diseases."

During the same year, *Health News & Review,* a bimonthly "health food" newspaper for the general public, reported "growing public recognition that AIDS, cancer, arthritis, even colds—very nearly the whole spectrum of infections and degenerative diseases—become manifest dangers only when the immune system is depressed. Strengthening the immune system . . . is clearly emerging as a health priority." The report then described how promoters of a wide variety of unproven nutrition practices related them to supposed immunological factors. Sugar, food allergies, and mercury fillings, for example, were said to weaken the immune system, while vitamin C, zinc, beta-carotene, and certain herbs were said to strengthen it. Although no scientific evidence supported any of these claims, "health food" marketers began marketing new products and recasting old ones as "immune boosters."

In 1989, volunteers of the Houston-based Consumer Health Education Council telephoned forty-one health-food stores and asked to speak with the person who provided nutritional advice. The callers explained that they had a brother with AIDS who was seeking an effective alternative against the AIDS virus. The callers also explained that the brother's wife was still having sex with her husband and was seeking products that would reduce her risk of being infected, or make it impossible. All forty-one retailers offered products they said could benefit the brother's immune system, improve the woman's immunity, and protect her against harm from the virus. The recommended products included vitamins (forty-one stores), vitamin C (thirty-eight stores), immune boosters (thirty-eight stores), coenzyme $Q_{10}$ (twenty-six stores), germanium (twenty-six stores), lecithin (nineteen stores), ornithine and/or arginine (nine stores), gamma-linolenic acid (seven stores), raw glandulars (seven stores), hydrogen peroxide (five stores), homeopathic salts (five stores), Bach Flower Remedies (four stores), blue-green algae (five stores), cysteine (three stores), and herbal baths (two stores). Thirty retailers said they carried products that would cure AIDS. None recommended abstinence or use of a condom.

In June 1993, the New York City Department of Consumer Affairs charged four supplement companies with deceptively promoting products characterized as "immune boosters." The action was taken under a city consumer protection law, passed in 1990, which regulates advertising of products and services claimed or implied to "boost, enhance, stimulate, assist, cure, strengthen or improve the body's immune system." Under this law, no such effect can be claimed without an accurate statement about whether or not the product or service is effective in preventing HIV infection or improving the health of an infected individual. The cited products were *Immune Protectors* (Twin Laboratories, Inc.), *Immunizer Pak Program* and *Immune Nectar* (Nature's Plus), *Pro-Immune Anti-Oxidant* (Nutritional Life Support Systems), and *Ecomer* (a shark liver oil capsule marketed by Scandinavian Natural Health & Beauty Products, Inc.).

The FDA has also acted against several companies that marketed bogus products with "immune" or "immu-" in their name. Despite these actions, however, many such products are still sold. In fact, since the potential market for "immune boosters" is everyone, supplement concoctions of this type will continue to be promoted even if a cure for AIDS is found.

# 12

# The Spine Salesmen

## Stephen Barrett, M.D.

Harriet Cressman was a lovely lady who lived with her husband on their farm in Pleasant Valley, Pennsylvania. One day, thinking that chiropractors were "bone specialists," she consulted one after developing a backache. He did not disappoint her. After examining her and taking an x-ray, he said that her spine was "tilted" but could be corrected by spinal "adjustments." The adjustments took place three times a week for several months. As Harriet's back symptoms improved, her treatment was reduced to twice a week, then once a week, and then once a month. At this point, although Harriet felt completely well, the chiropractor suggested that she continue adjustments regularly for "preventive maintenance." She did so faithfully for ten years and had no further trouble with her back—as far as she knew. Then, however, the chiropractor took another x-ray and gave her bad news: the x-ray showed "eighteen compressed discs and progressive osteoarthritis of the spine that was spreading rapidly." It would make her a helpless cripple if she did not have immediate treatment. He reassured her, however, that his new equipment could correct her disc problem and stop the spread of her arthritis.

Staggered by the news, Harriet went home to discuss the matter with her husband. But the chiropractor's receptionist had already telephoned Mr. Cressman to ask him to bring Harriet back immediately to the office. Because of the serious nature of the case, the chiropractor wished to begin "intensive treatment" that same day. The treatment would be in day-long sessions, alternating complete bed rest with spinal adjustments, acupuncture, and treatment with devices that would shock or stretch her muscles. The cost would be $11,000 but, with advance payment, the doctor would accept $10,000.

161

Because of her long association with the chiropractor, and because she was in no mood to trifle about her health, Harriet did not hesitate to raise the money. Supplementing her life savings with a bank loan, she paid in advance.

For the next few months, as far as she could tell, Harriet's treatment proceeded smoothly. Every week another full-spine x-ray was taken. Each time, the chiropractor pointed out on the x-ray film how she had improved. He also discussed other patients with her and asked her to help talk them into treatment with him. Advising Harriet that her condition might be hereditary, he suggested that other members of her family have spinal x-rays.

Harriet's son Donald did have an x-ray and was told by the chiropractor that he had a "pin dot of arthritis which, if untreated, would spread like wildfire and leave him crippled within a short time." Donald's cost? With the usual ten percent discount for advance payment—a mere $1,500.

A few months later, the chiropractor suddenly informed the Cressmans that he was moving to California. "What about us?" they asked. "Don't worry," he answered, but their worry increased and turned to suspicion when his answers became contradictory. Pressed by Harriet for the name of another chiropractor who could continue her treatment, the chiropractor named one. "Don't bother to call him before I leave," he said, "because he has already gone over your records and x-rays with me." Harriet did contact her chiropractor-to-be, however, and was told that her name had been mentioned, but that no record or x-ray review had taken place.

Shocked by the turn of events, the Cressmans consulted medical and legal authorities who suggested that they file criminal charges for "theft by deception." They did. Investigation by the Northampton County District Attorney's office uncovered other patients of the chiropractor who described similar experiences. A medical radiologist x-rayed the spines of Harriet and Donald and offered to testify at trial that neither had any condition which could possibly be helped by chiropractic treatment. When news of the arrest became public, a third patient filed a criminal complaint. The chiropractor, he claimed, had cheated him out of $2,075 by promising to cure his arm and leg, which had been paralyzed by a "stroke."

Now it was the chiropractor's turn to be stunned by the turn of events. He disappeared from public view and communicated through his attorney. He was innocent, he claimed, but was anxious to leave Pennsylvania as soon as possible. (He could not do so until the criminal cases were settled.) If the three complainants would drop their charges, he would return their money. Under a court-approved agreement, the $13,575 was returned and the charges were dropped.

Do you wonder whether Harriet Cressman had to be very gullible in order to part with $10,000 for such questionable treatment? Please let me assure you that she was a very intelligent person. *Until the chiropractor announced that he was leaving, she simply had no reason to be suspicious.* Though generally well-informed, she had never encountered criticism of chiropractic in any newspaper, magazine, book, or radio or television program. Like all chiropractors, hers was licensed by the State *as a doctor.* He seemed warm, friendly, and genuinely interested in her. And he did what she would expect a doctor to do: he examined her, took an x-ray, made a "diagnosis," and prescribed a "treatment" plan. She was happy to feel better and, like most people, gave no thought to whether the "treatment" had cured her or whether she would have recovered just as quickly with no treatment at all. Nor did she give any thought to the nature of chiropractic itself, how it began, how its practitioners are trained, or what they usually do. She certainly did not suspect that chiropractic is based on the mistaken beliefs of a grocer and his son.

## A Brief History

Chiropractic claims it began in 1895 when Daniel David Palmer (1845–1913) restored the hearing of a deaf janitor by "adjusting" a bump on his spine. Palmer fancied that he had helped the man by releasing pressure on the nerve to his ear. A grocer and "magnetic healer" by profession, Palmer did not know that the nerve from the brain to the ear does not travel inside the spinal column. But no matter—he soon knew that he had discovered *the* cause of disease: interference with the body's nerve supply caused by misaligned bones ("subluxations"). Palmer concluded that "about 95 percent of diseases are caused by subluxated vertebrae; the remaining 5 per cent by slightly displaced joints other than those of the backbone." He claimed that subluxations interfered with the body's expression of "Innate Intelligence"—the "Soul, Spirit, or Spark of Life" that controlled the healing process.

A few months after this revelation, Palmer set up the Palmer College of Chiropractic to convey his insights to others. One of his early pupils was his own son, Bartlett Joshua (1881–1961), better known as "B.J." The boy began to help run the school soon after it opened. Gradually, however, B.J. took over. In 1906, Daniel David was charged with practicing medicine without a license and went to jail. When he was released, B.J. bought out his interest in the school. Business boomed, and many Palmer graduates opened schools of their own. Cash was the basic entrance requirement for most of them, and some even trained their students by mail.

As competition among chiropractors grew, and as many were jailed for practicing medicine without a license, they began to pressure state legislators to license them. Responding to this pressure, perhaps with the hope that licensing would lead to higher standards of education and practice, states began to pass licensing laws. The first area to license chiropractors was the District of Columbia in 1896. Between 1913 and 1933, forty states passed licensing laws. The rest gradually followed suit, with Louisiana being the last to do so in 1974. Chiropractors may not prescribe drugs or perform surgery, but are permitted to "adjust" the spine. *But for what?* If all disease is caused by spines that need adjustment, can't chiropractors treat everything?

During the past twenty-five years, I have collected hundreds of brochures and newspaper advertisements relating "spinal problems" to virtually the entire gamut of disease. During the 1970s, for example, many chiropractors used charts that pictured a spine and claimed that more than one hundred diseases— including hernias, crossed eyes, whooping cough, pneumonia, anemia, gall- bladder conditions, hardening of the arteries and thyroid conditions—are related to nerve pressure at its various parts. The chart pictured on the next page was sent to me by a reporter who obtained it at the clinic of a chiropractic college.

Throughout the 1970s, pamphlets sold by Palmer College claimed that chiropractic could play an important role in treating appendicitis, bronchitis, tonsillitis, epilepsy, liver disease, kidney disease, diabetes, and a wide variety of other diseases. The liver pamphlet stated, "Chiropractic is the only science which seeks to find the basic cause producing the abnormally functioning liver." The gallstone pamphlet suggested that "the best approach to a permanent solution to gallstones or any other health problem is to see your chiropractor regularly." The kidney pamphlet concluded: "If you are suffering from kidney disease, the logical course is to visit your chiropractor. He will examine your spine to see where your trouble exists. A chiropractic adjustment will have you feeling better in no time." The diabetes pamphlet, however, paid modest tribute to the medical profession; it said that achieving metabolic balance required "a cooperative effort between the patient, his medical doctor, and his Doctor of Chiropractic." In 1979, my survey of thirty-five local chiropractic offices found that twelve used Palmer College pamphlets, eleven used equally outlandish ones from other sources, and five used pamphlets that were more subdued but still exaggerated what chiropractors could do.

In 1975, I initiated prosecution of a Bethlehem, Pennsylvania, chiroprac- tor who had advertised that "intense, fearful constricting chest pain" and "blurred vision" are reasons to see a chiropractor. Other ads in the case claimed that "pinched nerves" could cause abnormal blood pressure, hay fever, sinus trouble, arthritis, pleurisy, glandular trouble, goiter, bronchitis, and colds, as

# CHART OF EFFECTS OF SPINAL MISALIGNMENTS

"The nervous system controls and coordinates all organs and structures of the human body." (*Gray's Anatomy*, 29th Ed., page 4.) Misalignments of spinal vertebrae and discs may cause irritation to the nervous system and affect the structures, organs, and functions which may result in the conditions shown below.

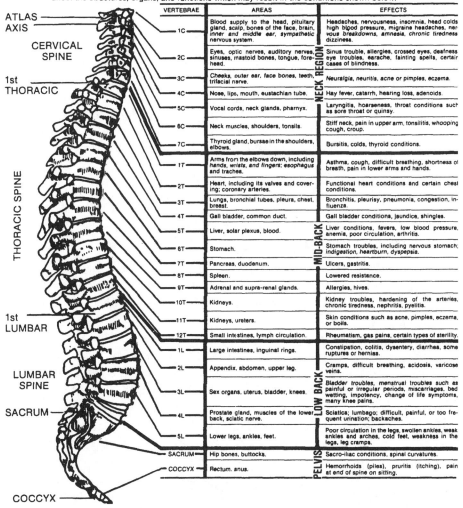

| VERTEBRAE | AREAS | EFFECTS |
|---|---|---|
| 1C | Blood supply to the head, pituitary gland, scalp, bones of the face, brain, inner and middle ear, sympathetic nervous system. | Headaches, nervousness, insomnia, head colds, high blood pressure, migraine headaches, nervous breakdowns, amnesia, chronic tiredness, dizziness. |
| 2C | Eyes, optic nerves, auditory nerves, sinuses, mastoid bones, tongue, fore-head. | Sinus trouble, allergies, crossed eyes, deafness, eye troubles, earache, fainting spells, certain cases of blindness. |
| 3C | Cheeks, outer ear, face bones, teeth, trifacial nerve. | Neuralgia, neuritis, acne or pimples, eczema. |
| 4C | Nose, lips, mouth, eustachian tube. | Hay fever, catarrh, hearing loss, adenoids. |
| 5C | Vocal cords, neck glands, pharynx. | Laryngitis, hoarseness, throat conditions such as sore throat or quinsy. |
| 6C | Neck muscles, shoulders, tonsils. | Stiff neck, pain in upper arm, tonsilitis, whooping cough, croup. |
| 7C | Thyroid gland, bursae in the shoulders, elbows. | Bursitis, colds, thyroid conditions. |
| 1T | Arms from the elbows down, including hands, wrists, and fingers; esophagus and trachea. | Asthma, cough, difficult breathing, shortness of breath, pain in lower arms and hands. |
| 2T | Heart, including its valves and covering; coronary arteries. | Functional heart conditions and certain chest conditions. |
| 3T | Lungs, bronchial tubes, pleura, chest, breast. | Bronchitis, pleurisy, pneumonia, congestion, influenza. |
| 4T | Gall bladder, common duct. | Gall bladder conditions, jaundice, shingles. |
| 5T | Liver, solar plexus, blood. | Liver conditions, fevers, low blood pressure, anemia, poor circulation, arthritis. |
| 6T | Stomach. | Stomach troubles, including nervous stomach, indigestion, heartburn, dyspepsia. |
| 7T | Pancreas, duodenum. | Ulcers, gastritis. |
| 8T | Spleen. | Lowered resistance. |
| 9T | Adrenal and supra-renal glands. | Allergies, hives. |
| 10T | Kidneys. | Kidney troubles, hardening of the arteries, chronic tiredness, nephritis, pyelitis. |
| 11T | Kidneys, ureters. | Skin conditions such as acne, pimples, eczema, or boils. |
| 12T | Small intestines, lymph circulation. | Rheumatism, gas pains, certain types of sterility. |
| 1L | Large intestines, inguinal rings. | Constipation, colitis, dysentery, diarrhea, some ruptures or hernias. |
| 2L | Appendix, abdomen, upper leg. | Cramps, difficult breathing, acidosis, varicose veins. |
| 3L | Sex organs, uterus, bladder, knees. | Bladder troubles, menstrual troubles such as painful or irregular periods, miscarriages, bed wetting, impotency, change of life symptoms, many knee pains. |
| 4L | Prostate gland, muscles of the lower back, sciatic nerve. | Sciatica; lumbago; difficult, painful, or too frequent urination; backaches. |
| 5L | Lower legs, ankles, feet. | Poor circulation in the legs, swollen ankles, weak ankles and arches, cold feet, weakness in the legs, leg cramps. |
| SACRUM | Hip bones, buttocks. | Sacro-iliac conditions, spinal curvatures. |
| COCCYX | Rectum, anus. | Hemorrhoids (piles), pruritis (itching), pain at end of spine on sitting. |

**This chart was in a brochure acquired in 1979 at a clinic at New York Chiropractic College. Many chiropractors have displayed charts like this to explain what spinal adjustments supposedly can do. Some still use them today.**

well as stomach, liver, kidney, and gallbladder problems. At a preliminary hearing, a medical cardiologist testified that severe chest pain could represent a heart attack requiring emergency care and that delay in getting such care could be fatal. Seven chiropractors testified in support of the advertising claims. Here is the testimony of one of them:

Q. Sir, if somebody came to you complaining of blurred vision, would you examine the eye?

A. I would examine the spine. I examine everyone's spine.

Q. If someone came to you complaining of goiter, would you examine the goiter?

A. I would examine the spine again.

Q. If someone came to you complaining of intense pain in the chest radiating down the left arm, would you examine, or would you attempt to examine the heart by using an electrocardiogram machine?

A. I only check the spine for vertebral subluxations.

Q. Would you use a stethoscope to check the heart pain at that point if somebody came to you with that complaint?

A. We don't use a stethoscope in checking the pain. We only check the spine for subluxations.

At a subsequent hearing, the chairman of the Pennsylvania State Board of Chiropractic Examiners and faculty members from three different chiropractic schools endorsed the ads as accurate and representative of what is taught in chiropractic schools.

One of the experts I had lined up was Edmund S. Crelin, Ph.D., a prominent anatomist from Yale University. During the early 1970s, he had actually tested Palmer's "subluxation" theory by studying the spines of three adults and three infants within a few hours after their death. While twisting each spine with a drill press, he observed the spinal nerves and the openings through which they passed. Even with greater force than could occur in a living person, no nerve compression took place. As the advertising case unfolded, it appeared that the courts might have to judge the validity of Palmer's theory itself. The case never came to trial, however, because the district attorney who was handling it left office, the chiropractor's lawyer was elected district attorney, and the judge refused to appoint someone else to carry the matter forward.

**Types of Chiropractors**

Although philosophy and treatment vary greatly from one practitioner to another, chiropractors may be divided into two main types: "straights" and "mixers." Straights tend to cling to Palmer's doctrine that almost all disease is caused by misaligned vertebrae ("subluxations") that may be correctable by spinal adjustment. Mixers acknowledge that factors such as germs and hormones play a role in disease, but they tend to regard mechanical disturbances of the nervous system as the underlying cause of lowered resistance to disease. In addition to spinal manipulation, mixers may use nutritional methods and various types of physiotherapy (heat, cold, traction, exercise, massage, and ultrasound). Straights tend to disparage medical diagnosis, claiming that examination of the spine is the proper way for chiropractors to analyze their patients. Mixers are more likely to diagnose medical conditions in addition to spinal abnormalities, and to refer patients to medical practitioners for treatment.

The largest chiropractic organization is the American Chiropractic Association (ACA), with about 22,000 members, including 6,000 students. Most ACA members adhere to a mixer philosophy. The second largest organization is the International Chiropractors Association (ICA), which has about 6,000 members, including 2,000 students. Its members tend to adhere to a straight philosophy. The two groups have considered merging, but have been unable to agree upon the definition and scope of chiropractic. In addition, there is considerable animosity between them.

In 1984, some clear-thinking chiropractors formed the National Association for Chiropractic Medicine with hopes that they could help place chiropractic on a sound, scientific basis. To gain admission to this group, applicants must sign a written pledge to "openly renounce the historical chiropractic philosophical concept that subluxation is the cause of disease," and to restrict their scope of practice to "neuromusculoskeletal conditions of a nonsurgical nature." So far about three hundred chiropractors and chiropractic students have joined.

Overall, during the past fifteen years, there appears to have been a gradual shift toward the mixer philosophy and away from literal beliefs in Palmer's dogma. Over half of the approximately 45,000 chiropractors now practicing graduated since 1980. Since the majority of schools espouse a mixer philosophy, chiropractic philosophy and practice are moving in that direction.

**The Accreditation Decision**

In 1968, after an extensive investigation of chiropractic schools, the U.S. Department of Health, Education, and Welfare (HEW) concluded:

> Chiropractic theory and practice are not based upon the body of basic knowledge related to health, disease, and health care which has been widely accepted by the scientific community. Moreover, irrespective of its theory, the scope and quality of chiropractic education do not prepare the practitioner to make an adequate diagnosis and provide

appropriate treatment. Therefore, it is recommended that chiropractic service not be covered under Medicare.

In 1972, while the U.S. Department of Education was still part of HEW, an accreditation official asked whether it would be appropriate to recognize an agency for chiropractic schools in light of this extremely negative report. HEW's Office of General Counsel replied that "the Commissioner of Education is not called upon to express his opinion as to the legitimacy or social usefulness of the field of training seeking recognition." Two years later, based on completion of the necessary paperwork, the U.S. Office of Education (USOE) approved the Council on Chiropractic Education (CCE) as an accrediting agency for chiropractic schools.

CCE follows a mixer philosophy. The few schools that still cling to a subluxation-based ("no diagnosis") philosophy have been unable to sustain USOE recognition of an accrediting agency of their own. Since graduation from an accredited school is necessary for licensure in most states, these schools face extinction unless they make a fundamental change in their teachings. Although the quality of education in the CCE-approved schools is much better than it was in 1968, chiropractic is still attached to its cultist roots and riddled with unscientific beliefs and practices.

## "Subluxations" and X-Rays

Most chiropractors claim that x-rays help them locate the "subluxations" that D. D. Palmer imagined were the cause of "nerve interference." But they do not agree among themselves about what subluxations are. Some chiropractors believe that subluxations are displaced bones that can be seen on x-rays and can be put back in place by spinal adjustments. Others define subluxations vaguely and say that they do not show on x-rays. But what chiropractors say about x-rays also depends in part upon who asks and how the question is posed.

In the early 1960s, when the National Association of Letter Carriers Health Plan included chiropractic, it received claims for treatment of cancer, heart disease, mumps, mental retardation, and many other questionable conditions. In 1964, chiropractors were asked to justify such claims by sending x-ray evidence of spinal problems. They submitted hundreds, all of which supposedly showed subluxations. When chiropractic officials were assembled to review them, however, they were unable to point out a single subluxation.

Older chiropractic textbooks show "before and after" x-rays that are supposed to demonstrate subluxations. In 1971, hoping to get a first-hand look at such x-rays, I challenged the local chiropractic society to demonstrate ten sets. They refused, suggesting instead that I ask the Palmer School to show me some from its "teaching files." When I did, however, Palmer vice-president Ronald Frogley, D.C., replied:

Chiropractors do not make the claim to be able to read a specific subluxation from an x-ray film. [They] can read spinal distortion, which indicates the possible presence of a subluxation and can confirm the actual presence of a subluxation by other physical findings.

Frogley might have answered more cautiously had he anticipated the wording by which Congress included chiropractic under Medicare. The law, passed in 1973, calls for payment for the treatment of "subluxations *demonstrated by x-rays to exist.*" To help chiropractors get paid, the American Chiropractic Association issued a *Basic Chiropractic Procedural Manual,* which defined subluxations as anything that can interfere with spinal function and said, "Since we are obligated to find subluxations before receiving payment, it behooves us to make an objective study of what films show in the way of subluxations." Referring to the Letter Carriers experience as an "unfortunate debacle which almost destroyed chiropractic credibility in Washington," it cautioned, in italics, *"The subluxations must be perfectly obvious and indisputable."* (These strategic comments were omitted from subsequent editions of the manual.)

In 1980, a prominent chiropractic educator asked one thousand chiropractors on the ACA mailing list to check whether they agreed with a series of statements related to chiropractic beliefs. Only thirty-seven of 268 respondents (14 percent) checked "I do not believe that the chiropractic subluxation is a significant cause of disease." Asked whether Palmer's monocausal theory is "scientifically supported," twelve out of 260 (5 percent) said "completely," 195 (75 percent) said "partially," and 53 (20 percent) said "not at all."

A 1986 report from the U.S. Department of Health and Human Services' Office of the Inspector General (OIG) noted that Medicare paid chiropractors more than $93 million during 1984, that the amount paid to chiropractors had expanded at the rate of 18.7 percent between 1975 and 1984, and that chiropractic manipulation was the ninth most frequently billed procedure under Medicare during 1983. When OIG investigators surveyed 145 chiropractors by telephone, 84 percent said that some subluxations do not show on x-rays, but nearly half responded that when billing Medicare, they "could always find something" (by x-ray or physical examination) to justify the diagnosis, or actually tailored the diagnosis to obtain reimbursement.

In 1990, Medicare paid about $181 million for chiropractic services. Do you know of any other law that requires the U.S. government to pay for treating something that doesn't exist?

### Spinal Roulette?

It should be obvious that to help someone, doctors must first be able to figure out what is wrong. Most patients protect themselves from misdiagnosis by consulting a medical doctor before they go to a chiropractor. Those who start with a chiropractor, of course, take a greater risk. Chiropractors are not well trained in diagnosis and are prohibited by law from doing some tests that might be crucial to a medical investigation.

Although spinal manipulation may be appropriate for the treatment of certain back disorders, in the hands of chiropractors it can be dangerous. I know of one man who was paralyzed from the waist down after a spinal manipulation. Unknown to his chiropractor, spinal cancer had weakened the patient's spinal bones so that the treatment had crushed his spinal cord. In another case I investigated, a patient who took anticoagulants (blood thinners) had serious bleeding into his back muscles after a manipulation. Surgery was required to remove the collected blood.

From time to time, broken bones, paralyses, and strokes have been noted in court cases and medical journals. So have deaths from cancer, infectious diseases, and other conditions where chiropractors did not know enough to refer the patient in time for proper medical treatment. Although such serious cases are relatively rare, they are inexcusable. Lesser complications such as sprains are more common, but statistics are hard to collect. Some patients are too embarrassed to publicize them. Some do not realize that their extra discomfort is the result of inappropriate treatment. And others are sufficiently fond of the chiropractor that they cannot believe they were mistreated.

Peter J. Modde believes that "malpractice is an inevitable result of chiropractic philosophy and training." A 1964 graduate of Palmer College, he practiced in Renton, Washington, and was president of his county chiropractic society and chairman of the public relations committee of his state association. Midway in his chiropractic career, Modde came to two painful conclusions— that chiropractic theory is a delusion, and that chiropractors are not adequately trained in diagnosis. For several years he limited his practice to physical therapy of patients who had been evaluated by medical doctors.

According to Modde, "The more the patient relies on a chiropractor for diagnosis of his case, the more vulnerable he will be. Patients who use chiropractors as primary physicians, either because they don't know any better or because they have been turned off by orthodox medical care, run the greatest risk." In an attempt to remedy this situation, Modde persuaded medical doctors in the Seattle area to offer a special 300-hour course in diagnosis, but his chiropractic colleagues rejected this idea. Thoroughly disillusioned, Modde began to publicize his views and make himself available for expert testimony in malpractice cases. He was expelled from his state and national associations, his malpractice insurance was canceled, and an unsuccessful attempt was made to revoke his license. He remained in practice for several more years and then switched to another occupation. Before he did so, however, he produced a lengthy book called *Chiropractic Malpractice.*

Among the cases that Modde reviewed is that of a forty-seven-year-old man who consulted a chiropractor for leg pain of three days' duration. The chiropractor did not remove the patient's trousers, shoes, or socks. Instead, he examined only his back, diagnosed "lumbalgia," and manipulated the man's spine. Three days later, when the patient's pain persisted, he consulted a medical doctor who realized that the problem was a blocked artery that had been cutting down circulation of blood to the leg. Had the problem been diagnosed earlier, surgery could have removed the block. By this time, however, amputation of the leg was necessary.

After this case was publicized, the largest chiropractic malpractice insurance company issued a statement to its policyholders that was later published in the ACA *Journal of Chiropractic*:

> It has been mentioned in various locations of the country that some chiropractors diagnose and treat patients through their clothing. Following discussion with legal counsel . . . it was determined by [our] Board of Directors that legal defense of this kind of case was more difficult and consequently more costly to our company. A frequent basis for claims against our insureds is failure to properly diagnose the patient's condition. A diagnosis or treatment should not be made through the patient's clothing if this will interfere in any way with giving proper care. We recommend that careful discretion concerning this procedure be exercised by all.

(In other words, *it wouldn't look good in court.*)

## "Chiropractic Pediatrics"

Many chiropractors encourage families to rely upon them for the *primary* care of children. The International Chiropractors Association (ICA) even holds an annual National Conference on Chiropractic & Pediatrics, at which chiropractors have described their experiences in treating epilepsy and ear infections. A 1990 ICA policy statement recommends "the earliest possible evaluation, detection and correction of chiropractic lesions (subluxations) in children, especially infants, to maximize the potential for normal growth and development."

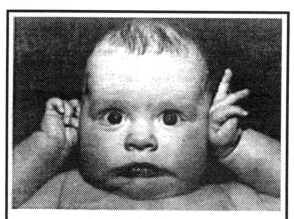

# MOMMY, MY EARS HURT!

**Did You Know?**

1. If left untreated, Ear Infections can cause permanent hearing loss.

2. The most common Antibiotic used is Amoxicillin. According to the *Journal of the American Medical Association* (Dec. 1991), this treatment is ineffective. In fact, occurrence of fluid in the middle ear is 2 to 6 times more likely after treatment.

3. The most common surgery is tympanostomy (tubes in ears). According to a British Study, these tubes can cause scars on the ear drum which can cause the very thing they are trying to avoid, permanent hearing deficit.

4. **The treatment of choice, Gentle Chiropractic Adjustments.** Adjustments correct misalignments of the spine, restoring normal function to the nervous system, in turn allowing normal drainage of the fluid in the middle ear. The inviting environment for the bacteria and viruses is removed, allowing the ears to **heal naturally and without side effects.**

5. **Drs. ▬▬ and ▬▬▬▬▬** at ▬▬▬▬ Family Chiropractic, on the corner of ▬▬ and ▬▬ Roads, are Experts in the care of Children with ear infections and many other problems. Mention this ad when you call and Drs. ▬▬ will check your child (at no charge) to see if they can be helped with Chiropractic.

## Call ▬▬▬▬▬

**This ad appeared in April 1993 in a newspaper in Pennsylvania. The *JAMA* article mentioned in item #2 was not about ear infections. It concerned serous otitis, a *painless* collection of fluid in the middle ear.**

In 1992, the ICA released a videotape called "Chiropractic and Your Child: A Partnership for the Future." Intended for viewing in chiropractic offices, it asserts that: (1) pediatricians typically diagnose and treat disease with little emphasis on prevention; (2) subluxations arise from "falls, blows, birth trauma, and normal daily living"; (3) standard medical treatment for middle ear infections is ineffective and can produce significant side effects; (4) middle ear infections are caused by subluxations of the bones of the neck and head; (5) chiropractic treatment can help prevent such infections; and (6) chiropractors are primary-care physicians who are able to determine what is wrong and what type of care is needed. These assertions are false—and potentially dangerous. The ad on the previous page illustrates how far some chiropractors go to solicit patients with ear infections.

On March 18, 1993, the chiropractic world was stunned by an article in *The Wall Street Journal.* The article described how a five-year-old boy and his four-year-old sister had developed mastoiditis, an infection of the middle ear so advanced that it invaded the skull. Both had been seen by a chiropractor who diagnosed the original infection and treated it with spinal manipulation. The children should have been referred to a medical doctor for antibiotic therapy. Instead, both became seriously ill, and the girl lost her hearing in one ear. The article noted that chiropractors were conducting marketing seminars, holding conventions, distributing pamphlets and coloring books, and pushing telemarketing scripts, all with the aim of drawing infants into their practices for basic health care. It also cited a 1991 newspaper ad placed by chiropractors in California to discourage parents from having their children immunized.

A few days later, following an emergency telephone conference, the American Chiropractic Association responded with a full-page ad in *The Wall Street Journal.* The ad, which cost $115,000, stated that "any doctor of chiropractic who would seek to substitute spinal manipulation for antibiotic therapy in the treatment of bacterial infections . . . is acting counter to accepted clinical practices." The ad also said that routine vaccinations have been proven effective in controlling many diseases and that chiropractic manipulation is not a substitute for them.

Despite these comments—which I believe were sincere—the ACA vigorously promotes the idea that chiropractors should treat children. Louis Sportelli, D.C., a former chairman of the ACA's board of governors. himself has written and published a booklet called *Introduction to Chiropractic,* which asserts that "regular spinal adjustments are a part of your body's defense against illness." Chiropractors have purchased more than two million copies of the booklet for distribution to the public. The ninth edition, which was also distributed by the ACA, states:

The strains to which children are subject can easily be a contributing factor in creating spinal malfunctions (subluxations) and/or nerve irritation. . . . Clinical evidence suggests that common disorders of childhood such as colds, constipation, asthma, and other conditions can be helped through spinal manipulations (adjustments) if they are the result of neurological irritations caused by spinal imbalances. . . .

If parents were as concerned about having their children's spines checked for minor derangements (subluxations) as they are about having their teeth checked for cavities, they would be helping their youngsters attain a healthier state of well-being. Proper spinal care is essential to your child's health.

On March 29, 1993, an ACA official informed the President's Task Force on National Health Care Reform that chiropractors are "trained, licensed, and obligated under state law to diagnose any and all health conditions." Shortly afterward, the Federation for Chiropractic Education and Research asked chiropractors to donate money for research that would "ensure chiropractic's status as a primary care provider." In April 1993, in the *ACA Journal of Chiropractic*, ACA officials explained why they had responded so vigorously to the article in the *Wall Street Journal*:

The . . . article could not have come at a worse time for the profession. The Clinton administration's health-care task force was literally making the cut on who was "in" and who was "out" of the minimum benefits package. . . . There was no way we could allow what amounted to a bunch of snake-oil salesmen to drag the entire profession down by trying to defend outrageous and indefensible conduct."

Two other chiropractors who think children should be treated early in life are Palmer and Jennifer Peet, who practice in South Burlington, Vermont, and operate The Baby Adjusters, a chiropractic supply firm. The Peets also teach in the certification program in chiropractic pediatrics co-sponsored by Life Chiropractic College and the International Chiropractic Pediatrics Association. In the *Wall Street Journal*, Jennifer stated that her clinic adjusts the spines of 150 to 200 patients a day, mostly children and some infants, and that "chiropractors are seeing that if you start young with a child you have a better chance to improve their well-being." Palmer's foreword to the second edition of Jennifer's 300-page *Chiropractic Pediatric & Prenatal Reference Manual* states:

In your practice right now, you probably have children that are developing colon cancer, that will manifest in 50 years if you don't adjust them now. . . . *Now* is the time to tell your patients that subluxations are slowly killing their children. The time is *now* to start adjusting children from birth. . . . One should never underestimate the power of the chiropractic adjustment. Use the information within this book to give your best adjustments to infants and children. Then all the power in heaven will break loose within them and miraculous healings will occur on a daily basis.

The book also claims that "the dangers of vaccinations to the young child are profound" and that "in some cases, the vaccine acts nonspecificly [*sic*] to increase a child's preexisting chronic disease tendency." The book concludes: "Every time a child receives a chiropractic adjustment it should be given as if their very life depends on it, because it does."

ICA officials are unhappy with both the *Wall Street Journal* article and the ACA's "apologetic" response. ICA's president stated that his group has launched a 300-hour Diplomate in Chiropractic Pediatrics program to provide "quality education in pediatrics." An ICA past president accused the ACA of abrogating chiropractic principles by inferring that chiropractic care of childhood infections is inappropriate. ICA's board chairman called the ACA response "spineless."

If a chiropractor limited his practice to musculoskeletal conditions such as simple backaches, if he were able to determine which patients are appropriate for him to treat, if he consulted and referred to medical doctors when he couldn't handle a problem, if he were not overly vigorous in his manipulations, if he minimized the use of x-rays, and if he encouraged the use of proven public health measures, his patients would be relatively safe. But he might not be able to earn a living.

## The Selling of the Spine

A chiropractor's income depends not only on what he treats but on how well he can sell himself. A survey by the American Chiropractic Association found that in 1991 its members had a median gross income of $179,706 with a net of $70,025. However, the meaning of this figure is not clear. Many chiropractic graduates do not remain in practice, and others are forced to practice part-time. Top chiropractic salesmen can earn a fortune.

Intensive selling of the spine begins in chiropractic school as instructors convey the scope and philosophy of chiropractic to their students. After graduation, chiropractors can get help from many practice-building consultants who offer seminars and ongoing management advice.

During the 1970s, flamboyant ads from practice-builders were much more common than they are today. The Drennan Seminar, for example, offered to "double your income and patient volume in 90 days" and said that one out of every ten registrants would receive a free Cadillac. The Stoner Chiropractic Research Foundation offered to "show you how to make $350,000 as easily as

$50,000"; promised "no more end-of-the-month jitters"; and depicted a chiropractor headed for the First National Bank, pushing a wheelbarrow overflowing with stacks of money. Dr. Robert A. Jarmain invited chiropractors to a three-day seminar to "build the $1,000,000 practice." The Yennie Chiropractic Success Seminar offered to "put you on the road to total success" and to "upgrade your practice into the $100,000—$200,000—$300,000 service levels." In 1978, Clinic Masters advertised that three thousand chiropractors had enrolled in its program and increased their incomes, on average, more than $50,000 a year. Its fee for a program of seminars and ongoing consultation was $20,000—$100 initially and the rest payable as income rose. Its seminars included "How To Increase Insurance Business $100,000 Or More A Year" and "How To Achieve The 'Optimum Gettable' With Every Patient." Santavicca and Associates charged $30,000 for its advice—$100 for an initial three-day seminar and the rest payable as income rose. Recent ads for Nikitow Training Seminars promise that they will reveal how "only 200 NP's [new patients] in one year yield you ONE MILLION DOLLARS – CASH COLLECTIONS."

The largest practice-building firm is the Parker Chiropractic Research Foundation of Fort Worth, Texas, founded by James W. Parker, D.C. A 1987 brochure for its Parker School of Professional Success Seminar claimed that "over 125,000 Doctors of Chiropractic, spouses and staff assistants worldwide—over two thirds of all practicing chiropractors—have attended nearly 300 Seminars more than 400,000 times. . . . Resulting in millions and millions of additional patients being served. . . . And surely resulting in at least a billion dollars of EXTRA CHIROPRACTIC EARNINGS!" Attendees receive a diploma for completing "the prescribed course of study at the Parker Chiropractic Research Seminar." In 1989, the fee for first-time chiropractors was $389 for the four-day course plus a gold-lettered plaque indicating membership in Parker Chiropractic Research Foundation.

Parker's basic course was built around a 335-page *Textbook of Office Procedure and Practice Building for the Chiropractic Profession.* Parker appears to believe that the scope of chiropractic is unlimited. The *Textbook* suggests that patients be offered a "free consultation" but led into an "examination" that costs them money. It suggests that "One adjustment for each year of age is a rough thumbnail guide of what people will willingly accept and pay for," but "If in doubt about the payment or the return of the patient, take only the smaller x-rays on the first visit but ostensibly x-ray fully."

Writing in a Parker publication, L. Ted Frigard, D.C., a prominent California chiropractor, has asserted: "A patient is much more satisfied if you give him an adjustment every time he comes into the office. If you do not . . . you will have to spend a lot of time explaining why you didn't."

Share International, Parker's sales organization, sells hundreds of educational items and other practice-building aids. One is a chart like that on page 165 of this book. Another is a "report of findings" on which chiropractors note "subluxations" and the (large) number of visits needed to correct them. A set of cassette tapes I acquired in the late 1970s included *Sentences that Sell,* in which Parker describes how chiropractors associated with him tested ideas scientifically and reported back to him how they worked. The set also included *Ways to Stimulate Referrals,* in which he tells how to steer conversations to sick people. "In a casual, natural way," patients should be asked about the health of their families, friends, and neighbors. Should any be ailing, patients should be urged to be "Good Samaritans" by telling them about "all the wonderful things" that chiropractic might do for them.

During the 1970s, for about $20, chiropractors could get copies of 107 advertisements to "guide" preparation of their own ads. Most of the ads were case histories. The instructions that accompanied them suggested: "Re-type each ad on your own stationery for presentation to the editor. This would indicate that they are your own creations, and that the cases mentioned . . . are from your own files." Sale of this advertising kit was discontinued after its instructions were exposed in Jack Anderson's syndicated newspaper column.

Despite the questionable methods Parker has espoused, he is a highly respected and integral part of the chiropractic world. He is president of the Parker College of Chiropractic in Dallas, Texas, which he founded in 1978. He has lectured at many other chiropractic schools, and school officials often attend ceremonies at his seminars.

Sid Williams, D.C., another leading promoter, has been president of the International Chiropractors Association and is president of Life Chiropractic College in Marietta, Georgia. His other enterprises have included Si-Nel (a chiropractic supply house), *Today's Chiropractic* (a journal), *Health for Life* (a testimonial newspaper), the Life Foundation (for public education), and the Life DE Meetings (at which Williams expounds on chiropractic's "Dynamic Essentials"). Williams appears to believe that virtually all health problems are caused by nerve interference and should be treated by chiropractic methods. In 1979, he appeared on CBS's "60 Minutes," adjusting the neck of an infant girl. When asked why, her mother said the adjustments (begun on the child's third day of life) were "preventative measures—to keep her healthy."

The Life DE meetings are intended to inspire chiropractors to greater income as well as greater self-confidence. During the late 1970s, the fee was $325 for a three-day program during which "the DE Team speakers will show you how to increase your practice with the secrets that have enabled them to build their practices into the $300,000–$500,000 range." Other ads for the seminars boasted that their top instructors saw 200 to 400 patients per day.

During the 1970s, William distributed two volumes entitled *Dynamic Essentials of the Chiropractic Principle, Practice and Procedure*. One volume, also called the "Doctors Red Senior Textbook," outlines his views on the importance of chiropractic. It states: "Life Foundation and the Life Principle offer the world its one hope for freedom from disease, self-annihilation and eventual oblivion." The volume also affirms that God told Williams "in very clear language on three different occasions during a five-month period" to commence the DE meetings.

The practice-building aspects of the DE meetings were centered around the other volume, which resembles Parker's textbook but is far more detailed in its instructions. The initial phase of patient contact is said to have three parts: the consultation, the examination (including an x-ray of every patient), and the report of findings. On page 129 we read:

> Every step of your procedure should be thorough enough to convince the patient that you are not overlooking anything. The sophisticated age in which we live prevents the simplicity of chiropractic from being understood by the average person. . . .
>
> The examination procedures are not diagnostic, they are to emphasize to the patient that a weakness exists in his body and that they have been caused by spinal fixations. By fortifying the patient's knowledge of the 'spinal cause' by the use of test instruments and graphs, the patient is able to see beyond any doubt that he is actually physically sick; that a spinal condition caused it, and that something needs to be done chiropractically to correct it.

Much of this volume is composed of statements for selling patients on chiropractic care. On pages 98–100, for example, Williams recommends that the doctor feel the spine for tender spots, "predict the conditions that might occur underneath," and ask whether various symptoms have yet occurred. If the patient answers no to any of them, say: "Well, Mrs. Jones, it certainly is a wonder. I must say you have a strong constitution in order to stand up under the many problems that you have. You have trouble in many areas, but you don't have many symptoms as of yet. But I would make the prediction that if you hadn't turned to chiropractic, you'd be a very sick girl shortly." Page 148 suggests telling patients: "Medicine is very effective in its place; however, it is a simple fact that it is becoming obsolete. The theory of medicine is false."

Williams's suggested goal was to convince patients to continue "preventive maintenance" once a month for life. (Page 75 notes that "once the patient has experienced relief through chiropractic adjustments, he will accept almost any reasonable recommendation.") If the patient asks, "But will I have to continue with chiropractic care as long as I live?" the recommended reply (page 175) is:

> (Chuckling) No ma'am, you won't have to continue it as long as you live. Only as long as you want to stay healthy. Every spine needs some maintenance, Mrs. Jones. My family and I are checked regularly on a monthly basis, and more often when we think that it is necessary. Yes, if you want to stay healthy, you will have to continue some chiropractic care.

Page 216 describes a technique called "sealing the patient in." First the patient is asked if various positive responses have occurred yet. If any have, he is told he even looks better. Then he is instructed to rest quietly in the chiropractor's office so he can get "filled up with the thought that he is better, looks better, and he will be able to tell all his friends how much better he is." But page 218 cautions: "Keep in mind that we don't want to feature 'Well' or 'Cure' too soon or too strongly because the patient won't show up for the next visit since he thinks 'I'm ready to quit; I am well.' He is never well—just better. Don't emphasize improvement too fast. Instead we say, 'We want to get you over on the good side of the ledger and keep you there.'"

During the late 1970s, I acquired a set of tape-recorded lectures from the April 1978 DE meeting. In *The Patient Report That Eliminates Premature Dropouts,* Williams advised using a magnifying glass to point out to patients the "fixations" on their x-rays. "If you'll remember the first time someone showed you an atlas and the condyles of an A-to-P cervical view, it looked like so much nothing. But you can get the magnifying glass out and . . . you'll say 'Here . . . here,' and they'll say 'Um hm . . . Um hm.' And they'll go home and they'll say, 'I saw it. He showed it to me!'" But if patients don't look convinced while listening to the report, Williams suggests in the tape called *Office Procedures of the Big Men,* "Tell 'em they ain't ready—you gotta re-x-ray 'em."

Singer Enterprises, a practice-management firm in Clearwater, Florida, offers additional insights in its bimonthly *Purpose Newsletter.* According to a recent issue:

> Patient retention comes as a result of education. . . . There is usually only one reason why your patients don't continue to receive the chiropractic care they need: They don't understand what a subluxation is and its effects. . . .
>
> We must educate patients so that they understand that chiropractic care is a part of life; once subluxations are corrected, the body will innately heal itself. . . .
>
> Only the consumer who understands nerve interference will pay cash after his symptoms are gone.

Curiously, Sid Williams has expressed concern about overutilization. In the January/February 1992 issue of *Today's Chiropractic,* he said:

> Unfortunately, some members of the chiropractic profession have been engaging in what amounts to "crime and wicked conduct" in their practices by jumping on the bandwagon of getting all they can from the insurance industry while the "getting" is good. They have been playing a numbers game of getting as many patient visits and as many dollars per visit by whatever means they (and often their practice consultants) can devise. . . . Some members of our profession have been engaging in outright fraud with too many examinations and inflated office fees—which include inappropriate and worthless therapies and x-ray procedures—that sometimes amount to $1,000 for the first visit before they've done anything at all for the patient!

### How to Attract Patients

Practice Management Associates (PMA), a Florida-based firm run by Peter Fernandez, D.C., advertised that chiropractors who followed its guidelines would gross an average of $240,000 in their first year of practice and that the average for all of their clients was about $350,000. The firm touted itself as "the world's largest full-service chiropractic management firm." An ad for one of its 1991 seminars stated: "We use an 'idea' factory approach which teaches a chiropractor every conceivable way that exists to attract new patients, from the most subtle to the most aggressive."

Fernandez has marketed a cassette tape series called "How to Keep Your Patients Coming Back," which included this inspirational message:

> Constantly educate your patients as to the value of chiropractic. . . . Get out there and beat the bushes, advertise, word-of-mouth, either way. But let's let the people in our country know what we can do. We only take care of four percent of the people. Guess what, gang? One hundred percent of the people out there have spines, 100 percent have subluxations. They all need adjustments. We have 95 or 96 percent of the people still to reach.

Fernandez has also produced a five-volume series called *Secrets of a Practice-Building Consultant.* The first (1981) edition of Volume I, *1001 Ways to Attract Patients,* included the following suggestions on how to build one's reputation when beginning chiropractic practice:

• Never go anywhere without being paged. This affixes your name in people's minds. . . . Whenever you're not busy, tell your receptionist that you are going to a certain supermarket, and . . . to have you paged as if for an emergency. . . . This paging procedure can be used 15 to 20 times a day very successfully.

• Your wife and/or receptionist can dial any phone number and say, "Is this Dr. So-and-So's, the chiropractor's office? I hear he is tremendous with treating headaches and I've got a terrible headache." . . . I know a doctor who employed a woman to make these calls eight hours a day. It was her only function on his staff! He built a large-volume practice in a short time using this technique.

• Write notes on good chiropractic literature . . . with a red pencil: "John, this man cured my headaches. Go to him!" or "Bob, this is the best doctor in the whole town! He cured the back problem that I have had for the past 15 years!" Then take this literature, with your name and location stamped on it, and lay it all over town.

The fifth volume in the series, published in 1990, is called *How to Become a Million Dollar a Year Practitioner.*

For several years, Fernandez published *Chiropractic Achievers*, a bimonthly magazine distributed free of charge to chiropractors throughout the United States. One thing it reported was the record set by clients during their first thirty business days—the highest of which was $91,000 in services to 177 new patients. A 1987 ad for Fernandez's school of patient longevity stated, "Once you've acquired a patient, keep him coming back because he wants to, because he believes in chiropractic and in you."

During the early 1990s, Fernandez and PMA became embroiled in a large number of lawsuits with clients who said they were dissatisfied. Another company has purchased the right to service PMA's clients, and Fernandez has dropped from the limelight.

### Bait-and-Switch?

A few years ago, Terence Rondberg, D.C., of Chandler, Arizona, launched the Vertebral Subluxation Research Institute (VSRI), which taught how to recruit volunteers for "research" and convert them into patients. For $2,500, it provided videotapes, detailed instructions, and a ready-to-frame "Research Associate" certificate. To attract chiropractors to its program, VSRI ran ads asking "Can you fit 20 new patients into your schedule this month?" Respondents received a videotape in which clients told how much the program had built their practice and how they had recovered their initial investment within a few weeks.

The program was based mainly on telemarketing to recruit "research volunteers," who would be converted into patients. According to VSRI's manual, "Every time someone enters your office—for any reason—you are given a valuable opportunity to introduce that person to the life-enhancing benefits of chiropractic and to the particular advantages of your care." A VSRI symposium taught how to convert the volunteers into "lifetime patients"—even if they had no symptoms.

During the first visit, patients completed a questionnaire that asked sketchy questions about emotional status, diet, exercise activities, alcohol and tobacco habits, health history, family data, and income. (The questions covered only a tiny portion of what a competent physician would ask in a medical or lifestyle history.) Next, patients were asked to read a brochure explaining the supposed dangers of subluxations ("The Silent Killer") and the chiropractor's role in correcting them. Then came the spinal examination, followed—in most cases—by an x-ray exam. The instructions stated that everyone should be x-rayed unless there were "counter-indications" or this was incompatible with the chiropractor's style of practice. The second visit was a "report of findings" to discuss the "subluxations or other spinal conditions for which chiropractic would be beneficial." Noting that people without symptoms often show "definite evidence" of subluxations, the manual suggested telling them that chiropractic treatment might prevent future trouble.

One investigator posing as a volunteer reported that a VSRI practitioner in California said her lumbar spine had "a distinct curve to the left." To avoid trouble, she was told, exercise might help, but chiropractic treatment three times a week for a month would be best. According to chiropractic sources, twelve visits is the "magic number," above which insurance companies look closely at whether treatment is necessary.

VSRI claimed that the purpose of its program was to explore possible connections between "subluxations" and various lifestyle factors. Even if this were true, the data generated by such a study would be meaningless because the participating chiropractors diagnosed "subluxations" in different ways. In October 1990, the International Chiropractors Association's board of directors denounced "patient research/solicitation schemes" as "inherently suspect" and "unethical," while the American Chiropractic Association's board called them "unacceptable and possibly illegal." Not long after these criticisms were publicized, VSRI disappeared from view.

### Care to Have A Check-Up?

How often should people who feel well have their spine examined and adjusted? In 1979, representatives of the Lehigh Valley Committee Against Health Fraud

(LVCAHF) posed that question to thirty-five local chiropractors in Allentown, Pennsylvania, and nearby communities. Almost all recommended at least one check-up per year. The majority gave answers in the range of four to twelve times a year.

The American Chiropractic Association says that one of the best ways to guard your health is through periodic spinal examinations. "Check your calendar and see how long it has been since you and every member of your family had a spinal examination. If several months have elapsed . . . make an appointment."

Some chiropractors have advertised that "chiropractic prolongs life." Yet inspection of the *ACA Journal of Chiropractic* suggests otherwise. From 1976 through 1981, the journal contained more than two hundred obituary notices that specified the age of death. The average was only sixty-six, about five years less than the national average for men.

If you go to a chiropractor, what should you expect? During the 1970s, LVCAHF sent a healthy four-year-old girl to five chiropractors for a "check-up." The first said the child's shoulder blades were "out of place" and found "pinched nerves to her stomach and gallbladder." The second said the child's pelvis was "twisted." The third said one hip was "elevated" and that spinal misalignments could cause "headaches, nervousness, equilibrium or digestive problems" in the future. The fourth predicted "bad periods and rough child-birth" if her "shorter left leg" was not treated. The fifth not only found hip and neck problems, but also "adjusted" them without bothering to ask permission. Unfortunately, the adjustments were so painful that we decided to postpone further investigation until adult volunteers could be found.

The next volunteer, a healthy twenty-nine-year-old psychologist, visited four more chiropractors for check-ups. The first diagnosed an "atlas subluxa-tion" and predicted "paralysis in fifteen years" if this problem was not treated. The second found many vertebrae "out of alignment" and one hip "higher" than the other. The third said the woman's neck was "tight." The fourth said that misaligned vertebrae indicated the presence of "stomach problems." All four recommended spinal adjustments on a regular basis, beginning with a fre-quency of twice a week. Three gave adjustments without warning—one of which was so forceful that it produced dizziness and a headache that lasted for several hours.

Another volunteer, a thirty-six-year-old housewife, visited seven other chiropractors. The first found "minor structural problems" in the neck, mid-back and lower spine regions and recommended four to six treatments. The second found nothing wrong. The third said the woman's left hip was lower than her right hip, adjusted a few areas of her spine (painfully) and suggested she return if she felt "sluggish." The fourth said her right hip and several vertebrae were "twisted." After pressing on the offending body parts, he suggested a return appointment in a week to see if the adjustments held. The fifth chiropractor thought there might be a serious problem with a "pinched nerve" in the neck that could cause "sinus trouble"—but he could not be sure without an x-ray. The sixth, who called himself a "herbologist," used muscle-testing to diagnose a "vitamin C deficiency" and indicated he could do extensive nutritional testing if requested. The seventh thought there was a hip problem, adjusted it, and recommended an x-ray for further diagnosis.

In 1981, Mark Brown, a reporter for the *Quad-City Times*, a newspaper in Davenport, Iowa, conducted a five-month investigation of chiropractors during which he visited about two dozen of them as a "patient." He reported that each one said he was a "chiropractic case," and that all but one insisted on x-rays before treatment. One chiropractor placed a potato and an egg on the reporter's chest to test the strength of his arms, held a magnet over his thymus gland, concluded that nutrient deficiencies were present, and sold him four bottles of "glandular" substances for $47.50. Another chiropractor was noted to diagnose patients by passing a cylindrical instrument over the patient's back and marking any spots over which the instrument makes a squeaking noise. Another claimed to diagnose subluxations by using an instrument that records temperature differences from one side of the spine to another. Another examined patients' eyes for markings he claimed would indicate what diseases were found within the body—a practice called iridology. Another told the reporter his ears were acting as "antennae for nerve energy" that had become congested in his diaphragm. Brown also reported that on one day during his investigation, one chiropractor told him his left leg was shorter than his right and another chiropractor told him just the opposite. Other chiropractors also told him that he suffered from hiatal hernia, "ileocecal valve syndrome," and "ocular lock."

During 1989, William M. London, Ed.D., assistant professor of health education at Kent State University, visited twenty-three chiropractors in Ohio and Florida who had advertised free consultations or examinations. Every one of them espoused subluxation theory either during the consultation or in waiting room literature, and all but two recommended periodic preventive maintenance. Seventeen performed examinations. Of these, three identified subluxations (at differing locations), three said his left leg was shorter than his right leg, and two said his right leg was shorter than his left one. Seven recommended treatment.

In 1993, a healthy twenty-five-year-old producer from WJW-TV in Cleveland, Ohio, visited three chiropractors who had advertised free examinations. The first one found nothing wrong (as had an orthopedist and a chiropractor used as consultants for the investigation). The second chiropractor, using a "biomagnetic scanner," diagnosed "underactive pituitary, underactive adrenal, underactive gallbladder, underactive kidney, and problems with the liver." The third chiropractor, whose comments followed a script distributed by a practice-building organization, told the producer he had "twisted vertebrae" and should have at least ten treatments. If he did not, the chiropractor claimed, the problem would insidiously get worse, "kind of like cancer. . . . You don't know it usually until it's the end."

Many chiropractors recruit patients by offering free spinal screenings at shopping malls, health expositions, and other public events. From what I have seen, everyone who gets screened is advised to have further services. Several years ago, one exhibitor who examined me recommended treatment for excessive tension of my neck (which, if it existed, did not bother me at all). More recently, a chiropractor stated that pains in my left shoulder were caused by a subluxation in my neck and that an immediate $5 deposit would cover the cost of a $75 visit to his office. The actual cause (which I knew) was tendinitis of a biceps muscle that would rub against a shoulder bone when I raised my arm. Soon afterward an orthopedist cured the problem by inserting an instrument into my shoulder and shaving the bone so that the tendon no longer encounters it.

Significant numbers of chiropractors use diagnostic methods that have no scientifically recognized validity. Practitioners of "applied kinesiology" claim that diseases throughout the body can be diagnosed fully, or in part, by testing muscle strength after placing various substances in the mouth. Followers of Activator Methods compare the lengths of the patient's legs to determine whether the patient's spine is properly aligned; the problems detected by this procedure are then corrected by small blows to the spine, or elsewhere, delivered with a hand-held spring-loaded hammer.

Followers of B.E.S.T. (Bio Energetic Synchronization Technique) claim that unequal leg length signifies an imbalance in the patient's electromagnetic field, which the chiropractor can correct with his own electromagnetic energy. According to this notion, two fingers on each of the chiropractor's hands are North poles, two are South poles, and the thumbs are electromagnetically neutral. When imbalance is detected, the hands are held at "contact points" until "pulsation" is felt and the patient's legs test equally long. Proponents of this technique recommend that testing be started early in infancy and continued periodically throughout life.

Information about applied kinesiology, Activator Methods, and B.E.S.T. is available from books, newsletters, audiotapes, and videotapes, and at seminars held frequently throughout the United States. Each of these systems is claimed by its leading proponents to have thousands of adherents.

### "Chiropractic Nutrition"

About fifty companies market supplements through chiropractic offices, where they typically are sold for two or three times their wholesale cost. Many of these products are intended for the treatment of disease even though they are unproven and lack FDA approval for this use. Since it is illegal to place an unproven therapeutic claim on a product label, claims of this type are conveyed separately through product literature distributed at chiropractic meetings, company-sponsored seminars, and by mail. A few companies distribute elaborate manuals listing the diseases their products can supposedly treat.

Regional distributors, who may handle the products of one company or several, mail information or visit chiropractic offices in much the same way that drug "detailers" attempt to educate physicians. However, the information delivered by legitimate drug company representatives is strictly regulated by the FDA and must be complete and based on well-designed scientific tests. The information conveyed to chiropractors has neither of these characteristics and is transmitted through channels that are intended to be hidden from the FDA.

The percentage of chiropractors engaging in unscientific nutrition practices is unknown, but several reports suggest that it is substantial. In 1988, 74 percent of about 2,400 chiropractors who responded to a questionnaire in the leading chiropractic newspaper reported using nutritional supplements in their practice. Not long afterward, researchers from San Jose State University's Department of Nutrition and Food Science mailed a survey to 438 members of the San Francisco Bay Area Chiropractic Society. Of the one hundred who responded, sixty said that they routinely provide nutrition information to their patients, thirty-eight said they provide it on request, sixty claimed that they treat patients for nutritional deficiencies, nineteen said they use hair analysis, and nine indicated that they use "applied kinesiology" for nutritional assessment. Neither hair analysis nor applied kinesiology is valid for nutritional assessment of patients.

Although some aspects of scientific nutrition are taught in chiropractic schools, many ideas that chiropractors absorb—in school and afterwards—are as unscientific as their basic theory of disease. Chiropractors who give nutritional advice typically recommend vitamin supplements that are unnecessary or inappropriate for treatment of the patient's health problem. Some chiropractors have charged thousands of dollars for treatment programs involving diagnostic evaluations, vitamins, adjustments, and massage over a period of several months.

Bruce West, a chiropractor who publishes a monthly newsletter called

*Health Alert,* also markets supplement products to his readers. In a recent mailing he plugged *Cardio-Plus* ("to protect against heart attacks, angina, and stroke"), *Chlorophyll Complex Perles* (a "super longevity product" to make you "look younger and feel more energetic"), *Catalyn* ("to improve your immune function and beat fatigue), and *Min-Tran* (to "easily combat stress" and help avoid kidney stones and cataracts). The products, for which West charges $64 for a month's supply, are manufactured by Standard Process Laboratories, a leading supplier to chiropractors and other unconventional health professionals. According to West:

> Catalyn is the most time-honored product ever made by Standard Labs. Like the company that produces it, it has been proven effective by withstanding the test of time. First produced in 1930, it has been utilized MILLIONS OF TIMES. In fact, more physicians who practice nutrition have utilized this product over ANY OTHER.

West's mailing did not specify the basis for this statement. Nor did it mention that it is illegal to claim that *Catalyn* boosts immunity. Nor did it reveal that the FDA had twice ordered the manufacturer (doing business as Vitamin Products Company) to stop making false claims for *Catalyn* and later obtained a criminal conviction against the company for marketing 115 products with illegal claims (see Chapter 28).

In another mailing, West urged his readers to buy a special filter to remove chlorine from their shower water in order to protect themselves and their children from skin difficulties and various other health problems. According to the flyer, "people who have suffered precancerous keratotic lesions on their skin for decades. . . . say their lesions clear up within a matter of weeks once the chlorine is removed from their shower."

Although some chiropractors give rational nutrition advice to their patients, chiropractic journals contain little or no discussion of what should be advised. Although patients have been seriously harmed by toxic doses of vitamin A prescribed by chiropractors, I have seen no case reports in chiropractic journals or warnings that high doses can be toxic. Nor has any prominent chiropractor or major chiropractic organization ever openly suggested that there is anything wrong with the way chiropractors "practice nutrition." The March 1993 issue of *ACA Journal of Chiropractic* even contains an article called "The Subluxation Complex: Nutritional Considerations," which states:

> Chiropractors can . . . greatly influence the production of chemical irritants through nutritional intervention. . . . Such an approach could significantly reduce the . . . reflexogenic activity that initiates/perpetuates the development of the subluxation complex.

### Don't Let Chiropractors Fool You

Three recent events have given chiropractic a boost. In 1987, a federal court judge ruled that the American Medical Association (AMA) had engaged in an illegal boycott. The AMA appealed, but was unsuccessful. In 1990, an article in the *British Medical Journal* said that certain patients treated by chiropractors did better than comparable patients treated at a medical facility. And in 1991, a RAND Corporation panel concluded that spinal manipulation is an appropriate treatment for low-back pain. Chiropractors would like you to believe that each of these events is evidence that chiropractic works. The issues involved, however, are not that simple.

The antitrust case was launched in 1976 when five chiropractors began a series of lawsuits against the AMA, other professional organizations, and several individual critics, charging that they had conspired to destroy chiropractic and to illegally deprive chiropractors of access to laboratory, x-ray, and hospital facilities. The suits were based on the theory that since chiropractors were licensed professionals, attempting to interfere with their activities violated antitrust laws.

During the 1960s and early 1970s, the AMA engaged in a wide variety of antichiropractic activities. These activities were intended to protect the public from unscientific and unethical practices that were rampant during those years. Under antitrust law, however, good intentions may not be adequate justification for a boycott. Faced with an uncertain outcome and the prospect of great legal expense, most of the defendant groups settled their cases out-of-court by agreeing that their members were free to decide for themselves how to deal with chiropractors. The AMA adopted a similar policy, but chose to meet the chiropractors in court.

Following a jury trial (won by the AMA), an appeal to a higher court (won by the chiropractors), and an agreement to narrow the scope of the proceedings, the case was retried in front of a federal judge. In 1987, the judge ruled in favor of the chiropractors. Her lengthy opinion, however, was not complimentary to chiropractic. For example, she said that during the 1960s, "there was a lot of material available to the AMA Committee on Quackery that supported its belief that all chiropractic was unscientific and deleterious." She noted that chiropractors still took too many x-rays. She concluded that the dominant reason for the AMA's antichiropractic campaign was the belief that chiropractic was not in the best interests of patients. But she ruled that good intentions did not justify attempting to contain and eliminate an entire licensed profession without first demonstrating that a less restrictive campaign could not succeed in protecting the public. The AMA appealed the decision to higher courts, but was not successful.

Although chiropractors trumpet the antitrust ruling as an endorsement of their effectiveness, it was not. The outcome was based on narrow *legal* grounds and not the merits of chiropractic.

In 1990, a British research team concluded: "For patients with low back pain in whom manipulation is not contraindicated, chiropractic almost certainly confers worthwhile, long term benefit in comparison with hospital outpatient management. . . . mainly in those with chronic or severe pain." The study involved 741 patients between the ages of eighteen and sixty-five who lacked signs of spinal nerve compression, infectious disease, or other conditions that require medical intervention. The chiropractic treatment spanned up to thirty weeks (versus twelve weeks for hospital-based treatment) and cost about 50 percent more. The outcome was measured by a self-administered questionnaire about pain intensity, not a clinical evaluation. Patients who had not previously had back pain showed no difference in outcome. Among patients with a prior history of back pain, those in the chiropractic treatment group scored significantly better than those in the hospital-based group at six-, twelve-, and twenty-four-month follow-up intervals. No clear relationship was found between the number of treatments and the extent of improvement for either chiropractic or hospital-based treatment.

The ACA claims that this study "confirms previous studies . . . that chiropractic procedure can relieve chronic and severe pain, both immediate and long-term, in half the time it takes medical physicians and physical therapists." But there are at least four reasons why this interpretation is overstated:

1. The researchers themselves cautioned that their findings may not apply to all patients with back pain.

2. The questionnaire used to evaluate pain intensity may not be a valid measure of outcome.

3. Some hospital physiotherapy departments may have been unable to provide optimum care because they had more work than they could handle.

4. The study was not applicable to chiropractic as practiced in the United States. All patients in the study were screened by doctors at *medical* facilities to be sure they did not require intervention by a physician. Most patients who go to chiropractic offices are not screened in the same way. And, as indicated throughout this chapter, many encounter practices that are unscientific and inappropriate.

The RAND Corporation has conducted a three-part study of the appropriateness of spinal manipulation for low-back pain. In the first phase, completed in 1991, a seven-member interdisciplinary panel identified sixty-seven relevant articles and nine books published between 1955 and 1989. From this review, the panelists concluded:

1. Data from twenty-two controlled studies support the use of manipulation for acute low-back pain in patients showing no signs of lower-limb nerve root involvement.

2. Scientific reports provide no help in deciding when spinal manipulative treatment should be stopped, with respect to either improvement or worsening of symptoms. It is not clear how many, if any, manipulations are necessary after a patient has become pain-free.

3. There has been no systematic study of the frequency of complications from spinal manipulation for low-back pain. Although the risk appears small when compared to the large number of manipulations performed, no firm conclusions may be drawn because there are few data in the scientific literature.

Although chiropractors have promoted the RAND study as an endorsement of chiropractic, it is not. It merely supports the use of manipulation for carefully selected patients. Very few of the reports identified by the RAND panel involved manipulations done by chiropractors; most were done by medical practitioners.

As far as I know, no study has assessed whether current chiropractic education prepares its graduates to make adequate diagnoses, provide appropriate treatment, and make appropriate referrals. There been no scientific study to measure the quality of care in typical chiropractic offices. Nor has anyone determined whether faith or greed is the major reason for frequent spinal adjustments for "preventive maintenance." My observations suggest that consumers should be wary of chiropractors, except for the few who belong to the National Association for Chiropractic Medicine.

Chiropractic has been described as the "greatest tribute to applied public relations that the world has ever known." Despite its shortcomings, millions of people have tried it. Chiropractic's ultimate goal is inclusion in national health insurance. Unless concerned citizens can find ways to organize and protest, your tax dollars will wind up paying for D.D. Palmer's dreams.

# 13

# Homeopathy: Is It Medicine?

## Stephen Barrett, M.D.

Homeopathy is based on the medically disputed concept that infinitesimal amounts of substances that can cause symptoms in healthy people can cure sick individuals with similar symptoms. The number of American practitioners is not large, but remedies for self-use—sold through health food stores and other channels—are being vigorously promoted. Their advocates state that they are safe, effective, natural remedies that have no side effects. This chapter summarizes my detailed investigation of the homeopathic marketplace.

## Homeopathy's Roots

Homeopathy dates back to the late 1700s when Samuel Hahnemann (1755–1843), a German physician, began formulating its basic principles. Hahnemann was justifiably distressed about bloodletting, leeching, purging, and other medical procedures of his day that did far more harm than good. He was also critical of medications like calomel (mercurous chloride), which was given in doses that caused mercury poisoning. Instead, he developed his "law of similars"—that the symptoms of disease can be cured by substances that produce similar symptoms in healthy people. The word "homeopathy" is derived from the Greek words *homeo* (similar) and *pathos* (suffering or disease).

Although ideas like this had been espoused by Hippocrates in the fourth century B.C.E., and by Paracelsus, a fifteenth-century physician, Hahnemann was the first to use them in a systematic way. He and his early followers conducted "provings" in which they administered herbs, minerals, and other substances to healthy people, including themselves, and kept detailed records of what they observed. Later these records were compiled into lengthy reference books called *materia medica,* which are used to match a patient's symptoms with a "corresponding" drug.

Hahnemann believed that diseases represent a disturbance in the body's ability to heal itself and that only a small stimulus is needed to begin the healing process. In line with this—and to avoid toxic side effects—he experimented to see how little medication could be given and still cause a healing response. At first he used small doses of accepted medications. But later he used enormous dilutions and concluded that the smaller the dose, the more powerful the effect—a principle he called the "law of infinitesimals."

That, of course, is just the opposite of what pharmacologists have demonstrated. As summarized in the 1977 report of an Australian Parliament committee of inquiry:

> For each [drug] property, there is a clearly defined dose-response relationship in which increasing the dose increases the effect. . . . There is not one example in the whole area of pharmacology in which simple dilution of a drug enhances the response it produces any more than diluting a dye can produce a deeper hue, or adding less sugar can make food sweeter.

## Homeopathy's Remedies

Homeopathic drugs are made from minerals, botanical substances, zoological substances, and several other sources. If the medicinal substance is soluble, one part is diluted with either nine or ninety-nine parts of distilled water and/or alcohol and shaken vigorously; if insoluble, it is finely ground and pulverized in similar proportions with powdered lactose (milk sugar). One part of the diluted medicine is diluted, and the process is repeated until the desired concentration is reached. Dilutions of 1 to 10 are designated by the Roman numeral X ($1X = 1/10, 2X = 1/100, 3X = 1/1,000, 6X = 1/1,000,000$). Similarly, dilutions of 1 to 100 are designated by the Roman numeral C ($1C = 1/100, 2C = 1/10,000, 3C = 1/1,000,000$, and so on). Most remedies today range from 6X to 30X.

According to the laws of chemistry, there is a limit to the dilution that can be made without losing the original substance altogether. This limit, called Avogadro's number ($6.023 \times 10^{23}$), corresponds to homeopathic potencies of 12C or 24X (1 part in $10^{24}$). Hahnemann himself realized there is virtually no chance that even one molecule of original substance would remain after extreme dilutions. But he believed that the vigorous shaking or pulverizing with each step of dilution leaves behind a "spirit-like" essence—"no longer perceptible to the senses"—which cures by reviving the body's "vital force." Hahnemann's theories have never been accepted by scientifically oriented physicians, who charge that homeopathic remedies are placebos (inert substances).

Because homeopathic remedies were actually less dangerous than those of nineteenth-century medical orthodoxy, many medical practitioners began using them. At the turn of the century, homeopathy had some fourteen thousand practitioners and twenty-two schools in the United States alone. But as medical science and medical education advanced, homeopathy declined sharply, particularly in America, where its schools either closed or converted to modern methods. The last pure homeopathic medical school in America closed during the 1920s, but Hahnemann Medical College (Philadelphia) continued to offer homeopathic courses on an elective basis until the late 1940s. A few graduates from other modern medical and osteopathic schools later became homeopaths by taking courses here or abroad or by training with a practicing homeopath.

Homeopathic remedies were given legal status by the 1938 Federal Food, Drug, and Cosmetic Act, which was shepherded through Congress by Senator Royal Copeland (D-NY), a prominent homeopathic physician. One provision of this law recognized as drugs all substances included in the *Homeopathic Pharmacopeia of the United States.*

The basis for inclusion in the *Pharmacopeia* is not modern scientific testing, but homeopathic "provings" conducted as long as 150 years ago. The current (ninth) edition describes how more than a thousand substances are prepared for homeopathic use. It does not identify the symptoms or diseases for which homeopathic products should be used; that is determined by the practitioner. A 1982 supplement to the eighth edition states:

> Homeopathic drugs are safe, effective, and compatible with all types of medical, surgical, psychological, physical, and nutritional therapy. Since sensitivity reaction seldom occurs, Homeotherapeutics is the safest method of treating infants, children, elderly patients, and individuals who have an allergic diathesis or history of previous drug reactions, whether iatrogenic or from poisoning.

## Today's Marketplace

The 1993 directory of the National Center for Homeopathy, in Alexandria, Virginia, lists about three hundred licensed practitioners, about half of them physicians and the rest mostly naturopaths, chiropractors, acupuncturists, veterinarians, dentists, nurses, or physician's assistants. But Jay P. Borneman, whose family has been marketing homeopathic remedies since 1910, believes that several hundred more consider themselves homeopaths and that many conventional physicians utilize one or a few homeopathic remedies for specific conditions. Larger numbers of homeopaths practice in England, France, India, Germany, parts of the former Soviet Union, and several other countries where homeopathy is more popular.

Laypersons are also involved in practicing homeopathy. Some operate offices, which may not be legal. A few nonaccredited schools have offered correspondence courses leading to certificates or "degrees" in homeopathy. Consumers interested in homeopathic self-treatment can obtain guidance through lay study groups, books, and courses sponsored by the National Center for Homeopathy. Membership in the center, open to anyone, costs $35 per year and includes a subscription to its monthly newsletter *Homeopathy Today*. The center now has about 8,000 members. A similar organization, the International Foundation for Homeopathy, is located in Seattle, Washington.

Most homeopathic practitioners still rely on *materia medica* in choosing among the thousands of remedies available. "Classical" homeopaths—who follow Hahnemann's methods closely—take an elaborate history to fit the remedy to the individual. The history typically includes standard medical questions plus many more about such things as emotions, moods, food preferences, and reactions to the weather. The remedy for symptoms on one side of the body may differ from that for identical symptoms on the other side of the body. Classical homeopaths prescribe one substance at a time, while nonclassical homeopaths may prescribe several. Several computer programs are available to help practitioners select their remedies.

Homeopathic remedies are available from practitioners, health-food stores, and drugstores, as well as from manufacturers who sell directly to the public. Products are also sold person-to-person through multilevel marketing companies. Several companies sell home remedy kits. The size of the homeopathic marketplace is unknown because the largest manufacturers keep their sales figures private. However, *Health Foods Business* has estimated that 1992 sales through health-food stores totaled about $160 million.

FDA officials have noted that homeopathic remedies used to be marketed on a small scale by a few long-established companies, mainly to serve the needs of licensed practitioners. The products bore little or no labeling for consumers because they were intended for use by homeopathic physicians who would make a diagnosis and either compound a prescription, dispense the product, or write a prescription to be filled at a homeopathic pharmacy. During the past fifteen years, however, the homeopathic marketplace has changed drastically. New firms have entered the field and sold all sorts of products through health-food stores and directly to consumers. In 1986, Jay Borneman readily admitted to me:

> There is a lot of insanity operating under the name of homeopathy in today's marketplace. Companies not committed to homeopathy's principles have been marketing products that are unproven, untested, not included in the *Homeopathic Pharmacopeia,* and combination products that have no rational or legal basis. Some are simply quack products called homeopathic for marketing purposes.

Perhaps the most blatant promotion was that of Biological Homeopathic Industries, Albuquerque, New Mexico, which, in 1983, sent a 123-page catalog to almost two hundred thousand physicians nationwide. Among its products were *BHI Anticancer Stimulating, BHI Antivirus, BHI Stroke*, and fifty other types of tablets claimed to be effective against serious diseases. In 1984, the FDA forced the company to stop distributing several of the products and to tone down its claims for the rest.

In 1985, agents of the FDA and Pennsylvania Health Department seized some $125,000 worth of drugs sold person-to-person by Probiotic, Inc., of Reading, and Homerica, Inc., a subsidiary. The products were called *Skin Relief, Human Power Recharger,* and *Pain Control,* but their labels did not state what they were for, what was in them, or how to use them.

In 1988, the FDA took action against companies marketing "diet patches" with false claims that they could suppress appetite. The largest such company, Meditrend International, of San Diego, instructed users to place one or two drops of a "homeopathic appetite control solution" on a patch and wear it all day affixed to an "acupuncture point" on the wrist to "bioelectrically" suppress the appetite control center of the brain.

During the past few years, at least ten other companies have offered dubious homeopathic products for over-the-counter sale. Some examples are: *Arthritis Formula, Bleeding, Kidney Disorders, Flu, Herpes, Exhaustion, Whooping Cough, Gonorrhea, Heart Tonic, Gall-Stones, Prostate Pain, Candida Yeast Infection, Cardio Forte, Thyro Forte,* and *Worms.*

Natra-Bio's fanciful products have included *Bedwetting, Chest Cold, Hemorrhoids, Nervousness, Smoking Withdrawal Tablets,* and *Detoxification* ("for the relief of constipation, lack of energy, and headaches due to overindulgence in food and alcohol"). The company's *Homeopathic Reference Manual* for retailers states:

Unlike any other form of medicine, the patient can confidently listen to their own body and determine for themselves what they need to do. In homeopathy, there is no harm in taking the wrong medicine or too much medicine.

In the United States, homeopathy's most prolific publicist is probably Dana Ullman, M.P.H., president of the Foundation for Homeopathic Education and Research. In a magazine article, Ullman reported that homeopathic practitioners are treating AIDS patients and believe that their methods are effective against immunosuppression in patients whose disease is in its early stages. But he noted that "no carefully controlled research has yet definitely shown the efficacy of homeopathy" for AIDS patients. At a recent meeting, Ullman informed me that his foundation, despite its name, does not fund research because he does not have sufficient time for fundraising.

In 1992, Nature's Way, of Springville, Utah, began marketing a line of homeopathic remedies formulated by Ullman. The products include: *Insomnia, Sinusitis,* and *Migraine Headache* for families; *Vaginitis* and *Menopause* for women; and *Earache* for children. The company has promised an "aggressive marketing strategy"—with ads in healthcare, women's and parenting magazines—intended to "make homeopathy a household word." Its ads claim that "homeopathic medicine offers a significant advantage over its orthodox counterparts."

## Homeopathy's Legal Status

In most states, homeopathy can be practiced by any physician or other practitioner whose license includes the ability to prescribe drugs. Three states—Arizona, Nevada, and Connecticut—have separate homeopathic licensing boards. The Nevada situation is notable because some of its practitioners acquired their homeopathic license after another state had revoked their medical license for cancer quackery.

Arizona's licensing boards are subject to "sunset" review, which means they will be abolished unless reauthorized by the Arizona legislature. In 1985, as the expiration date for the homeopathy board drew near, the state's homeopaths joined forces with health-food stores to lobby vigorously. To counter the idea that a board might not be needed because there were only a handful of homeopaths in the state, the American Institute of Homeopathy (a group of about one hundred classical homeopathic physicians) urged its members to apply for licensure in Arizona "to show that there are doctors interested in practicing homeopathy today." According to the National Health

Federation, a health-food industry group that helped with the campaign, close to two thousand supporters attended hearings and state legislators got hundreds of handwritten letters supporting homeopathic licensing. The reauthorization bill passed unanimously.

In January 1986, the North Carolina Board of Medical Examiners revoked the license of George A. Guess, M.D., the state's only licensed homeopathic physician, after concluding that he was "failing to conform to the standards of acceptable and prevailing medical practice." Dr. Guess is a 1973 graduate of the Medical College of Virginia and was board-certified in family practice from 1976 through 1983. But in 1978 he began practicing homeopathy. During hearings held by the board, another family practitioner testified that although Guess was intelligent and well trained in scientific medicine, "homeopathy is not medicine."

Guess appealed and was successful in lower court rulings; but in 1990 the North Carolina Supreme Court upheld the board. Although no one at the board's hearing had testified that Guess's homeopathic treatment had ever harmed a patient, the Supreme Court reasoned that a general risk of endangering the public is inherent in any practice that fails to conform to "acceptable and prevailing" medical standards. Guess then appealed through the federal courts, and a group of his patients joined in a class-action suit supported (free-of-charge) by the North Carolina chapter of the American Civil Liberties Union. In 1992, after the appeals had failed, Guess relocated his practice to Virginia.

Most pharmacy school educators seem to share the North Carolina board's feelings about homeopathy. In 1986, I sent a questionnaire to the deans of all seventy-two U.S. pharmacy schools. Faculty members from forty-nine schools responded. Most said their school either didn't mention homeopathy at all or considered it of historical interest only. Hahnemann's "law of similars" did not find a single supporter, and all but one respondent said his "law of infinitesimals" was wrong also. Almost all said that homeopathic remedies were neither potent nor effective, except possibly as placebos for mild, self-limited ailments. About half felt that homeopathic remedies should be completely removed from the marketplace.

Public protection regarding drugs is based on a framework of federal laws and regulations which require that drugs be safe, effective, and properly labeled. However, the FDA has not demanded that homeopathic remedies be proven *effective* in order to remain on the market. Its current guidelines, issued in 1988, state:

> Homeopathic drugs cannot be offered without prescription for such serious conditions as cancer, AIDS, or any other requiring diagnosis and treatment by a licensed practitioner. Nonprescription homeopathics

may be sold only for self-limiting conditions recognizable by consumers. . . . [Their] labeling must adequately instruct consumers in the product's safe use.

Of course, if products don't work, there is no such thing as safe use.

The health-food industry is well aware of the unique regulatory status of homeopathic remedies. (While it is illegal to make unproven therapeutic claims for dietary supplements, the FDA tolerates most such claims for nonprescription homeopathic remedies.) A recent article in a trade publication said that "there is more freedom in selling homeopathy than most other categories." Another article even suggested that "when a customer comes into your store complaining of an earache, fever, flu, sore throat, diarrhea, or some other common health problem . . . one word that should immediately come out of your mouth is 'homeopathy.'" A third article said that, because of an FDA crackdown on several nutritional supplements, "more and more companies were turning to herbs and homeopathy to regain sales." Yet another article stated: "Homeopathy is natural medicine's favorite son in the 1990s. Suddenly the category is appearing everywhere—in newspapers, on radio talk shows, on special television programs. . . . For natural products retailers, it can be a dream come true." In the latter article, a marketing manager for a homeopathic manufacturer stated: "Retailers can say exactly what's on the package—if it's to alleviate sinusitis or influenza, they can say that too. It doesn't matter if they are selling directly to an FDA agent."

### Homeopathic Research

Since many homeopathic remedies contain no detectable amount of active ingredient, it is impossible to test whether they contain what their label says. They have been presumed safe, but unlike most potent drugs, they have not been proven effective against disease by double-blind testing.

Probably the best review of homeopathic research is the two-part article by A.M. Scofield, Ph.D., a British biochemistry professor. Published in 1984 in the *British Homeopathic Journal*, the article concludes:

Despite a great deal of experimental and clinical work there is only a little scientific evidence to suggest that homeopathy is effective. This is because of bad design, execution, reporting or failure to repeat promising experimental work and not necessarily because of the inefficacy of the system which has yet to be properly tested on a large enough scale. . . . It is hardly surprising in view of the quality of much of the experimental work as well as its philosophical framework, that this system of medicine is not accepted by the medical and scientific community at large.

In 1986, the British journal *Lancet* published a report that fifty-six hay fever patients who were given a homeopathic preparation of mixed grass pollens had fewer symptoms than a comparable group of fifty-two patients who received a placebo. In 1989, *Lancet* reported another study in which a homeopathic remedy showed modest benefit for flu-like symptoms. Future studies should include an independent laboratory analysis to ensure that the homeopathic products have not been adulterated with therapeutic amounts of drugs known to be effective.

In 1990, an article in *Review of Epidemiology* analyzed forty randomized trials that had compared homeopathic treatment with standard treatment, a placebo, or no treatment. The authors concluded that all but three of the trials had major flaws in their design and that only one of those three had reported a positive result. The authors concluded that there is no evidence that homeopathic treatment has any more value than a placebo.

Proponents trumpet the few "positive" studies as proof that "homeopathy works." Even if their results can be consistently reproduced (which seems unlikely), the most that the study of a single remedy for a single disease could prove is that the remedy is effective against *that* disease. It would not validate homeopathy's basic theories.

## "Electrodiagnosis"

A few physicians who consider themselves homeopaths use "electrodiagnostic" devices to help select the remedies they prescribe. This approach was developed during the 1950s by a German physician named Reinhold Voll and is sometimes called electroacupuncture according to Voll (EAV). The devices are galvanometers, which measure changes in the skin's electrical resistance. One wire from the device goes to a brass cylinder covered by moist gauze, which the patient holds in one hand. A second wire is connected to a probe that the doctor touches to "acupuncture points" on the patient's other hand or foot. This completes a low-voltage circuit and the device registers the flow of current.

Voll postulated that "electromagnetic energy" originating from body organs could be measured along "acupuncture meridians." When diseased organs were detected, low-voltage currents were applied until "electromagnetic energy balance" was achieved. Later, vitamin injections and homeopathic remedies were added to the treatment regimen.

The leading proponent of "electrodiagnosis" in the United States is F. Fuller Royal, M.D., owner and medical director of The Nevada Clinic in Las Vegas. The facility opened in 1980 as The Nevada Clinic of Preventive Medicine, but in 1983 its name was shortened because insurance companies would not honor claims from a "preventive medicine" clinic. ("With the name change," the clinic newsletter has noted, "more patients' insurance claims are being paid.") During a recent interview on NBC's "Dateline," Dr. Royal was asked, "Is there any disease, malady, illness that cannot be treated by homeopathy?" He replied, "I personally don't think so."

At The Nevada Clinic all patients are diagnosed with a "modern" version of Voll's device called the Interro. Pressing the probe to the patient's skin causes a band to rise from 20 to up to 100 on a scale on its computer screen. The less the electrical resistance, the higher the score. Readings over 60 are said to represent "inflammation," readings of 48 to 60 are "normal," and readings below 48 represent "degeneration," which may signify cancer or atherosclerosis. The device makes a whining noise resembling that of an electrical motor; the higher the number, the louder the noise.

The Interro is programmed so that charts and tables can be placed on the screen to help the doctor select from approximately 1,700 homeopathic remedies. One or more remedies are then placed in a tray attached to the computer to receive an "energy transfer." Other "electrodiagnostic" devices are used to diagnose allergies, determine whether patients should take dietary supplements, or should have their mercury-amalgam fillings removed.

In 1986, at Dr. Royal's invitation, I underwent all of the electrodiagnostic tests except for vitamin testing. After utilizing the Interro, he said I had a number of "electromagnetic blockages" that could be removed by injecting my scars with vitamin $B_{12}$ prepared "electromagnetically" with the device. Royal also said I had "temporomandibular joint stress, probable subclinical allergies, and possible mild early preclinical arthritis." He prescribed five homeopathic remedies for home use and advised having my dentist replace one of my mercury fillings with another material.

During the testing, I noticed that the harder the probe was pressed to my finger or toe, the higher the reading on the Interro screen. Royal readily acknowledged this, but said, "that's why it takes a lot of training to use the equipment properly."

Royal called his approach "bioenergetic medicine" and said it was the wave of the future. He was introduced to it by Floyd Weston, a former insurance executive who had investigated its use in Germany while conducting a worldwide search for "the answer to good health." Royal told me that Weston had investigated the situation in Nevada and reported that influential persons were interested in having another type of tourist industry besides gambling and had promised him that Royal would not be bothered there by medical authorities. The Governor of Nevada subsequently appointed Royal to a homeopathic advisory board, and a homeopathic licensing law was passed which included "noninvasive electrodiagnosis" as part of the definition of homeopathy. Royal became a member of Nevada's homeopathic licensing board and was its president from 1983 to 1985.

Several other practitioners in Nevada and elsewhere are using the Interro or an earlier version such as the Dermatron or the Accupath 1000. When I asked an FDA official whether they were legal under federal law, she replied that the agency considered them a "significant risk," had prosecuted one manufacturer, and had tried to block importation by other manufacturers. "But once a device is in the hands of a medical practitioner," the official said, "we are dependent, to a large extent, on State Medical Boards to initiate legal actions." Under Nevada law, of course, the devices are legal. Insurance companies that have balked at paying for treatment by Nevada homeopaths have even been threatened with sanctions by the state's insurance commissioner!

In 1988, after an extensive investigation, the *Las Vegas Review-Journal* urged the Nevada legislature to transfer homeopathic regulation to the Nevada Board of Medical Examiners. The newspaper reported that at least ten of the thirty-two people licensed by the board had been in hot water with medical boards in other states for questionable or unlawful practices—and that four licenses had been obtained by submitting "phony credentials from imaginary schools or licensing boards."

Harvey Bigelson, M.D., a former president of Arizona's homeopathic board, may also be in hot water. In December 1992, a federal grand jury accused him of one count of conspiracy to defraud the United States; sixty-three counts of false, fictitious, or fraudulent claims; forty-four counts of mail fraud; one count of conspiracy to commit an offense against the United States; and eight counts of obstruction of proceedings before departments, agencies and committees. The indictment states that he attempted to collect about $8,000 for colonic therapy, massage therapy, and chiropractic services (including acupuncture)—which he knew were not covered under Medicare—by submitting claim forms on which they were represented by procedure code numbers for services covered under "physical medicine." The indictment also charges that Bigelson and two associates attempted to evade prosecution by changing data in the computer account histories of several patients and by submitting altered and falsified progress notes in response to a grand jury subpoena.

## Overview

During my lengthy investigation of homeopathy, I met many of its leaders and was impressed with their warmth and sincerity. But the key question is whether homeopathy is effective. In January 1987, *Consumer Reports* concluded:

> Unless the laws of chemistry have gone awry, most homeopathic remedies are too diluted to have any physiological effect. . . . CU's medical consultants believe that any system of medicine embracing the use of such remedies involves a potential danger to patients whether the prescribers are M.D.'s, other licensed practitioners, or outright quacks. Ineffective drugs are dangerous drugs when used to treat serious or life-threatening disease. Moreover, even though homeopathic drugs are essentially nontoxic, self-medication can still be hazardous. Using them for a serious illness or undiagnosed pain instead of obtaining proper medical attention could prove harmful or even fatal.

Homeopathic leaders insist that their remedies are effective and that studies do support this viewpoint. They also suggest that homeopathy's popularity and long survival are evidence that it works. But the only way for homeopathy to gain acceptance by the scientific community would be to demonstrate positive results through repeated experiments designed with the help of critics and carried out with strict safeguards against experimenter bias and fraud.

If the FDA required homeopathic remedies to be proven effective in order to remain on the market—the standard it applies to other remedies—homeopathy would face extinction in the United States. But no indication exists that the agency is considering this. FDA officials regard homeopathy as relatively benign and believe that other problems should get enforcement priority. If the FDA attacks homeopathy too vigorously, its proponents might even persuade Congress to rescue them. Regardless of this risk, the FDA should not permit worthless products to be marketed with claims that they are effective.

# 14

# Genuine Fakes

**Thomas H. Jukes, Ph.D.**
**Stephen Barrett, M.D.**

Foods labeled "organic" or "organically grown" usually cost more than "regular" or "conventionally grown" foods. Sometimes they cost twice as much—or more. Are they worth their extra cost? Are they any different from other foods?

Let's begin our inquiry by asking what the "organic" label means. The most representative definition still is the one given at a public hearing in 1972 by the late Robert Rodale, one of the nation's most active promoters of "organic agriculture." He stated:

> Organically grown food is food grown without pesticides; grown without artificial fertilizers; grown in soil whose humus content is increased by the additions of organic matter; grown in soil whose mineral content is increased with applications of natural mineral fertilizers; and has not been treated with preservatives, hormones, antibiotics, etc.

Let's look closely at the components of this definition to see whether they make sense.

### "Without Pesticides"

Organic promoters imply that the use of pesticides is bad and dangerous, and that foods grown under "organic" conditions will contain no pesticides. Although Rodale's definition did not actually state this, many retailers claim that organically grown foods are free of pesticides. The truth is they are not.

Over the years, laboratories have found little difference in the level of pesticide residues between foods that are labeled "organic" and those that are not.

Thus, if you buy "organic" foods with the hope of avoiding all pesticides, you are not likely to be successful. But don't let this trouble you. The pesticide content of today's food poses no threat to our health. Indeed, some amounts are so small that they would not even be detectable were it not for the exquisite sensitivity of modern equipment that can measure some substances in parts per *trillion.* (A part per trillion is the equivalent of a single drop of water for 1,000 swimming pools.) Moreover, pesticides have a greater margin of safety than many other substances found naturally in foods we eat all the time without worry. The residue limits set by the Environmental Protection Agency are often several hundred times lower than the level that causes no effect in test animals.

Under its regulatory monitoring program, the FDA collects samples from individual lots of both domestically grown and imported food and analyzes them for pesticide residues. The FDA likewise does a Total Diet Study (also called a Market Basket Study) to estimate the dietary intakes of pesticide residues for eight age-sex groups from infants to senior citizens.

To obtain the samples, FDA personnel purchase foods from local supermarkets or grocery stores four times a year throughout the United States. Each "market basket" contains 234 individual items judged through nation-wide dietary surveys to represent what Americans eat. The foods are prepared for eating and then analyzed for pesticide residues. These results are combined with food consumption data to estimate the actual amounts of pesticide residues in foods as they are usually eaten. During the past several years, about 1 percent of the samples have contained residues exceeding regulatory limits, and the Total Diet Study has shown that the dietary intake of pesticide residues was only a small fraction of acceptable limits.

### "Without Artificial Fertilizers"

Many organic advocates suggest that "natural" fertilizers are better able to nourish plants and produce more nutritious foods. They also suggest that natural fertilizers contain some ingredient found in nature but lacking in artificial fertilizers. These ideas are good sales gimmicks, but nothing more. From the plant's point of view, it makes no difference where its food comes from. Chemicals are taken up and used by the plant in their inorganic chemical state whether they are fed to the plant in manure, compost, or manufactured fertilizer. All plants care about is whether they have enough food. If they do, they will grow. If not, they won't.

Experiments conducted for many years at the Michigan Agricultural Experimental Station, the U.S. Plant, Soil and Nutrition Laboratory at Cornell University, and the British Experimental Farm all indicate that there is no difference in major nutrient content whether foods are grown on soils fed with animal or synthetic plant foods. The amount of vitamin C in apples, for example, cannot be made equal to that in oranges by the addition of any amount of fertilizer. This is because nutritional content (other than minerals) is controlled by hereditary factors (genes). Fertilizers can, however, influence the mineral composition of plants. The iodine content, for example, may vary with the iodine content of the soil, and the same may be true of other elements such as zinc, cobalt, and selenium. These variations are rarely significant in the diet, except that toxic levels of selenium occur naturally in some soils. (Selenium is not added to "chemical" fertilizers.)

The fact that mineral content of soil can affect mineral content of plants encourages the organic food industry to suggest that its recommended fertilizers are the best way to supply minerals. "After all," they say, "we return to nature what belongs to nature. Animals that eat plants nourished by soil return the elements to the soil via their manure. Nothing is lost." This reasoning is faulty. If a soil is deficient in a nutrient, use of manure from animals fed from that soil guarantees that the nutrient will remain missing. Moreover, some nutrients entering animals will not return to the soil because they meet other fates, such as becoming part of the human food supply. The best way to ensure proper plant growth is to determine by analysis what the soil needs and to add the needed chemicals.

**"Additions of Organic Matter"**

The implication here is that organic matter alone conditions soil best for plants. It has long been standard agricultural practice to plow crop residues and "green-manuring crops" back into the soil. This makes the soil easier to work and can improve the seedbed for the coming crop. This practice works well together with the use of fertilizers. Composts and animal manures can also help the physical characteristics of the soil; in fact, there are times when the so-called mulching process is necessary and highly advantageous. Scientific farmers can easily determine and supply whatever their soil needs. Incidentally, it is possible to grow vigorous, healthy plants with no soil at all, simply by adding chemical nutrients to water. This method is called hydroponics.

Low availability and high distribution costs make it clear that the world cannot rely on animal-produced fertilizers to grow its food. It takes twenty pounds of manure to supply the same amount of nutrients as one pound of synthetic fertilizer. More often than not, the wastes from farm animals accumulate at great distances from food-growing areas. It is expensive to collect and haul manures great distances and then spread them on fields. Manure has another disadvantage: it can contaminate plants with Salmonella germs that cause dysentery, a serious diarrheal illness. Manure can also spread intestinal parasites.

### "Not Treated with Preservatives, Hormones, Antibiotics"

Here the organic and natural food promoters suggest that all chemicals associated with food production are bad. But they don't tell you that without the use of additives it would be impossible to feed large populations. They also don't mention that preservatives have been used for centuries to prevent foods from spoiling. The salting of meat and the pickling of cucumbers are familiar examples. Hormones are present naturally in all animals and plants. Antibiotics are valuable in controlling diseases of farm animals—some of which are dangerous to humans. Some antibiotics fed to farm animals travel through their intestines without getting into their meat. Those that do enter the meat are destroyed by cooking.

Most additives are used—in tiny quantities—to enhance food colors and flavors. Additives also perform vital functions in food preservation and enrichment. The World Health Organization estimates that almost a quarter of the food produced is lost each year before it gets into consumer hands as a result of infestation by insects and rodents and because of spoilage. Food additives slow down deterioration considerably and, as a result, make the food supply more plentiful.

Permitted preservatives prevent spoilage by bacteria, molds, fungi, and yeast. They also extend shelf life and protect natural food color or flavor. Antioxidants delay or prevent rancidity or enzymatic browning. Calcium propionate, which is used to prevent bread from getting moldy, is normally produced, as well as used, in the human body. Leaving it out of bread will do the consumer no good whatsoever; it will, however, result in a lot of moldy bread being thrown out in the garbage. And, as indicated in Chapter 2, people who eat a Swiss cheese sandwich consume enough calcium propionate from one ounce of natural cheese to preserve two loaves of bread.

These facts should make it clear that sweeping general attacks on food additives make no sense at all. The only proper way to evaluate food additives is to do so individually. A few additives—most notably sulfites—can cause adverse effects in sensitive individuals. But scientific evaluations, including data from FDA market basket studies, indicate that the benefits of using additives far outweigh the risks.

## "Etc."

The term "etc." is not defined. Presumably, this allows the definition to be expanded at will to keep pace with the imagination of "organic" producers. For example it has been applied to the eggs of chickens allowed to roam free with the roosters and to fish "caught in the pollution-free, mineral-rich Atlantic Ocean."

In 1971, shortly before his death, organic guru J.I. Rodale (Robert Rodale's father) told a *New York Times Magazine* reporter that "organically grown food" contains "things you don't even know exist" and that "a little gleam of something" is missing from chemical fertilizers. When asked what this "gleam" might be, he replied:

> Who knows? It may be a form of matter that we don't know yet. Maybe something that's excreted by enzymes, or bacteria. Maybe the bacteria who live off these things are healthier and can work like they used to work in the old days, and they've lost this ability through the artificialization of the soil and whatnot.

In 1980, a team of scientists appointed by the U.S. Department of Agriculture (USDA) to study "organic farming" concluded that there was no universally accepted definition of the term. Their report stated:

> The organic movement represents a spectrum of practices, attitudes, and philosophies. On the one hand are those organic practitioners who would not use chemical fertilizers or pesticides under any circumstances. These producers hold rigidly to their purist philosophy. At the other end of the spectrum, organic farmers espouse a more flexible approach. While striving to avoid the use of chemical fertilizers and pesticides, these practitioners do not rule them out entirely. Instead, when absolutely necessary, some fertilizers and also herbicides are very selectively and sparingly used as a second line of defense. Nevertheless, these farmers, too, consider themselves to be organic farmers. Failure to recognize that the organic farming movement is distributed over a spectrum can often lead to serious misconceptions.

It certainly can! Many members of the "industry" consider themselves "organic" whether they actually follow the definition or merely do the best they can. Undaunted by these realities, the USDA Study Team recommended that certification programs be established "to assure that organically produced foods are properly labeled" and that local USDA representatives should help organic producer associations develop criteria for certification standards!

## Taste

Three factors affect the taste of fruits and vegetables: their genetic makeup, how ripe they are when harvested, and how fresh they are when eaten. "Organic" advocates maintain that their foods taste better, arguing that since their produce comes from small farms, it is more likely to be sold locally in fresh condition. They also claim that supermarket produce is bred for shipping and preservation qualities rather than for flavor.

Many years ago, these claims were scientifically tested by research at the University of Florida. In this experiment, twenty men and women met several times a week for three months to compare twenty-five "health foods" with their supermarket cousins. Color, flavor, texture, odor, and general acceptance were rated. None of the "health foods" was found to be superior on the basis of general acceptance. However, many of the regular foods were rated better for color, flavor, texture, and general acceptance. Regular foods that were scored higher than health foods by the panel included dried apples, apple juice, applesauce, cashews, cereal, Swiss cheese, coconut, corn chips, ice cream, mayonnaise with tomato, peanut butter, sesame chips, and tomato juice. The only health-food qualities that were scored higher than those of regular foods were the odors of apple butter and pizza and the color of ketchup. A recent study, performed in Israel, obtained 460 assessments of nine different fruits and vegetables and found no significant difference in taste quality between "organic" and conventionally grown samples.

"Organic chickens" were said by J.I. Rodale to yield meat with a "hearty flavor" because they are "allowed to scratch in the ground and eat the worms, bugs, and other critters." They eat chicken droppings, too—and these help "flavor" the meat.

## Cost

Many studies have shown that foods labeled "organic" cost more than conventionally grown foods. The weekly *Organic Wholesale Market Report* indicates that for most fruits and vegetables, retailers pay 50 to 100 percent more for "organically grown" products than for conventionally grown products.

Consumer Alert, a nonprofit consumer educational group based in California, has compared the cost of an average weekly basket of organic groceries with that of traditional items in six major U.S. cities. In 1989, it reported that the organic basket averaged $96.97, while the regular basket averaged $77.90—a 24 percent difference that would amount to $1,000 per year for a family of four. The group also reported that less variety was available among "organically grown" foods.

### The Debate over "Consumer Protection"

The lure of extra profits tempts many enterprising merchants to label regular foods "organic." Calling this practice deceptive, promoters of "real" organic food want government agencies to "protect" their customers from "fake" organic food. Over the years, various growers' associations have developed programs whereby farmers who follow their guidelines can identify their products as "certified." Ignoring the fact that "real" organic food is identical or inferior to regular food, they suggest that their customers should be able to get "what they think they are paying for"—that is, foods produced by "genuine" organic methods.

### The FTC's Near-Debacle

In 1974, the Federal Trade Commission (FTC) began a rulemaking proceeding concerned with food advertising claims. The original FTC staff proposal included a ban on the terms "organic," "organically grown," and "naturally grown." The agency noted that these terms were not clearly defined and were also used interchangeably by both sellers and buyers of these products.

FTC Commissioner William Dixon presided over the agency's inquiry. In 1978, after several periods of public comment and fifty days of testimony by interested parties, he concluded that foods labeled "organic" or "natural" were neither safer nor more nutritious than their ordinary counterparts. Indeed, Dixon said, some "natural" foods may be less safe or nutritious than foods that have been fortified or highly processed.

Although Dixon reached the correct scientific conclusions, he thought that public confusion pointed to a need for more regulation rather than a ban. He stated that the term "health food" ought to be banned as inherently misleading, but the terms "organic" and "natural" should be officially defined by the FTC. During the proceedings, one proponent had presented a 600-word "definition" of "natural" foods. Although the definition was filled with inconsistencies, Dixon regarded it as "among the most constructive received" and said it could well "form the basis for a final solution."

The FTC staff then issued its recommendations for a final rule. No food could be advertised as a "health food," but the term "health food store" would still be permitted. "Organic" and "natural" would be redefined by the FTC. The organic definition would be similar to that propounded by Robert Rodale, and "natural" would mean "minimal processing." But in 1980, the full commission decided not to prohibit health food claims or adopt standards for organic foods. It also instructed the staff to consider further the standards for "natural" foods. In 1982, the commission voted to terminate the entire rulemaking procedure in favor of a case-by-case approach. One commissioner who dissented warned that this would "invite a free-for-all for deceptive health claims for food."

### "Alternative Agriculture"

During the 1980s, "organic food" advocates became associated with another loosely defined philosophy called "alternative" agriculture. This, according to a 1989 National Academy of Sciences report, is:

> a spectrum of farming systems, ranging from organic systems that attempt to use no purchased synthetic chemical inputs to those involving the prudent use of pesticides or antibiotics to control specific pests or diseases. Alternative farming encompasses, but is not limited to, farming systems known as biological, low-input, organic, regenerative, or sustainable. It includes a range of practices such as integrated pest management; low-density animal production systems; crop rotations designed to reduce pest damage, improve crop health, decrease soil erosion, and, in the case of legumes, fix nitrogen in the soil; and tillage and planting practices that reduce soil erosion and help control weeds.

Of course, many of these practices are a legitimate part of scientific agriculture. But the "organic food" industry developed political allies who, while they did not necessarily believe in the organic mythology, wanted to increase government support for research. (These allies included agricultural and business interests, biotechnology companies, and various environmental and consumer groups which are concerned that pesticides may have adverse effects on human health and the environment.) In 1990, their combined lobbying efforts resulted in a federal law calling for the establishment of standards for "organically produced" foods. Although the standards have not yet been proposed, a committee has been appointed to draft them.

## Overview

Two hundred years ago, the average family in the Western world had to spend most of its time grubbing for a meager living from the soil. The lack of fertilizer, the presence of pests that demolished crops, and the absence of knowledge about plant breeding, all combined to keep most people hungry. Then chemists discovered that plants were actually nourished by inorganic chemicals, including phosphate, potash, nitrate, and ammonia. These could come either from the breakdown of manure by soil bacteria, or from rock phosphate, inorganic potash, nitrates, and ammonia salts. The agricultural revolution thus began.

Little more than a century ago, farmers were helpless against the fungus blight that turned their potatoes into a black slime. With no pesticides available to control the blight, one million people had starved to death during the Irish potato famine of 1846. But as agricultural knowledge increased by leaps and bounds, farming became increasingly more scientific. Plant and animal breeding gave us fine new strains of grains, vegetables, fruits, poultry, pigs, and cattle. More efficient fertilizers and a wide variety of pesticides were developed. Thanks to these advances, once rare delicacies became commonplace as farmers were able to feed larger and larger urban populations.

The new chemical methods required careful regulation to see that farmers used them properly. Pure food laws were passed to make sure that only insignificant traces of unwanted pesticide residues were present in foods. These laws appear to be working well: there has not been one documented case of illness in the United States that can be attributed to a scientific agricultural procedure. By contrast, in countries where "organic" fertilizers (such as human waste) are used, food poisoning from disease organisms is quite common.

As scientific agriculture developed, so did methods of processing, preserving, and distributing foods. Yet even in the face of such fantastic scientific progress, the voices of quackery have decried our food supply as neither safe nor nutritious. They either ignore or fail to understand scientific thought. At the same time, they profit greatly by frightening the public into buying their ideas, their publications, and their overpriced or unnecessary "health" products.

Many Americans, worried about pollution and food safety, are responding to the quacks. Although "organic" foods can neither be defined meaningfully nor told apart from "regular" foods, some people are willing to pay more for them. But the ultimate irony is that the "organic food" industry, which itself preys on confusion and false hopes, has gained passage of a federal law that will endorse its products. Rather than protecting consumers, this will encourage the purchase of "genuine" fakes—whose only "extra" is extra cost.

# 15

# The Overselling of Herbs

## Varro E. Tyler, Ph.D., Sc.D.

Rational herbalism encompasses scientific testing, honest reporting of the results, and safe use of effective herbs by informed practitioners and the public. It also includes the production and ethical marketing of herbal products. Rational herbalism, which brings honor to the wonder-filled world of plants, does exist as part of the science of pharmacognosy. However, there is a dark side to herbalism which I call *paraherbalism.*

Rational herbalism and paraherbalism can be compared to Dr. Jekyll and his evil self, Mr. Hyde. As with these famous fictional characters, there is ever-present danger that the good of herbalism will be destroyed by the evils of paraherbalism. That would be tragic because herbalism based on scientific research could play a useful role in health-care.

### Paraherbalism Is a Pseudoscience

Pseudoscientists typically fail to use rigorous experimental methods, lack a coherent conceptual framework, and claim positive results not corroborated by impartial observers. The fact that paraherbalists fail to develop or accept accurate information about their recommended remedies and simply reassert untested dogma clearly identifies their field as pseudoscientific. These problems are rampant in herbal literature, both old and new.

• The leading seventeenth-century astrologer and apothecary, Nicholas Culpeper, said, in reference to the common weed burdock, "the root beaten with a little salt, and laid on the place, suddenly easeth the pain thereof, and helpeth those that are bit by a mad dog." Maud Grieve repeated this advice without a word of caution in her 1971 book, *A Modern Herbal*. In fact, there is no scientific evidence that burdock has any useful therapeutic activity against rabies—or any other disease.

• Homeopath Edward Bach, who developed the Bach Flower Remedies more than fifty years ago, believed that sun-warmed dew absorbs vital healing powers from plants. Thus, if flowers are placed in pure spring water in a glass bowl in full sunlight, healing energy is transmitted to the water, which can be used in tiny doses to treat patients. Bach claimed that while his remedies did not cure disease, they increased the condition of health of the user. He offered no scientific explanation for this, preferring to keep his remedies "free from science, free from theories." Recent promoters have postulated that Bach's remedies work through a "nonphysical" energy field emanating from the plants.

• Dorothy Hall, a third-generation Australian herbalist, claims that herbs can be matched to personality traits as well as to health problems. Her book *Creating Your Herbal Profile* (1991) contains "person-pictures" for about fifty herbs. It suggests, for example, that the "mugwort" person is often "highly intelligent with great acuity of the senses," while the "celery" person is "busy and conscientious" and "finds it unpleasant to be idle."

• Since the early 1960s, sassafras oil and safrole, which is obtained from it, have been recognized as carcinogens in rats and mice. Their use as flavors or food additives is now forbidden by the FDA under the Delaney Clause of the amended Food, Drug, and Cosmetic Act. Nevertheless, sassafras is still considered an unexcelled home remedy by paraherbalists who never mention its toxicity or who, at best, discount this risk substantially.

• In 1974, a dubious journal article concluded that yucca is useful in the general management of the various forms of arthritis. Although the Arthritis Foundation dismissed the study's design as invalid, it is still cited by paraherbalists as evidence that yucca is effective. In 1979, for example, John Heinerman wrote in *Science of Herbal Medicine*: "Yucca root contains special steroid saponins which have been successfully tested under clinical conditions to determine its effectiveness in treating acute forms of arthritis."

• One of the most common herbs marketed in the United States is comfrey, some species of which contain pyrrolizidine alkaloids that are toxic to the liver. Paraherbalists praise its supposed virtues and usually fail to mention the scientific evidence of its harmful nature.

• No scientific evidence supports the use of alfalfa for arthritis, spirulina for weight loss, Mormon tea for venereal disease, damiana for sexual stimulation, eyebright for loss of vision, or borage for melancholy. Yet paraherbalists, either ignoring contrary evidence or parroting the claims of Culpeper and others, advocate such use.

**False Tenets**

Paraherbalism is characterized by at least ten false tenets. While not every paraherbalist embraces them all, enough do to warrant the conclusion that all ten are characteristic of the field.

• *Tenet #1: A conspiracy by the medical establishment discourages the use of herbs.* One forceful statement of this tenet is Heinerman's assertion: "A large percentage of this suspicion of herbs and natural healing methods is due to the unmitigated prejudice and slanderous opposition posed by the regular medical community at large. Quite often they are joined in this harmful conspiracy by the pharmaceutical industry." Others have suggested that herbalists (and other health food industry "pioneers") are automatically branded as quacks and charlatans by the "FDA-AMA combine."

I have met very few physicians who knew enough about herbs to voice any opposition. Indeed, very few doctors give herbal medicine any thought at all. Physicians are taught nothing about the subject in medical school. If they become curious and purchase a popular book on the subject, reading that yucca roots are "mashed and boiled to make a tea for treating diabetes" might inspire them to shelve the volume among others devoted to superstition and witchcraft. They might even throw the book away, but they would not stop using insulin, which they know has been proven effective.

Inquisitive physicians might even look up the credentials of some of those whose writings on herbal remedies are widely distributed. If so, they might find that Sybil Leek is described in *Who's Who in America* as an astrologer who wrote several books on witchcraft, including *Diary of a Witch*. They might also learn that Richard Passwater and Earl Mindell obtained their "Ph.D." degrees from nonaccredited correspondence schools (see Chapter 27). Such credentials are not likely to inspire scientifically trained physicians to have much confidence in the paraherbal advocates.

In the pharmaceutical industry, another attitude prevails. Here it is recognized that plants have yielded effective drugs such as opium, digitalis, ergot, and belladonna.. But there is insufficient profit potential to stimulate much research into new plant drugs. With the cost of developing a new chemical entity into a marketable drug now over $200 million, pharmaceutical manufacturers focus on products where patent protection can be achieved rather than on widely used plant remedies that probably cannot become patentable drugs. Again, there is no conspiracy involved, but simply a lack of expected profit.

• *Tenet #2: Herbs cannot harm, only cure.* It is ancient dogma—repeated in modern paraherbals—that drugs of vegetable origin are automatically good, while those derived from minerals or petroleum are necessarily bad. William

Smith, for example, states in *Wonders in Weeds* : "It cannot be emphasized too highly that herbal medicine is 'safe medicine,' a claim that cannot be applied to orthodox remedies."

This thesis denies the fact that some plant constituents are among the most toxic substances known. Acutely toxic alkaloids, ranging alphabetically from aconitine to zygadenine, are abundant. Other constituents, such as the peptide amatoxins in certain fungi, can also kill. Even so, consumers are probably less likely to suffer from acute strychnine poisoning by eating *Nux vomica* seeds than they are to receive exposure to milder and less obvious toxins through repeated use of such remedies as sassafras or comfrey. Treatises by Culpeper and sixteenth-century herbalist John Gerard are still widely cited, although some of the herbs they recommend contain cancer-causing compounds.

• *Tenet #3: Whole herbs are more effective than their isolated active constituents.* As medical science developed, it became apparent that most herbs were not as effective or as easy to administer in controlled amounts as their purified active constituents and, further, that the action of the latter could be improved, in many cases, by chemical modification or the production of synthetic analogs. Yet many modern paraherbalists maintain that plants are not only the safest way to administer medicine but also the most effective. They claim that apart from their active principles, plants may contain other substances that enhance their therapeutic action by some sort of a synergistic process.

Perhaps the most persistent advocate of this doctrine has been Andrew T. Weil, M.D., who argues: "In the case of drug plants, the whole forms, being complex mixtures and therefore impure, tend to be safer than their unmixed derivatives, freed from diluents and made available in highly refined form." Weil also argues that the lesser concentration of an active constituent present in plant tissue renders such a drug safer to use. Finally, he contends that the various active constituents in a plant work synergistically to produce a total effect greater than the mere sum of the individual component activities.

Weil's first two points can be dismissed simply by pointing out that dosage, which governs a drug's safety and efficacy, is much more readily controlled with purified constituents. Synergism occasionally occurs, but for every case where a desirable action is enhanced, there is one where undesirable actions are produced. For example, cinchona bark contains some twenty-five closely related alkaloids, but the only one recognized as useful in the treatment of malaria is quinine. A person who took powdered cinchona bark would also ingest the alkaloid quinidine, a cardiac depressant, and cinchotannic acid, which would induce constipation.

An even more significant example is comfrey, whose leaves and underground parts are widely recommended by modern herbalists as wound healers. Whatever activity of this sort the plant possesses is due to its content of allantoin, an agent that apparently promotes cell proliferation. However, some species of comfrey also contain carcinogenic pyrrolizidine alkaloids, including echimidine and symphytine. Purified allantoin, free from accompanying carcinogens, would obviously be safer to use.

• *Tenet #4: "Natural" and "organic" herbs are superior to synthetic drugs.* Paraherbalists claim that products made by the metabolic processes of plants or animals possess an innate superiority over identical products synthesized in a chemical laboratory. The falsity of this claim was demonstrated as long ago as 1828 when the German chemist Friedrich Wöhler synthesized urea from inorganic materials. Wöhler's synthetic urea was identical in every respect to the urea biosynthesized and excreted by animals or biosynthesized and accumulated by many species of higher fungi. Thus, such statements as "The pharmaceutical industry needs to stop fooling around with dangerous synthetic chemicals and return, once again, to the more natural substances God has placed upon this earth for our health and benefit" are derived from baseless belief rather than scientific methodology.

The term "organic" is used to describe plants grown without pesticides or synthetic fertilizers. Materials made from such plants are believed to be superior in some way to those produced by conventional agriculture. This belief is based on a complete misunderstanding of plant nutrition and physiology. Plants require inorganic nutrients such as nitrogen, phosphorus, and potassium for normal growth. They obtain these elements from the soil and have no mechanism for distinguishing their original source. If adequate amounts are present, plants grow normally. If they are not present, growth does not occur.

Pesticides are a slightly different matter. Appropriate safety limits have been established, and some pesticides have been banned. It is possible to grow plants without using pesticides, but pests cause damage and yields per acre are much diminished. So one either trusts conventional farmers and the regulatory process or one pays considerably more for food because less is produced.

• *Tenet #5: The "Doctrine of Signatures" is meaningful.* The three most popular aphrodisiacs sold in the Orient owe their alleged properties to the so-called Doctrine of Signatures—the ancient belief that the form and shape of a drug source determine its therapeutic virtue. Thus, rhinoceros horn, deer antlers, and ginseng root with their phallic resemblance—or bifurcated ginseng with attached rootlets, because of its similarity to the human body complete with phallus—are all highly esteemed as agents of virility. In Chinese pharmacies, antlers are typically displayed on velvet mats in glass showcases and sold at prices comparable to that for fine pearls.

Deer antler and rhinoceros horn have never been proven to contain any constituent that stimulates libido or cures impotence; any activity must be attributed to the placebo effect. Ginseng does contain triterpenoid saponins to which various physiological activities have been attributed. However, no substantial evidence that ginseng enhances human sexual experience or potency has been published in the scientific literature.

The Doctrine of Signatures is not unique to the Orient. Herbalist John Gerard reported in 1597 that eyebright juice applied to the eyes "taketh awaie the darknesse and dimnesse of the eies and cleereth the sight." Variations of this advice are duly repeated by most present-day paraherbalists.

Actually, no constituent of eyebright is known to be effective against any eye disease. Medieval herbalists assumed it was effective because the white to bluish corolla of its flower bears a bright yellow spot, making it resemble an eye with its pupil. Believing that this structure renders the plant effective against eye disease makes as much sense as believing that walnuts are good for mental illness because their kernels resemble the brain, or that liverworts are good for jaundice because their leaves resemble the shape of the liver.

• *Tenet #6: Reducing the dose of a medicine increases its therapeutic potency.* This, like the Doctrine of Signatures, is a principle espoused by homeopaths (see Chapter 13). Preparations described in *The Homeopathic Pharmacopoeia of the United States* are recognized as drugs under federal laws, a fact appreciated by paraherbalists. Some of the listed substances, such as cinchona, digitalis, and opium, are effective in appropriate dosage. But homeopathy advocates high dilution for maximal effect. In fact, many homeopathic remedies are so dilute that they are statistically unlikely to contain a single molecule of the original active substance. Homeopathy's supposed safety, "holistic" orientation, and vast materia medica of vegetable drugs appeal to many paraherbalists.

• *Tenet #7: Astrological influences are significant.* In his recent book, *Herbs, Health and Astrology,* Leon Petulengro comments, "Knowing as we do that planets and stars emit their own individual signals or vibrations, how can we disbelieve that ancient lore was right and that herbs and plants, and indeed humans, are ruled by these various vibrations or force fields?"

How, indeed? Just compare drugs with similar physiological effects and the different planets to which they are assigned. For example, broom, digitalis, lily-of-the-valley, and black hellebore all yield drugs that can slow the heartbeat, make it more regular, or otherwise strengthen it. But they look quite different from one another and belong to different plant families. Probably for this reason, Culpeper assigned each to a different "governing" planet, a classification repeated by Sybil Leek.

Culpeper assumed that diseases caused by a certain planet are cured by herbs of the same planet or the "opposite" planet. For example, since diseases of the heart and blood vessels are caused by the sun, they should be cured by herbs dominated by the sun or ruled by Saturn. If this were true, black hellebore would be the only herb in either of the above categories that is effective against heart disease. Actually, it is probably the least effective cardiotonic drug considered by Culpeper and was dropped from the *United States Pharmacopoeia* in 1882. Broom was listed in the official compendia until 1936 (and its active principle until 1950), and lily-of-the-valley root appeared until 1950. Digitalis is still listed, together with its constituent glycosides, but physicians now prescribe synthetic drugs that are more reliable and versatile than digitalis-leaf preparations. Thus, astrological reasoning classified only one out of four correctly and selected the least potent.

• *Tenet #8: Physiological tests in animals are not applicable to human beings.* When it suits their purposes, paraherbalists typically complain that the results of animal experiments should not be applied to herbs. Heinerman has said, for example, that sassafras was removed from the marketplace "because a bunch of 'puny, sickly, all-around crummy rats' just happened to get cancer when this plant was injected into them by their larger, less intelligent relatives."

It is true that great differences exist among various animal species and between animals and humans. However, there is a high probability of significance when diverse species show similar effects. For this reason, new drugs should be evaluated in several animal species, preferably from different orders. Herbs do need to be tested for safety and effectiveness. Animal testing may not be acceptable to paraherbalists, but the only alternative—initial screening of drugs in humans—is even less acceptable to the public.

• *Tenet #9: Anecdotal evidence is highly significant.* A century ago, glowing testimonials were widely used to sell patent medicines. Today, similar endorsements are used for herbal remedies. For example, *Herbal Success Stories,* published in 1980, recounts "actual case histories" of those who "either experienced the problem and cure themselves or helped a family member or friend with the ailment or cure." According to its author, readers can "use this book with assurance that successes related there are true."

Unfortunately, in individual cases, it is difficult or impossible to tell whether a reported cure resulted from the treatment, a placebo effect, or the body's ability to heal itself. It may also be difficult to tell whether an anecdote has been reported accurately or was even fabricated. Anecdotal evidence can provide leads for research, but it is not reliable for establishing therapeutic utility of an herb. That requires preliminary investigations in laboratory animals followed by randomized, double-blind clinical trials in humans.

• *Tenet #10: Herbs were created by God specifically to cure disease.* Many paraherbalists claim that God has provided a remedy for every ailment. Although this claim may appeal to deeply religious people, it is not testable and is therefore not a legitimate substitute for scientific evidence.

### The Current Marketplace

Americans spend well over a billion dollars per year for herb teas, bulk herbs, and other herbal products. Although many of these items are consumed for their flavor, most are probably used for supposed medicinal qualities.

In the United States, herbs marketed with therapeutic claims would be regulated as drugs under federal laws. To market an effective herb as a drug, a manufacturer would have to spend many millions of dollars on research that demonstrates safety and effectiveness. Since traditional herbal remedies are not patentable, manufacturers see little sense in doing research on herbs that might gain FDA approval. Instead, herbal products are marketed under the guise of foods or nutritional supplements, without therapeutic claims on their labels. No legal standards of quality exist or are now enforced, and, with some herbal products (particularly those with expensive raw ingredients), consumers have less than a 50 percent chance that the contents and potency are accurately disclosed on the label.

Although little or no information about herbal products is now found on their labels, it is readily offered through other channels of communication. In fact, more misinformation about the safety and efficacy of herbs is reaching the public currently than at any previous time, including the turn-of-the-century heyday of patent medicines. The literature promoting herbs includes pamphlets, magazine articles, and books ranging in quality from cheaply printed flyers to elaborately produced studies in fine bindings with attractive illustrations. Some of the unsubstantiated claims made in such publications for popular herbs are quoted and discussed in the tables on the following pages. Practically all of these writings recommend large numbers of herbs for treatment based on hearsay, folklore, and tradition. The only criterion that seems to be avoided in these publications is scientific evidence. Some writings are so comprehensive and indiscriminate that they seem to recommend everything for anything. Even deadly poisonous herbs are sometimes touted as remedies, based on some outdated report or a misunderstanding of the facts. Particularly insidious is the myth that there is something almost magical about herbal drugs that prevents them, in their natural state, from harming people. Herbs are also marketed by naturopaths, acupuncturists, iridologists, and chiropractors, many of whom prescribe them for the entire gamut of health problems.

Many herbs contain hundreds or even thousands of chemicals that have not been completely catalogued. Some of these chemicals may turn out to be useful as therapeutic agents, but others could well prove toxic. With safe and effective medicines available, treatment with herbs rarely makes sense. Moreover, many of the conditions for which herbs are recommended are not suitable for self-treatment. In a market dominated by paraherbalism, consumers are less likely to receive good value for money spent on herbal "remedies" than for almost any other health-related product.

The tables below compare facts about the more popular herbs with some of the specious claims made for them.

## Bloodroot, Damiana, Garlic, and Milk Thistle

| Claims | Facts |
|---|---|
| Bloodroot is "so effective . . . in treating skin cancers that four separate U.S. patents exist for this express purpose. . . . We make no 'drug' claims on this product." | If U.S. patents were any criterion for the validity of product claims, perpetual motion machines would be a reality. Asserting that bloodroot cures cancer is a "drug" claim in spite of the disclaimer. Such a claim is supported primarily by popular use in the 1850s, not by modern evaluation. Self-treatment of any type of cancer is unwise. |
| "Damiana leaves have been exalted for their aphrodisiac and tonic effects. They are respected as a palliative for male impotence." Damiana "tends to encourage amorous dreams." | There is no scientific evidence that damiana is an effective aphrodisiac. |
| Deodorized garlic "retains all the traditional well known medicinal and nutritional properties of raw garlic, without garlic's odor. . . . These studies show that allicin, an enzyme found in raw garlic, is responsible for these healthful effects." | Most authorities believe that totally odorless garlic preparations are ineffective. Enteric-coated garlic tablets are an exception because they release the active principles in the small intestine without causing an odor problem. Allicin is not an enzyme; it is one of the odorous active principles of garlic produced from alliin by the enzyme alliinase. |
| "Milk thistle exerts a protective effect and a regenerative action on the liver. Milk thistle tea is recommended for liver illness or liver sensitivities. The damage is soon repaired and the feeling of well being is increased." | Milk thistle may well contain constituents capable of exerting a protective effect on the liver, but they are practically water-insoluble. Studies show that ordinary tea preparation extracts only about 10 percent of the active principles from the herb. Obviously, it is not a suitable method of administration. |

## Echinacea, Ginseng, and "Siberian Ginseng" (Eleutherococcus)

| Claims | Facts |
|---|---|
| "Echinacea is one of the best blood cleansers .... It is good for blood poisoning, carbuncles, all pus diseases, abscesses of the teeth, gangrene, all lymph swellings, snake and spider bites. . . . It has a history of being used against syphilis and gonorrhea." | The use of echinacea as a nonspecific stimulator of immunity and its effectiveness in preventing or treating such conditions as the common cold is supported by substantial evidence. It is not, however, useful for blood poisoning (tetanus), lymph swellings (which could be malignant), the bites of poisonous animals and insects, or the like. "Use against a disease" does not ensure that a product is effective. |
| Ginseng is said to counteract stress; enhance memory; stimulate the immune system; spur production of both interferon and antibodies; reduce blood cholesterol levels; produce an anticlotting (anti-platelet) effect; help to control diabetes; exert an antioxidant effect that can prevent cancer; help protect the liver from . . . drugs, alcohol, and other toxins; minimize cell damage from radiation; counteract fatigue; increase intestinal absorption of nutrients; and act as a mild aphrodisiac. | Proof of these assertions is lacking because carefully controlled studies in human beings have simply not been carried out. The only one reported, a 1982 study of mood changes and body feelings in females, proved inconclusive, possibly because it lasted only two weeks. Until adequate tests have been conducted, claims that ginseng has medicinal value should be considered unproven. Cautious observers should note that no other known drug has all of the salubrious properties that are attributed to ginseng. The existence of a true panacea must be considered unlikely. One thing about ginseng is certain, however: moderate doses taken for reasonable periods of time appear to be reasonably safe for consumption by normal (non-pregnant, non-elderly) adults. |
| "Siberian ginseng" (Eleutherococcus) is "a botanical cousin of the true ginsengs. The Panax [ginseng] and Eleutherococcus species contain similar active constituents. And studies show they have similar effects. As a result, they are used interchangeably in the West, and all are called 'ginseng.'" | Ginseng and Siberian ginseng (preferably called eleuthero to avoid confusion) are entirely different plants with different constituents and modes of action. Scientifically, the designation ginseng, even with the qualifying geographical adjective, Siberian, is a misnomer. The name was apparently first used in 1971 by a trade group in an effort to associate the glamour and mystique of its more valuable cousin, ginseng, with this cheaper product, eleuthero. The deception was successful and the appellation Siberian ginseng is widely used in this country. It is not ginseng, however. |

## Pau d'Arco, Sassafras, Saw Palmetto, and "Cho Low Tea"

| Claims | Facts |
|---|---|
| Pau d'arco. "Could an ancient South American Indian folk medicine cure many types of cancer? Physicians and former cancer patients say yes. . . . The bark cured everything. Cancer, Ulcers, Diabetes, and Rheumatism—the medicine cured them all. And what was impressive was the time it took to achieve the cure. ALMOST ALWAYS LESS THAN ONE MONTH." | These therapeutic claims are based on the herb's content of lapachol, a naphthoquinone. It seemed to show promise as an anti-tumor agent but was abandoned after effective doses proved to be toxic. Analysis of thirteen commercial pau d'arco products in Canada showed that only two of them contained even traces of lapachol or related compounds; further, teas prepared from those two samples contained no detectable amounts of the relatively water-insoluble naphthoquinones. |
| "Sassafras is a spring tonic. It will thin the blood after a heavy winter. It stimulates and cleans the liver of toxins. Given during painful mentsruation [sic], it will relieve the suffering and is effective in afterpains from childbirth. Sassafras is usually combined with other alterative herbs when used to purify the blood." | Science has not verified any of these claims. Sassafras does not thin the blood or remove toxins from the liver. It does not relieve menstrual cramps or postpartum pain. It does not purify the blood (an old term indicating that it cures venereal disease). In fact, it is toxic, producing cancer of the liver in small animals. Human consumption, therefore, is imprudent. |
| Saw palmetto is said to be "valuable in all diseases of the reproductive organs, ovaries, prostate, testes, etc." and a sex-life rejuvenator. "At the local health food store they sold me some saw palmetto berry to make into a tea, and promised if I drank it three times a day, I could start buying bigger bras after awhile. However, I haven't seen much progress." | Saw palmetto berries contain beta-sitosterol, which has a feeble estrogenic activity. It is, however, relatively water-insoluble and is poorly absorbed from the gastrointestinal tract. No wonder little progress was noted by the woman who wished to enlarge her breasts. Unidentified chemicals in the berries do possess androgenic (male-hormone) activity. However, the FDA has banned the sale of saw palmetto for the treatment of benign prostatic hypertrophy. |
| "New tea from China reduces cholesterol. Medical studies prove it! Just drinking this refreshing tea every day is as effective as medically prescribed drugs in reducing cholesterol." | No matter where it is grown, tea (black or green) has no proven cholesterol-lowering properties in human beings. The mail-order company that advertised in this manner actually had no tea to send to customers (see Chapter 20). |

## Comfrey, Gingko, Smilax Officinalis, and Suma

| Claims | Facts |
|---|---|
| "Comfrey is a cell proliferator and will help heal broken bones . . . . It is one of the best remedies for internal bleeding anywhere in the body. Use a strong decoction for bleeding and to build new flesh during wasting diseases." | The myth that comfrey promotes bone-healing comes from a misunderstanding of its common name, knitbone. It was once used as a poultice on the flesh around simple fractures to reduce swelling. People with internal bleeding or a wasting disease should certainly consult a physician. Depending on the exact source, comfrey (particularly the root) may be toxic. It cannot be recommended for internal use. |
| Gingko "may help reverse the aging process of the brain. . . . When you purchase this hard-to-find product, you can look forward to a healthier and possibly even longer life." | There is considerable evidence that gingko has a beneficial effect on cerebral blood flow, particularly in geriatric patients. It also may have useful properties as a free-radical scavenger. However, there is absolutely no evidence that it can reverse the aging process or prolong life. Gingko products are available in most health food stores and are not hard to find. |
| Smilax officinalis is "an herb that naturally increases testosterone levels in the body." It is "the only true source of testosterone. In fact pharmaceutical testosterone (anabolic steroids) are actually made from Smilax." | There is no evidence that Smilax contains testosterone or that it serves as a source of testosterone in the human body. It does contain chemicals that serve as precursors for the semisynthetic production of certain steroids in vitro, but this conversion takes place only in the chemical laboratory or factory, not in the human being. |
| "Suma has been used in the Amazon for at least three centuries as a tonic, aphrodisiac (increased well-being!) and as a treatment for diabetes, tumors, and skin problems of all kinds, including wounds." It is "particularly effective in tumor-remission and in cases of diabetes." Suma "from the moisture rich rain forest is . . . in a unique night cream. . . . Its nutrients smoothe and protect your skin" and makes it feel "younger, more supple, and revitalized." | If suma was used in the Amazon for the last 300 years, it was a well-kept secret. Until recently, it was not listed in any of the standard reference works on medicinal plants. An aphrodisiac would increase sexual pleasure, not one's feeling of well-being. There is no evidence that suma does either of these things. Preliminary tests have found that suma's constituents inhibited the growth of cultured cell melanomas. However, this is not unusual for plant constituents and does not mean suma is able to cause tumor remission in humans. The implication that because the plant grows under moist conditions it is a useful skin moisturizer is far-fetched. There is no evidence that suma "nourishes" or "revitalizes" the skin. |

# 16

# Vitalistic Gurus and Their Legacies

### Jack Raso, M.S., R.D.

This chapter describes several "healing" systems based on vitalism—the doctrine that an invisible, intangible, nonmaterial form of energy is responsible for all the activities of a living organism. In addition to a score of generic names, such as "vital force," this "energy" has many nicknames, including "*Ch'i*" or "*Qi*" (Chinese), "*ki*" (Japanese), "*prana*" (Hindu), and "the Innate" (fundamentalist chiropractic). Some vitalists hold that the "vital force" can exist independently of the human organism. Some claim or suggest that food can be "dead" or "living," and that "living" (or "live") foods contain a dormant or primitive "life force" that humans can "assimilate." Proponents of many "alternative" methods assert that the "vital force" can be utilized to prevent, diagnose, and treat disease; to improve health and physical fitness; and to prolong life. These approaches are not based on science but on superstition. The table on the next page compares the five vitalistic systems featured in this chapter.

## Macrobiotics

Macrobiotics is a quasi-religious movement and health-centered lifestyle founded by George Ohsawa (1893–1966) and popularized in the United States by Michio Kushi. Its centerpiece is a semivegetarian diet in which animal foods are used sparingly or not at all. Macrobiotic nutrition is focused on regulating the intake of two alleged elementary forms of energy: yin and yang. Whether a food is categorized as yin or yang is based largely on sensory characteristics and is unrelated to nutrient composition.

The earliest version of the diet, called the "Zen macrobiotic diet," was claimed to cure airsickness, bedwetting, cataracts, retinal detachment, near-sightedness, epilepsy, baldness, gonorrhea, syphilis, hemophilia, leprosy, polio, schizophrenia, and many other health problems. Proponents ascribed all these conditions to a dietary imbalance of yin and yang. In *Zen Macrobiotics* (1965), Ohsawa wrote that dandruff is "the first step toward mental disease."

The Zen macrobiotic diet involved seven classes of food and ten progressively restrictive dietary stages, termed "ways to health and happiness." The lowest stage comprised 10 percent grains, 30 percent vegetables, 10 percent soup, 30 percent animal products, 15 percent fruits and salads, and 5 percent desserts. In each "higher" (supposedly more healthful) stage, the percentage of grains increased by ten and percentages from the "animal" and "salad/fruit" categories decreased. The fourth stage eliminated fruits, the sixth stage all animal products, and the "highest" stage everything except grains. In all stages, fluid intake was discouraged.

In 1966, the Passaic (New Jersey) Grand Jury reviewed three cases of death and two cases of near-death from malnutrition among Zen macrobiotic adherents and concluded that the diet "constitutes a public health hazard." In 1967, the *Journal of the American Medical Association* reported how one of

## Five Vitalistic Systems

| System | Basis for Diet | Primary Foods | "Vital Principle" |
|---|---|---|---|
| Macrobiotics | George Ohsawa's version of traditional Chinese cosmology | Grains, especially brown rice | Ch'i, ki |
| Naturopathy | | "Natural" foods | Vis medicatrix naturae |
| Natural Hygiene | Herbert Shelton's food categories | Raw vegetables, raw fruits, and raw nuts | Essence, life force, vital force, nerve force, nerve energy |
| Ayurveda | So-called constitutional types | Grains, ghee (clarified butter), and specific vegetables, all preferably heated or cooked. Maharishi Amrit Kalash is advertised as "the perfect nutritional food." | Prana |
| Edgar Cayce tradition | Cayce's "psychic readings" | All foods of the plant kingdom | Spirit, soul |

these adherents had developed scurvy within ten months of starting the diet. These cases set the tone for scientific medicine's view of macrobiotics. In 1971, the AMA Council on Foods and Nutrition stated that followers of the diet, particularly the highest level, stood in "great danger" of malnutrition.

In *Macrobiotics: Yesterday and Today* (1985), macrobiotics insider Ronald Kotzsch, Ph.D., describes how a young woman in New York who had followed the diet's highest stage died in 1965—apparently of malnutrition and dehydration. Later that year, Ohsawa was sued for malpractice and the Ohsawa Foundation in New York was closed after a raid by the FDA. The East Coast hub of macrobiotics then shifted to Boston and its resident Ohsawa disciple, Michio Kushi.

Michio Kushi was born in Japan in 1926 and studied political science and international law before coming to the United States in 1949. In 1965, he moved from New York to Cambridge, Massachusetts, and founded the Erewhon Trading Company, which operated a small basement retail outlet for macrobiotic foods in nearby Boston. The store grossed about $200 to $300 weekly in 1967, but with increasing attendance at macrobiotic lectures, the business expanded into "nonmacrobiotic" foods (such as dairy products and honey) and "organically grown" foods. By the time it filed for bankruptcy in 1981, Erewhon encompassed more than ten stores, a large wholesale warehouse, and a macrobiotic rural community called Erewhon Farms.

In the 1970s, Kushi helped organize *East West Journal*, the East West Foundation, and the Kushi Institute. In 1981, the Kushi Foundation was established as the parent organization for the institute and the magazine. A few years later, One Peaceful World—a society dedicated to "planetary health"—was formed under the foundation's aegis. (*East West* was sold to outside investors in 1989, was renamed *East West Natural Health* in 1992, and is now called *Natural Health*.)

The Kushi Institute is located on six hundred acres in Becket, Massachusetts. In addition to holding lectures, seminars, and conferences, the institute markets more than a hundred books, audiocassettes, and videotapes about macrobiotics and other topics consistent with its beliefs. There are affiliated institutes in Amsterdam, Antwerp, Barcelona, Florence, Lisbon, London, and Kiental (Switzerland), and about six hundred independent macrobiotic "centers" located in many parts of the world. The institute reportedly has provided thousands of people with instruction in macrobiotic principles and techniques. Its Leadership Studies Program, with extension programs in several American cities, comprises three five-week tiers, each focused on personal, societal, or planetary health. Core subjects include Oriental diagnosis and *ki* development ("energy adjustment"). The current cost of this program is $8,250.

*Natural Health*, published bimonthly, contains about 150 pages per issue and has a circulation of about 175,000. Its editorial philosophy is leery of scientific medicine and supportive of vitalistic systems and methods, including: acupuncture, homeopathy, kundalini meditation, naturopathy, past-life therapy, and rolfing (a massage method for which vitalistic claims are made). Products that typify advertisements in *Natural Health* include: an "oxygen supplement" (supposedly furnishing vitamin "O"), a "multivitamin skin cream" ("the perfect skin food"), "guided imagery" audiotapes for cancer and AIDS, "music composed in a trance," an "elemental diode" that allegedly shields its wearer from electromagnetic fields, and Vedic horoscopes.

### What Is Macrobiotics?

The word "macrobiotic" derives from two Greek words: *makros*, meaning "large," and *biotos*; meaning "life." A Kushi Foundation pamphlet translates these Greek words as "great life." In *Zen Macrobiotics*, Ohsawa called macrobiotics "the medicine of longevity and rejuvenation." *Webster's Dictionary* defines macrobiotics as "the art of prolonging life." *The New Age Dictionary* (1990)—edited by Alex Jack, former editor-in-chief of *East West*—includes a definition ascribed to Michio Kushi:

> the way of health, happiness, and peace through biological and spiritual evolution and the universal means to practice and harmonize with the Order of the Universe in daily life, including the selection, preparation, and manner of cooking and eating, as well as the orientation of consciousness toward infinite spiritual realization.

However, Ronald Kotzsch has observed:

> There is no explicit, generally accepted understanding of what it means to be "macrobiotic." Macrobiotics is many-faceted. It includes a diet, a system of medicine, a philosophy, a way of life, a community, and a broad social movement.

According to ancient Chinese cosmology, yin and yang are the opposite but complementary cosmic principles or "energy modes" that compose the *Tao*. The word "Tao" is derived from a Mandarin word meaning "way"; it stands for ultimate reality, universal energy, and living in harmony with the universe. In Chinese tradition, the sky (the generator of all phenomena) exemplifies yang—the active, bright, male principle; the earth exemplifies yin—the passive, dark, female principle. Citing yin-yang theory, macrobiotics can categorize any phenomenon or concept as either yin or yang. However, while the Chinese theory (which includes acupuncture) distinguishes by function, macrobiotics distinguishes according to structure. For example, macrobiotics categorizes the earth as yang because it is denser than the sky (that is, the rest of the universe); Chinese cosmology takes the opposite view. Kotzsch notes that "while Ohsawa purports to present an ancient Oriental way of thinking, in practice his [system] does not correspond to the classical Chinese system."

A Kushi Foundation pamphlet states: "Macrobiotics is understanding the energetics of food and how to make the choices which can lead you in a more centered and positive direction. . . . As your body and mind become healthier and clearer, you will joyfully realize the boundless energy that lies within us all." Theoretically, macrobiotic assignment of "yin-ness" or "yang-ness" to foods is based on the food's color, pH, shape, size, taste, temperature, texture, water content, weight, and the region and season in which the food was grown. Furthermore, the "yin/yang-ness" of any food is affected by how it is prepared and eaten.

In *Zen Macrobiotics*, Ohsawa advised that "principal foods"—cereals (grains), sautéed vegetables, and soup—constitute at least 60 percent of one's diet. By itself, this recommendation does not sound unreasonable. But he further advised consuming foods within his seven classes that are at or "reasonably near" the midpoint of yin and yang—"unless there is a *specific* reason for another choice." Ohsawa's "reasons" included schizophrenia (a "yin disease" for which he recommended "all yang drinks") and kidney disease (for which he recommended brown-rice juice and azuki-bean juice with a pinch of salt). Moreover, several pages later Ohsawa defined "principal foods" as "only" cereals.

Yin-yang theory, religious underpinnings, and a Japanese culinary bias complicate macrobiotics. But its diet is reducible to the consumption of unprocessed or minimally processed foods, primarily whole grains and vegetables, which, ideally, should be grown "organically" in the region where the consumer lives and eaten in season. Kushi advises chewing food slowly and quietly at least fifty times per mouthful or until it liquefies. His "Standard Macrobiotic Diet"—designed primarily for residents of temperate regions—encompasses:

- Cooked, "organically grown," whole grains—an average of 50 percent of the volume of each meal

- Soup made with vegetables, seaweed, grains, or beans, usually seasoned with miso or soy sauce—about 5 to 10 percent of daily food intake

- "Organic" vegetables, preferably grown locally, mostly cooked—about 20 to 30 percent of daily food intake

- Cooked beans, soybean-based products, and seaweed—about 5 to 10 percent of daily food intake

- Beverages: "traditional," nonstimulating, non-aromatic teas (such as roasted brown rice tea); and water—preferably spring water or "quality" well water—not iced, and in moderation

- Fresh, white-meat fish—5 to 15 percent of food intake on one to three days each week, "if needed or desired"

- Fresh, dried, and cooked fruit, preferably grown locally and "organically"—two or three servings per week

- Occasional snacks: lightly roasted nuts, peanuts, and seeds

- Condiments: unrefined sesame oil, unrefined corn oil from stone-ground corn, sea salt, soy sauce, miso, gomashio (a mixture of dry-roasted and crushed sesame seeds and sea salt), seaweed powder, pickles such as umeboshi (a Japanese plum), tekka (a mixture of minced lotus root, burdock root, carrot, ginger, and miso), and sauerkraut.

"Food to avoid for better health" include meat, poultry, dairy products, refined sugars, molasses, honey, vanilla, tropical and semitropical fruits and fruit juices, coffee, mint teas, potatoes, sweet potatoes, yams, tomatoes, eggplant, peppers, asparagus, spinach, avocado, hot spices, refined grains, and all canned, frozen, or irradiated foods. Nutritional supplementation is discouraged, and fluid restriction is common. Kushi has proposed adaptations of his "standard diet" for various types of cancer.

But, as a Kushi Foundation pamphlet states, "macrobiotics is more than a hill of beans." Besides liberalizing Ohsawa's diet, Kushi spiritualized and "paranormalized" Ohsawa's already supernaturalistic philosophy, merging into the macrobiotic mainstream such matters as: Oriental physiognomy (including "diagnosis" of beauty marks), palmistry, Japanese astrology ("nine star ki"), dream interpretation, karma, chanting, shiatsu, ghosts, the "macrobiotic lifestyle" of Jesus Christ and his disciples, extraterrestrial encounters, exploring unexplained "other dimensions," and "seeing harmony in dualism." In the introduction to *Standard Macrobiotic Diet* (1992), Kushi states: "The goal of macrobiotics is to preserve the human race and to create a new species—*homo spiritus*." One of his "timeless and universal" teachings is that a depressed navel indicates a yang constitution and a protuberant navel signifies a yin constitution. The latter, Kushi says, may be the result of excessive fluid intake by one's mother during pregnancy.

According to the macrobiotic "way of life," one should: feel grateful toward nature and one's ancestors; walk barefoot daily, in simple clothing, on grass, soil, or the beach; use only "natural" and "organic" cosmetics; minimize the use of color televisions and computers; and sing a happy song every day. And one should refrain from: wearing synthetic clothing directly on the skin (it supposedly interferes with the body's "energy flow"); taking long, hot baths or showers unless one has consumed too much salt or animal food; and using electrical cooking appliances.

## A Seminar for Professionals

Throughout the year, the Kushi Institute conducts residential seminars ranging from weekend workshops to its Leadership Studies Program. In June 1989, I attended the five-day Michio Kushi Seminar for Medical Professionals, held in Becket. The seminar cost $450, which covered tuition, room, and board. However, upon registering, I was charged an additional $30 for membership in One Peaceful World—required for participation in all institute programs.

Eighteen people other than myself attended the seminar: twelve medical doctors, two registered nurses (one a nurse practitioner), an osteopath, an endodontist, a chiropractor, and a nutrition researcher with a doctorate. The M.D.s included a homeopath, an orthopedist, and a physician identified as a pioneer "clinical ecologist." The orthopedist complained that Western medicine was "so minutia-oriented." Two of the attendees were visibly overweight. One of the physicians said he had cancer. The attendees' experience with macrobiotics ranged from dabbling to ten years, but most had been involved for more than six months.

Each of us received a packet containing information on the diet, macrobiotic seminars and publications, traditional Oriental "arts of diagnosis," the Kushis' nearby "natural food" store, and their macrobiotic Japanese restaurant in Stockbridge, Massachusetts.

On the third day of the seminar, Kushi lectured on diagnostic principles. His broken English often made him unintelligible. "Modern medicine is physical, material way, analytical way," he said, "therefore overlooking this universe's force coming in, and the earth force go up, coming in constantly, constantly, constantly." To demonstrate this alleged force, Kushi produced nail clippers suspended from a dark thread. "This is no gimmick," he assured us. "It's a nail clipper. . . . This is just thread only." Kushi dangled the clippers over a supine doctor and the clippers began to move in circular fashion. He claimed that "chakras" were responsible for this movement—but close observation revealed that the circling was caused by motions of his arm.

In yoga philosophy, chakras are vortices that penetrate the human body and its "aura"; they are the means by which *prana* (the Hindu equivalent of *Ch'i*) is transformed and distributed (analogous to the "energy pathways" of acupuncture). Although hypothetically there are only five to seven major "body chakras," there is no consensus on the total number of chakras; hundreds of minor ones are said to exist. Neither is there any consensus on their location or alleged functions. In any case, there is no scientific evidence that chakras exist.

The methods espoused by Kushi are part of what he calls natural medicine, "the medicine of energy and vibrations." The diagnostic "arts" he employs include visual diagnosis, pulse diagnosis, meridian diagnosis, pressure diagnosis, voice diagnosis, behavioral diagnosis, psychological diagnosis, astrological diagnosis, environmental diagnosis, parental and ancestral diagnosis, aura and vibrational diagnosis, consciousness and thought diagnosis, and spiritual diagnosis—all of which were defined in the information packet we received.

Voice diagnosis supposedly identifies disorders of "certain systems, organs or glands." Kushi said, for example, that a "watery voice " signifies that the patient's "natural kidney-bladder," blood, and heartbeat are "overworked."

Astrological diagnosis is based on the time and place of birth, where one is raised, and current astrological and astronomical conditions. It is used to "characterize the basic constitutional tendencies of the body and the mind as well as the potential destiny of the current and future life of the subject." After outlining nine Oriental "astrological types," Kushi summoned volunteers representing "opposite" types, compared their smiles, and commented that some were "very idealistic, very romantic, uplifted" and fond of theatrics, while their supposed opposites were "gentle" and "more reserved."

Behavioral diagnosis supposedly reveals dietary imbalances impacting on behavior. For example, Kushi stated that fishy movements manifest overconsumption of fish. He illustrated this behavior by sitting in a chair and moving his knees repeatedly apart and together.

Environmental diagnosis involves an examination of atmospheric conditions and "celestial influences." It is used to reveal the "environmental cause" of physical and psychological disorders. Kushi said that, during sleep, one's head should lie to the north if one lives in the northern hemisphere and to the south if one lives in the southern hemisphere.

Lawrence Lindner, executive editor of the *Tufts University Diet and Nutrition Letter,* had a private consultation with a certified senior macrobiotics counselor at the Kushi Institute as part of an assignment for *American Health* magazine. In the May 1988 issue, Lindner reported that the counselor told him: (1) his heart was somewhat enlarged because he ate too much fruit, (2) his kidneys were weak, (3) he was slightly hypoglycemic, (4) deposits of fat and mucus were starting to build up in his intestines, (5) cold drinks could freeze the deposits and cause kidney stones, and (6) he should avoid eating chicken because it is linked with pancreatic cancer and melanoma. The consultation cost $200. Lindner concluded: "The macrobiotic lectures, courses, books and tapes . . . besides running into hundreds or thousands of dollars, teach a philosophy of life, not nutrient interactions." In a subsequent interview, he added, "Some people are attracted to macrobiotics because, like a typical cult, it seems to offer simple solutions to a variety of life's problems."

### Possible Dangers

Many reports have noted iron and vitamin $B_{12}$ deficiencies, rickets, retarded growth, and below-normal stature among children on the macrobiotic diet. Moreover, macrobiotic adults were found to have low serum concentrations of $B_{12}$. Several lawsuits have claimed that cancer patients who relied on macrobiotic methods instead of proven therapy met with disaster. (As far as I know, no such case has come to trial. They are either still pending or were settled out of court with an agreement not to disclose settlement terms.) The diet poses significant risks for persons with cancer or AIDS who use it in addition to scientific treatment.

Proponents of macrobiotics respond to these criticisms in several ways. They say that nutritional deficiencies result only from following the diet incorrectly—in an overly restrictive fashion. They claim they do not try to lure patients away from medical treatment with promises that the diet will cure them. And they point to research findings suggesting that macrobiotics is protective against coronary heart disease. (A study by William Castelli, M.D., for example, found that over a hundred followers of the macrobiotic diet in the Boston area had an average blood cholesterol level of 125, while control-group members of similar ages averaged 185.) However, they are not likely to mention that other approaches to disease prevention, such as the Pritikin program or well-rounded vegetarianism, are nutritionally superior and easier to maintain.

No long-range study has attempted to determine whether macrobiotic devotees wind up, on balance, better off than their nonmacrobiotic counterparts. Since macrobiotics is a lifestyle—and an ill-defined one—such a study could be difficult to construct; and if its results showed that devotees fared better, the reasons for their success might be extremely difficult to identify.

Although macrobiotic eating might improve the health of many American adults, it carries a significant and unnecessary risk of nutritional deficiencies. Nutrient supplementation, lab tests, and consultations with a qualified nutrition professional could minimize this risk. But macrobiotic philosophy discourages the use of such safeguards.

**Naturopathy**

Naturopathy—so-called natural therapeutics or natural medicine— is a composite "healing" tradition touted as "drugless" and reliant solely upon "natural" powers. Yet it is distinguished by a hodgepodge of vitalistic approaches such as acupuncture (including ear acupuncture and electroacupuncture), *jin shin* (a form of acupressure), *tui na* (Chinese "bodywork"), Chinese herbalism, zone therapy (reflexology), homeopathy, orthobionomy, and Jungian psychotherapy. Although naturopathy did not spring from a unified doctrine and is poorly organized in both theory and practice, naturopaths generally agree that a "life force" or "vital curative force"—misrepresented as the Hippocratic *vis medicatrix naturae*—normally flows through the body in various channels, and that blockages cause "imbalances" leading to disease. Literature from Bastyr University, the leading school of naturopathy, states:

> Naturopathic physicians seek to restore and maintain optimum health in their patients by emphasizing nature's inherent capacity to heal, the vis medicatrix naturae. . . . Naturopathic medicine recognizes an inherent ability in the body which is ordered and intelligent. Naturopathic physicians act to identify and remove obstacles to recovery, and to facilitate and augment this healing ability.

Naturopaths claim to remove or treat the "underlying causes" of disease on physical, mental/emotional, spiritual, social, and other levels; and to facilitate the response of the "life force" to illness through "cleansing" and "detoxification." Anything that supposedly dampens the "life force" is deemed an "underlying cause." The American Association of Naturopathic Physicians states: "Naturopathic medicine has its own unique body of knowledge, evolved and refined for centuries." In a 1991 article, naturopath Robert H. Sorge—founder of the Abunda Life Health Hotel in Asbury Park, New Jersey—states that the major contributors to an elevated cholesterol level include "devitalized foods," worry, fear, anxiety, autointoxication, "metabolic imbalance," "colon toxicity," malabsorption, and "liver sluggishness." Sorge's "N.D." degree came from a nonaccredited correspondence school that promoted "spondylotherapy"—emptying the stomach by concussion to affect, for example, bust development, syphilis, and impotence.

Most naturopaths believe that virtually all diseases are within their scope of practice. They offer treatment at their offices and at spas where patients may reside for several weeks. In addition to the approaches listed above, their methods include: hypnotherapy, biofeedback, Natural Hygiene (see below), fasting, nutritional supplementation, exercise, colonic enemas and other forms of hydrotherapy, ultrasound, diathermy (heat treatment), spinal manipulation, "natural childbirth care," and minor surgery. Naturopaths may use x-rays for diagnosis but not for treatment. The most comprehensive naturopathic publications, *A Textbook of Natural Medicine* (for students and professionals) and the *Encyclopedia of Natural Medicine* (for laypersons), recommend dietary measures, vitamins, minerals, and/or herbs for more than seventy health problems ranging from acne to AIDS.

The term "naturopathy" was coined in 1895 by Dr. John Scheel—a German-born homeopath who practiced in New York City—to describe his methods of health care. In 1902, he sold the rights to the name to Benedict Lust, who had come to the United States in 1892 to promote hydropathy ("water cure"). Lust was largely responsible for naturopathy's growth in this country. He acquired degrees in chiropractic, homeopathy, naturopathy, and osteopathy, and a medical license based on his homeopathy degree, which had taken less than two years to earn. Another prominent developer of naturopathy was Bernarr Macfadden, who promoted "physical culture."

In the United States, the heyday of naturopathy occurred during the 1920s and 1930s. But its popularity waned over the next three decades as scientific medicine developed and chiropractic schools stopped granting naturopathy diplomas.

Perhaps the severest critic of naturopathy in its early days was Morris Fishbein, M.D., editor of the *Journal of the American Medical Association*. In *Fads and Quackery in Healing* (1932), Fishbein stated:

> Naturopathy and the allied cults represent capitalization for purposes of financial gain of the old advice that outdoor life, good diet, enough exercise, and rest are conducive to health and longevity. When these simple principles can be linked with the printing of worthless pamphlets, intricate apparatus, or faith cures, the formulas yield gold. . . .
>
> The real naturopaths . . . advocated natural living and healed by the use of sunlight, baths, fresh air, and cold water, but there is little money to be made by these methods. Hence the modern naturopath embraces every form of healing that offers opportunity for exploitation.

In 1968, the U.S. Department of Health, Education, and Welfare (HEW) recommended against coverage of naturopathy under Medicare. HEW's report concluded:

> Naturopathic theory and practice are not based upon the body of basic knowledge related to health, disease, and health care which has been widely accepted by the scientific community. Moreover, irrespective of its theory, the scope and quality of naturopathic education do not prepare the practitioner to make an adequate diagnosis and provide appropriate treatment.

The doctor of naturopathy (N.D.) degree is now available from three full-time schools of naturopathy and a few correspondence schools. The curriculum at the full-time institutions includes two years of basic science courses such as human anatomy and physiology and two years of clinical naturopathy. In 1987, the U.S. Secretary of Education approved the Council on Naturopathic Medical Education (CNME) as an accrediting agency. Unfortunately, accreditation is not based on the soundness of what is taught, but on such factors as record-keeping, physical assets, financial status, makeup of the governing body, catalog characteristics, nondiscrimination policy, and self-evaluation system. CNME's recognition prompted the National Council Against Health Fraud to warn that "the accreditation process is defective at its core. . . . Many will be shocked to learn that no health care guild is legally required to be scientific."

Bastyr University, in Seattle, Washington, is accredited by the CNME. In addition to its N.D. program, Bastyr offers a B.S. degree program in Natural Health Sciences with majors in nutrition and Oriental medicine, and M.S. programs in nutrition and acupuncture. Bastyr also provides health-food retailers and their employees with home-study programs that promote "natural" approaches for the gamut of disease. The other four-year schools are the National College of Naturopathic Medicine in Portland, Oregon, and the recently opened Southwest College of Naturopathic Medicine and Health Sciences in Scottsdale, Arizona. Most of the latter's initial funding came from companies that market dietary supplements, homeopathic products, and/or herbal remedies. They apparently consider the school a good investment.

Naturopathic licensing laws exist in only seven states and the District of Columbia. Several other states have laws that permit naturopaths to practice, but in most states they are not officially allowed to do so. A directory in the January/February 1992 issue of *East West Natural Health* lists nearly four hundred naturopaths with practices in twenty-seven states, the District of Columbia, and Puerto Rico. The total number of practitioners is unknown but includes chiropractors and acupuncturists who practice naturopathy. Naturopathic services are not covered under Medicare or most health insurance policies.

**Natural Hygiene**

Natural Hygiene, a Spartan form of naturopathy, is a comprehensive philosophy of health and "natural living" whose ideal diet is restricted to vegetables, fruits, nuts, and seeds—all uncooked and minimally processed. Natural Hygiene recommends fasting whether one is sick or healthy, and denounces virtually all medical treatments—including herbal remedies and nutritional supplements. *Health Science,* the official membership journal of the American Natural Hygiene Society, summarizes the Hygienic philosophy on its masthead:

> Health is the result of natural living. When people live in harmony with their physiological needs, health is the inevitable result. By supplying the organism with its basic requirements (natural, unadulterated food; sunshine; clean, fresh air; pure water; appropriate physical, mental and emotional activities; and a productive lifestyle) while simultaneously eliminating all harmful factors and influences, the self-constructing, self-regulating, self-repairing qualities of the body are given full rein.

*Health Science* states that the Hygienic movement was founded during the 1830s by Sylvester Graham, "America's first crusader for healthful living in diet, exercise, sleep, bathing, clothing, and sexual, emotional and mental expression." The movement enjoyed considerable popularity, declined, and was revived by Herbert M. Shelton (1895–1985), who co-founded the American Natural Hygiene Society in 1948. "Today," Shelton said in a 1978 interview, "thanks to my untiring effort and the efforts of those who joined me in the work, men that were dead live again, principles that were forgotten have been refurbished, and a whole literature has been salvaged." In a 1982 interview, he claimed to have "brought order out of chaos."

To what principles and to whose order did Shelton refer? In the 1963 edition of *An Introduction to Natural Hygiene,* he stated that a loss of "nerve force" attends sexual orgasm, causing weakness; that sexual intercourse should not be indulged in for pleasure or relief, but only for procreation; that nature or God intended humans to go nude; that "whatever is natural is right"; and that our "natural (unperverted) instincts" can lead us correctly.

Shelton described his educational background in the 1978 interview. At age sixteen, having undergone "the usual brainwashing process of the public school system in Greenville, Texas," he "revolted against the whole political, religious, medical, and social system." After serving in the Army during World War I, he obtained a "Doctor of Physiological Therapeutics" degree from the Macfadden College of Physcultopathy. Next, Shelton took a postgraduate course at the Lindlahr College of Natural Therapeutics in Chicago—founded by iridology proponent Henry Lindlahr, M.D., N.D., who professed that "all disease is caused by something that interferes with, diminishes or disturbs the normal inflow and distribution of vital energy throughout the system."

From Chicago, Shelton went to New York, where, "after nine months of brainwashing," he received doctoral degrees from schools founded by Benedict Lust, one in naturopathy and another in chiropractic. Then he returned to Chicago to do postgraduate work at another chiropractic college, which was "accompanied and succeeded by thirty-one months of apprenticeship in four different institutions, where the most valuable thing I learned was what not to do."

The first of Shelton's approximately forty books, *Fundamentals of Nature Cure*, was published in 1920. In 1928, he opened Dr. Shelton's Health School in San Antonio, Texas, which operated at seven different locations until 1981. From 1934 through 1941, Shelton produced a seven-volume series called *The Hygienic System*. In 1949, he launched *Dr. Shelton's Hygienic Review*, a monthly magazine that was published for about forty years.

In 1982, a federal court jury awarded $873,000 to the survivors of William Carlton, a forty-nine-year-old man who had died after undergoing a distilled-water fast for thirty days at Shelton's Health School. An article in the *Los Angeles Daily Journal* stated that Carlton had died of bronchial pneumonia resulting from a weakened condition in which he lost fifty pounds during the last month of his life. The article also noted that he was the sixth person in five years who had died while undergoing "treatment" at the school. Shelton and his associate, chiropractor Vivian V. Vetrano, claimed in their appeal that Carlton had persisted in fasting after Vetrano had advised him to stop. However, the verdict was upheld by the Fifth Circuit Court of Appeals, and the U.S. Supreme Court declined further review.

Headquartered in Tampa, Florida, the American Natural Hygiene Society (ANHS) is the fountainhead of today's Natural Hygiene activity. Regular ANHS membership costs $25 and includes a subscription to *Health Science,* a thirty-two-page bimonthly magazine. The March/April 1993 issue states that ANHS has over eight thousand members. The group has actively promoted certification of "organic" foods and vigorously opposed compulsory immunization and food irradiation.

Each issue of *Health Science* includes a referral list of members of the International Association of Professional Natural Hygienists. The July/August 1993 issue lists thirty-three individuals; most are chiropractors, but a few hold a medical, osteopathic, or naturopathic degree. The list includes thirteen "certified" and eight "associate" members in the United States, and others in Australia, Canada, England, Greece, Israel, Japan, and Poland. Certified members include ANHS founders and "subsequent members who have successfully completed an internship (or its equivalent) in Natural Hygiene care with an emphasis on Fasting Supervision."

According to an ANHS brochure:

A thoroughgoing rest, which includes fasting, is the most favorable condition under which an ailing body can purify and repair itself. Fasting is the total abstinence from all liquid and solid foods except distilled water. During a fast the body's recuperative forces are marshaled and all of its energies are directed toward the recharging of the nervous system, the elimination of toxic accumulations, and the repair and rejuvenation of tissue. Stored within each organism's tissues are nutrient reserves which it will use to carry on metabolism and repair work. Until these reserves are depleted, no destruction of healthy tissue or "starvation" can occur.

ANHS publications promote fasting for children as well as for adults. The brochure also states:

Natural Hygiene rejects the use of medications, blood transfusions, radiation, dietary supplements, and any other means employed to treat or "cure" various ailments. These therapies interfere with or destroy vital processes and tissue. Recovery from disease takes place in spite of, and not because of, the drugging and "curing" practices.

Another conspicuous component of Natural Hygiene is its pseudo-scientific system of "food combining." In *Food Combining Made Easy* (a "nutrition classic," according to its cover), Shelton wrote: "To a single article of food that is a starch-protein combination, the body can easily adjust its juices ... to the digestive requirements of the food. But when two foods are eaten with different ... digestive needs, this precise adjustment of juices to requirements becomes impossible." A Natural Hygienist might claim, for example, that consuming a high-protein food and a high-carbohydrate food at the same meal, at the very least, taxes the body's enzymatic capacity. Such ideas were shown to be false more than fifty years ago, but the Hygienic faithful still hold them dear.

In *Food Combining*, Shelton grouped foods "according to their composition and sources of origin": (1) "proteins," including nuts, peanuts, and avocados; (2) "starches" and sweet fruits, including peanuts (again), chestnuts, pumpkin, bananas, and mangoes; (3) "fats," including most nuts (again) and avocados (again); (4) "acid fruits," including citrus fruit and tomatoes; (5) "sub-acid" fruits, including pears and apricots; (6) non-starchy and green vegetables, including lettuce, broccoli, and watercress; and (7) melons, including water-melon, honeydew, and cantaloupe. Hygienic classification schemes differ somewhat, but certain listed foods, such as garlic (an "irritant") and all animal-source foods, are not recommended under any circumstances.

Two bestsellers by Harvey and Marilyn Diamond—*Fit for Life* (1985) and *Living Health* (1987)—sparked a renaissance for Natural Hygiene. Harvey Diamond received his "Ph.D. in nutritional science" from the American College of Health Science, a correspondence school in Texas that has offered— under a half-dozen names—courses detailing the views of its administrator,

T.C. Fry. Marilyn holds a "master's degree" from the school, which is now called Health Excellence Systems. However, Fry's school has never been accredited or legally authorized to grant degrees. In 1986, Mr. Fry agreed to a permanent injunction barring him from representing his enterprise as a college or granting any more "degrees" or "academic credits" without authorization from the Texas Department of Higher Education. Fry's book *Laugh Your Way to Health* (1991) states that he did not complete high school, but attended college for three months—then dropped out "because they had nothing of significance to teach." The Diamonds quote him in *Living Health*: "On the day of reckoning, I doubt we will be judged by what certificates we have on the wall, but rather by the scars incurred in the battle for humanity."

Natural Hygiene advocates have written two other popular books: *The Beverly Hills Diet* (1981), by Judy Mazel, and *Unlimited Power* (1986), by Anthony Robbins.

Natural Hygiene is dangerous because it trivializes nutrient needs, encourages prolonged fasting, and discourages medical interventions almost across the board. While the Hygienic diet is admirably low in fat and high in fiber, the proscription of both dairy products and supplements in the context of a primarily raw-food diet is an invitation to osteoporosis. No scientific study has ever compared the disease and death rates of Hygienists with those of non-Hygienists. But it seems to me that the hazards of Natural Hygiene significantly outweigh the possible benefits.

### Ayurveda and Ayur-Ved

*Ayur* comes from the Sanskrit "ayus," meaning "life" or "life span." *Veda* has been interpreted as "knowledge," "science," and "sacred lore." Thus, Ayurveda is supposedly the science of life or longevity. Ayurvedic medicine is rooted in four Sanskrit books called the Vedas—the oldest and most important scriptures of India, shaped sometime before 500 B.C.E. The Vedas were thought to have been revealed by the godhead to sages, who passed them on by word of mouth. They consist of hymns, prayers, curses, incantations, and magico-religious poems. Vedic medicine developed as a combination of religious, magical, and empirical views and practices. The causes of disease include sin, violation of a norm, the unjust cursing of a fellow man, and the wrongs committed by one's parents or by "oneself" in a previous incarnation. Disease is either punishment meted out by the gods, directly or through demons, or is the result of witchcraft. Remedies include prayer, sacrifice, magic, exorcism, and water as a "purifier."

According to the principal Ayurvedic theory—called *tridosha*—the human body is composed of five "elements": earth, air, fire, water, and ether.

The preponderance of these elements determines various constitutional types, each prone to ailments due to a deficiency or excess of one or more elements. The fundamental constitutional types are *pitta*, *kapha*, and *vata*. These terms also designate the fundamental physiological forces—"humors" (body fluids) or *doshas*—postulated to characterize the types. *Pitta*—"fire" or "bile"—said to be a combination of fire and water, is analogous to the Chinese yang. *Kapha*—"mucus," "phlegm," or "water humor"—said to be a combination of earth and water, is analogous to the Chinese yin. *Vata*—"wind" or "air humor"—said to be a combination of air and "space," is believed to mediate between *pitta* and *kapha*. The *doshas* were identified with the three supposed universal forces: sun, moon, and wind.

The symptoms of excessive *pitta* are said to include anemia, cachexia (severe weight loss), diarrhea, fainting, fever, indigestion, nausea, vomiting, and generalized weakness. Insufficiency of *pitta* supposedly results in slowed digestion. Excessive *kapha* is said to cause anorexia, asthma, bronchitis, drowsiness, emaciation, fever, and vomiting, while excessive *vata* allegedly results in anorexia, diarrhea, fever, and generalized weakness. Fever and weakness thus are common to all excesses. The *doshas* purportedly can be balanced through meditation, diet, botanicals, specific exercises, and other means. According to Ayurveda, *prana*—the "life force"—is obtained from both food and the atmosphere. The Ayurvedic diet consists mainly of grains, ghee (a semifluid clarified butter), and certain vegetables.

Ayurvedic nutrition is concerned with "constitutional type," specific food characteristics, and the season of the year. Significant food characteristics include taste, temperature, oiliness/dryness, and liquidity/solidity. By Ayurvedic standards, foods capable of intensifying a particular *dosha* should not be consumed during the season in which the *dosha* predominates: Consuming spicy, pungent foods in summer is thought to intensify *pitta*; dry fruits and high-protein foods in autumn, *vata*; and cold drinks and dairy products in winter, *kapha*. For excess of *pitta*, astringent, bitter, and sweet foods are prescribed—e.g., beans, wheat and other grains, sweet milk, and bitter herbs. For excess of *kapha*, astringent, bitter, and pungent foods are prescribed—e.g., beans (again), hot spices, and acidic fruits. For excessive *vata*, acidic, salty, and sweet foods are prescribed—e.g., wheat (again), milk (again), acidic fruits (again), warm drinks, and sweet vegetables.

Traditionally, if diet therapy proved ineffective or the illness was severe, fasting, emetics, "drastic" purgatives, and bloodletting were used. Indeed, they were considered preventive medicine: an emetic biweekly, a purgative every month, and bloodletting twice a year. In traditional Ayurveda, alcoholism, anorexia, nausea, indigestion, ascites (fluid accumulation within the abdomen), and edema are treated with goat feces washed with urine; constipation is treated with a mixture of milk and urine; impotence is treated with 216 kinds of enemas (some including the testicles of peacocks, swans, and turtles); and epilepsy and insanity are treated with ass urine.

### "Spiritual Regeneration" and TM

Ayurvedic medicine's chief patron, the Maharishi Mahesh Yogi, was born in India in 1911. After attending Allahabad University, he became a monk and for thirteen years studied mysticism in the Himalayas. After his guru's death in 1953, he retreated to a cave, where he lived for two years.

The transcendental meditation movement began in India in 1955. According to *TM: Discovering Inner Energy and Overcoming Stress* (1975), by Harold H. Bloomfield, M.D., and associates, in 1958 the Maharishi "proclaimed the possibility of all humanity's attaining enlightenment" and inaugurated a "World Plan" intended to encompass "every individual on earth." Shortly thereafter, he embarked upon a world tour to spread his teachings. His world headquarters is now in the Netherlands.

The practice of TM (transcendental meditation) involves sitting in a comfortable position with one's eyes closed for fifteen to twenty minutes twice a day, mentally repeating a mantra—a "secret" magic word said to be chosen expressly for the meditator by a TM teacher.

In the 1970s, sociologist Eric Woodrum investigated the TM movement as a participant and divided it into three phases: During the "Spiritual-Mystical Period" (1959–1965), TM, under the auspices of the Spiritual Regeneration Movement, was considered the centerpiece of a "traditional" Hindu program leading ultimately to nirvana (extinction of the ego). During the "Voguish, Self-Sufficiency Period" (1966–1969), the movement became nontraditional and countercultural, and the goal of nirvana receded. During the "Secularized, Popular-Religious Period," which began in 1970, the movement shifted its public emphasis from "spiritual" goals to the alleged physiological, material, and social benefits of TM for conventional people. It produces a steady flow of "scientific validation" through an organizational arm, Maharishi International University.

In the mid-1970s, the Maharishi began professing he could teach advanced meditators to levitate. In the Spring 1989 issue of *Skeptical Inquirer*, Indian magician B. Premanand reported that in 1977 he had challenged the Maharishi to fly by his own power over a distance of about two miles. The Maharishi said he would do so if paid the equivalent of about $1,000, which he believed Premanand and his skeptics group could not afford. However, when they returned the next day with the money, the Maharishi declined to take flight, declaring that TM is not for demonstration purposes. Actually, "yogic flyers" become "airborne" only by hopping and do not reach an altitude of more than a foot.

In 1987, a federal court jury awarded $137,890 to an ex-devotee who contended that TM organizations had falsely promised that he could learn to levitate, reduce stress, improve his memory, and reverse the aging process. In 1988, an appeals court ordered a new trial. On June 20, 1991, the *Des Moines Register* reported that the case had been settled out of court for about $50,000.

According to the National Council Against Health Fraud's March/April 1991 newsletter, "Paraplegics have been bilked by promises that with enough TM training they would eventually rise from their wheelchairs by levitation." Other alleged benefits of TM and TM-Sidhi (advanced TM) have included elephantine strength, perfect health, immortality, "mastery over nature," "naturally correct" social behavior, and the powers of invisibility, immateriality, and telepathy.

### The Maharishi's Chief Messenger

Deepak Chopra, M.D., was born and raised in New Delhi, India, and attended the All India Institute of Medical Sciences. After graduation, he moved to the United States and completed residency training in internal medicine and endocrinology. According to a 1993 lecture pamphlet, after becoming chief of staff at the New England Memorial Hospital and establishing a large private practice, Chopra "noticed a growing lack of fulfillment and the nagging question, 'Am I doing all that I can for my patients?'" These problems, the pamphlet states, inspired him to learn TM and meet the Maharishi. The May/ June 1990 issue of *In Health* relates that in 1985 the Maharishi persuaded Chopra to found the American Association of Ayurvedic Medicine and become medical director of the Maharishi Ayur-Veda Health Center for Behavioral Medicine and Stress Management in Lancaster, Massachusetts.

Chopra calls himself the "chief messenger" of Ayurvedic medicine. In an audiotaped interview, he stated:

> According to Maharishi Ayur-Veda, it is consciousness which conceives, constructs, and actually becomes the physical body. . . . Our thoughts are really processes that become molecules. If you have happy thoughts, then you make happy molecules. On the other hand, if you have sad thoughts and angry thoughts and hostile thoughts, then

you make those molecules, which may depress the immune system and make you more susceptible to disease.

In *Perfect Health: The Complete Mind/Body Guide* (1990), Chopra asserts that attaining perfect health "is only a question of following the silent river of intelligence to its source." He advocates TM, aromatherapy, and "purification" programs. Early in 1991, it was reported that *Perfect Health* had sold eighty thousand copies, that the Lancaster center was booked up to a year in advance, and that thirteen similar centers in the United States had served more than a hundred thousand clients since 1985. A profile of Chopra in the January/February 1992 *American Health* stated that twelve to fourteen new patients per week underwent diagnosis and treatment at his facility, at a cost of $2,500 to $4,300 or more per person.

In 1985, the Maharishi began marketing a variety of products and services under the trademark "Maharishi Ayur-Veda" (changed to "Maharishi Ayur-Ved" in January 1993). These now include *Maharishi Amrit Kalash* ("the perfect nutritional food"); *rasayanas* ("rejuvenating" herbs); herbal teas, seasonings, aromatic oils, herbal cleansing bars, shampoos, and cosmetics related to Ayurvedic "mind-body types"; sweetened nut-butter spreads with herbs ("traditional health treats"); books and videotapes "of timeless knowledge"; and Vedic music cassettes and compact discs that are "in alliance with natural law" and "designed to be played at specific times of the day." *Maharishi Amrit Kalash* is said to increase stamina, happiness, and well-being; to improve mental clarity; and to protect "brain receptors from harmful chemicals while allowing the binding of naturally occurring neurochemicals associated with positive emotions." Two "complementary" formulations are available: "M4" (also called *Nectar*) is a combination of herbs and gooseberry-fruit concentrate; it costs $49.50 for twenty-one ounces. "M5" (also called *Ambrosia*) costs $45 for sixty "herbal tablets."

For health maintenance, proponents also recommend training courses in TM and TM-Sidhi for a total cost of $3,400, instruction in the Maharishi Psychophysiological and Primordial Sound Techniques for $1,400, and three weeks of *panchakarma* annually for $2,700 to $6,600. In *Perfect Health*, Chopra defines *panchakarma* as "purification treatment," the goal of which is to rid the body of *ama* ("residual impurities deposited in the cells as the result of improper digestion"). Chopra lists six steps of *panchakarma*: (1) "oleation," the ingestion of clarified butter or a medicated oil "to soften up the *doshas* and minimize digestive action"; (2) administration of a laxative to reduce *pitta*; (3) oil massage, the oil "herbalized" according to constitutional type; (4) "herbalized" steam treatments; (5) administration of medicated enemas (Ayurveda "lists well over a hundred") to "flush the loosened *doshas* out through the intestinal tract"; and (6) "inhalation" of medicinal oils or herbal mixtures.

Maharishi Ayur-Ved products are not only prescribed by Ayurvedic physicians, but are marketed by mail and at health fairs. Magazine ads, for example, have invited readers to have their body type determined by completing a questionnaire and submitting it with $14.95—for which they receive an analysis, "personalized dietary recommendations," and product literature. Similar questionnaires have been used at health fairs, where no fee is involved but respondents are urged to buy an herbal tea to balance their *doshas*. The questions involve, for example, hair texture, mental activity, memory, size of teeth, kind of dreams, and reactions to weather. In the January/February 1991 *Nutrition Forum*, Dr. Stephen Barrett reported an amusing experience at the Ayur-Veda booth at Whole Life Expo in New York City:

> I was informed by a Maharishi Ayur-Veda exhibitor that my "doshas" were imbalanced, and he offered to sell me a tea to correct this. When I indicated that my health was good, he replied that achieving balance through Ayurvedic measures would prevent *future* trouble.

One goal of Maharishi Ayur-Ved is "to achieve world peace by creating peace on the level of the individual." In 1992, TM proponents launched the Natural Law Party and fielded a presidential candidate and many candidates for state and federal offices. Its platform was expressed in a twenty-four-page advertisement, in tabloid format, distributed shortly before the November election. The health section stated:

> The Natural Law Party envisions a disease-free society, in which every American enjoys a long life in perfect health. By bringing life into accord with natural law, the prevention programs proposed by the Natural Law Party will eliminate disease and culture ideal health and vitality for everyone. . . .
>
> Research suggests that implementing the programs proposed by the Natural Law Party could cut healthcare costs in half, saving an estimated $400 billion annually for the nation.

Ayurveda proponents use a language of their own to describe practices that are not grounded in scientific knowledge. The diet they espouse appears innocuous, but it is based on religious, not scientific, principles.

## Edgar Cayce

Edgar Cayce (1877–1945), dubbed the "Sleeping Prophet" by biographer Jess Stern, was a precursor of "New Age" trance channeling, giving well over fourteen thousand "psychic readings" between 1910 and his death. A poorly educated photographer and Sunday-school teacher with no medical training whatsoever, Cayce gained nationwide renown for diagnosing illnesses and prescribing dietary and other remedies while in a self-induced hypnotic state. His current promoters claim:

> He could see into the future and the past . . . describe present far-off events as they were happening; and . . . astound doctors with his x-ray vision of the human body. His readings—his words while in this state—were carefully transcribed while they were spoken. He is undoubtedly the most documented psychic who ever lived. And the accuracy of his predictions has been put at well over ninety percent! At his death, he left a legacy of thousands of case histories that science is still at a loss to explain completely.

Cayce's career as a clairvoyant began in 1901 after a hypnotic session with a "magnetic healer." In a trance, Cayce supposedly diagnosed the source of—and prescribed a cure for—his own persistent case of laryngitis. According to *Mysteries of Mind, Space & Time—The Unexplained* (1992), Cayce similarly helped the hypnotist, who proposed that they use this method to cure others. When Cayce refused, his laryngitis recurred. Interpreting the recurrence as a divine gesture, he formed a partnership with the hypnotist. *Mysteries* states that whenever Cayce decided to quit giving "readings," he lost his voice or developed a severe headache. As news of the "healings" spread, thousands sought his help. Cayce offered guidance both to persons in attendance and to distant correspondents; he supposedly needed only the person's name and address. Allegedly drawing upon a "cosmic hall of records," Cayce revealed "facts" about mythical civilizations, astrological influences, "past lives," and future events. In *The Outer Limits of Edgar Cayce's Power* (1971), Cayce's sons stated that the transcripts of the readings comprise over fifty thousand single-spaced typewritten pages and more than ten million words.

### Cayce's Legacies

Five organizations have grown up around Cayce's work. The headquarters of the Association for Research and Enlightenment (A.R.E.), which occupies an entire city block in Virginia Beach, is home to four of them: Atlantic University, the Harold J. Reilly School of Massotherapy, the Edgar Cayce Foundation, and A.R.E., Inc.

According to its 1993–94 catalog, Atlantic University opened in 1930, closed two years later, and reopened in 1985. Although not accredited, it awards a master of arts degree in "transpersonal studies"—a term described in the catalog as "an interdisciplinary field which includes psychology, philosophy, sociology, literature, religion, and science." The courses cover astrology, dream work, *I Ching,* Jungian psychology, palmistry, psychometry, tarot, and processes to "balance and transform" human "energies." Students may pursue the master's degree largely by correspondence.

The Reilly School, which operates under the auspices of the university, was founded in 1931 and reopened in 1986. Certified by the Commonwealth of Virginia, the school offers a 600-hour diploma program in massage therapy. The program includes instruction in shiatsu, foot reflexology, hydrotherapy, diet, and preventive healthcare based on the Cayce readings. The school also offers workshops on biofeedback and Cayce home remedies.

The Edgar Cayce Foundation, chartered in 1948, was formed to preserve the Cayce readings and supporting documentation.

The A.R.E., which Cayce's son Hugh Lynn Cayce co-founded in 1931, functions as an eclectic "New Age" nerve center, from which emanates a steady flow of seminars and publications. A 1991 brochure describes it as "a living network of people who are finding a deeper meaning in life through the psychic work of Edgar Cayce." In 1976, Hugh Lynn became board chairman and his son, Charles Thomas Cayce, became president. The A.R.E. headquarters, a modern three-story building in Virginia Beach, includes a visitor/conference center, a library, and the A.R.E. bookstore. It receives more than forty thousand visitors and conference attendees annually. With more than fifty thousand volumes, the library has one of the world's largest collections of parapsychological and metaphysical literature.

Standard A.R.E. membership costs $30 per year, but nine-month "introductory" memberships are available for $15 or $20. Members receive the bimonthly magazine *Venture Inward* and can borrow books from the A.R.E. Library, join a study group, and attend or send their children to A.R.E.'s summer camp in the Appalachian foothills. They are also entitled to referrals to over four hundred practitioners who use the Cayce approach. In September 1992, an A.R.E. representative informed me that membership was approximately thirty-nine thousand, plus about a thousand subscribers.

Members are also invited to participate in "home research projects," in which they perform activities pertaining to such matters as astrology and numerology and report the results. Participation is free for some projects, but others cost from $17 to about $30 per person. A 1991 issue of the *Home Research Project* bulletin states: "The main commitment of A.R.E. as a research organization is to encourage you to test concepts in the Cayce readings and to look for—and expect—results." Study groups center on such concerns as diet, the laws of reincarnation (karma), metaphysical dream interpretation, and the spiritual legacies of ancient Egypt and Atlantis. According to an A.R.E. letter, "Thousands gather together in small groups all over the country to study and apply spiritual principles in daily living." A.R.E. mailings to prospective members state: "There is no human problem for which the Cayce predictions do not offer hope." A.R.E. "research reports," based on the Cayce readings, are available on a wide variety of topics, including scar removal, warts, arthritis, diabetes, and multiple sclerosis.

Each year, A.R.E. holds dozens of conferences in Virginia Beach and various other cities. They have covered such subjects as angels, astrology ("the key to self-discovery"), chakra healing, "intuitive healing," reincarnation, UFOs, weight control, and "holistic" financial management. A flyer for a 1992 "psychic training" seminar states: "You are already psychic.... You only need to become aware of it!"

Many of Cayce's remedies are sold through the mail by Home Health Products, Inc., also in Virginia Beach. Home Health specializes in "natural products for a holistic approach to health care" and bills itself as an "official supplier of Edgar Cayce products for health, beauty, and wellness." Its own products include skin conditioners, laxatives, and a few supplements, but its catalog also offers supplements made by other companies. Products advertised therein have included: (1) *ANF-22*, touted as "powerful relief from the pain, swelling and stiffness of arthritis"; (2) *Aphro* "Herbal Love Tonic"; (3) *Bio Ear*, said to provide "all-natural relief for ringing, buzzing, and noise in the ear"; (4) *Brain Waves*, described as a mental stimulant; (5) *Cata-Vite* (formerly *Cata-Rx*), said to be "a safe non-prescription formula which counteracts nutritional deficiencies associated with age-related cataracts"; (6) *His Ease*, alleged to "increase seminal fluid and sexual virility"; (7) *Kidney Flush*, claimed to "help flush away urinary infections"; (8) *Liva-Life*, for "toxic overload"; (9) *Liver Tonic Detoxifier*, "an all-natural mixture that detoxifies and cleanses the liver"; (10) *Prostate Plus*, proposed as an alternative to surgery; (11) *Ribo Flex*, "muscle/joint nourishment that reduces painful muscle spasms and enhances natural flexing action"; (12) *Sugar Block*, said to "prevent absorption of unwanted sugar"; (13) *Thyro-Vital*, claimed to "improve thyroid function"; (14) Jerusalem Artichoke Capsules, an Edgar Cayce product described as "a natural equivalent to insulin injections"; and (15) *Mummy Food* (nuggets composed of figs, dates, and cornmeal). The Winter 1992 catalog states:

> Mummy Food has a fascinating history. In a dream that Edgar Cayce had concerning the discovery of ancient records in Egypt, a mummy came to life to help him translate these records. This mummy gave directions for the preparation of food that she required, thus the name

"mummy food.". . . For particular individuals [Cayce] stated that it was "almost a spiritual food."

The company's brochure states: "In addition to changes in diet, Edgar Cayce frequently recommended specific remedies and treatments. Many of these had to be custom-formulated from herbs, oils, and other naturally occurring substances." An A.R.E. videotape describes Cayce's home remedies, a collection of sixteen methods that include: castor-oil packs ("to help with arthritis, colds, gallstones, ulcers, and more"), peanut-oil massages ("to prevent arthritis"), potato poultices ("to relieve tired or strained eyes"), castor-oil liniments ("to remove warts"), and coffee-ground foot baths ("to soothe sore feet and improve circulation in the legs").

The A.R.E. Bookstore, which sells direct and by mail, features many books by or about Cayce, including *The Complete Edgar Cayce Readings* on CD-ROM, priced at $500. It also carries a large selection of uncritical books and videotapes on paranormal and supernaturalistic topics, including guardian angels, "magic" flower remedies, "money magnetism," Japanese astrology ("nine star ki"), the souls of animals, chakras, the "human energy field," reincarnation, crystal healing, the healing "art of bioenergy," and the "healing power of prayer."

Another item sold by the bookstore is the *Physician's Reference Notebook*, by William A. McGarey, M.D., and associates. The book offers treatment recommendations based on the Cayce readings for over fifty diseases and conditions, including baldness, breast cancer, color blindness, diabetes, hemophilia, hydrocephalus, leukemia, multiple sclerosis, muscular dystrophy, stroke, stuttering, and syphilis. In the 1980s, an A.R.E. mailing to chiropractors stated:

> This book is a "magic tool" to be used in conjunction with your professional skill and knowledge in healing some of your more difficult cases. One of our colleagues, using the information in our commentaries, has cured dozens of psoriasis cases. . . . Even some of the neurological degenerative conditions, such as M.S. [multiple sclerosis], A.L.S. [amyotrophic lateral sclerosis], or even . . . [foot drop] have responded exceptionally well to these recommendations.

According to the *Notebook*: (1) baldness is most often caused by glandular insufficiency and spinal lesions (subluxations); (2) color blindness is caused by the conduct of the afflicted person in a past life, and treatment should include spinal adjustments and a diet consisting mostly of alkali-producing foods; (3) hemophilia is correctable, "a simple case of a deep-seated defect in the assimilations of the body," and treatment of newborns so afflicted should consist primarily in the addition of blood pudding to the diet; (4) obesity is caused principally by an excess of starches in the diet, and treatment should include the elimination of most starches; and (5) psoriasis is caused by a thinning of the intestinal walls, which "allows toxic products from the intestinal tract to leak into the circulatory system and find their way into the lymph flow of the skin."

### The A.R.E. Clinic

In 1970, William A. McGarey, M.D., and his wife, Gladys McGarey, M.D., founded the A.R.E. Clinic in Phoenix, Arizona. According to *Medical World News*, they opened the facility to offer "comprehensive care to patients seeking holistic medical alternatives." Later, Gladys McGarey resigned as clinic co-director and set up another "holistic" practice in Scottsdale, Arizona, with their physician-daughter.

A founding member of the American Holistic Medical Association, William McGarey is currently board chairman of the clinic. In an interview in *Health Talks* (1989), he said that the clinic had a staff of forty-five or fifty persons, including five physicians (one an osteopath), a chiropractor, and a psychologist with a doctoral degree. An advertisement for the clinic in the January/February 1992 issue of *East West Natural Health* names two naturo-paths.

In the *Health Talks* interview, McGarey denied any conflict or contradiction between his Cayce-based practices and his medical education. "The philosophy behind the A.R.E. clinic," he said, "is that everyone is a whole human being . . . created in the image of God." According to McGarey, the clinic consists of a general practice, a "brain injury center," and an "energy medicine center that looks at the biomagnetic energies of the body." The clinic offerings include "electromagnetic field therapy," relaxation training, the laying on of hands, and the residential Temple Beautiful Program. McGarey described this as an eleven-day "rejuvenation program" that includes dream analysis, stress reduction, visualization, biofeedback, exercise, nutrition, and supplementation. A 1991 brochure stated that the program had been conducted more than two hundred times over the past decade, accommodates ten to fifteen participants, and costs $4,100. In 1990, the clinic began offering telephone consultations, which cost $50 per session of fifteen to sixty minutes.

In *Health Talks*, McGarey lamented: "When doctors fail to recognize the spiritual aspect of the human being, they miss the most important part." When one recognizes our destiny as "getting back to our spiritual origin," he said, "there is a different kind of emphasis on healing; you do not get tied up with modalities. Healing is more of a spiritual event." McGarey also stated that when treating someone, "we cannot consider ourselves as the healer. We are only the . . . channel of the Great Healer." In *Edgar Cayce Remedies* (1983), McGarey advocates application of potato poultices to the eyes for cataracts, monthly "high-colonic" enemas for angina pectoris, and castor-oil packs for epilepsy and cat bites.

### Diet Basics

Parapsychology popularizer Hans Holzer, Ph.D., has called Cayce the "greatest of all dietetic healers." In *Beyond Medicine* (1987) he writes: "Edgar Cayce abundantly made clear in his writings [that] certain combinations of foodstuffs are chemically incompatible in the human system [and] can create damage or at the very least ill health." Holzer gives two examples: coffee should be taken black or with hot milk, but not with cold milk; and tea with sugar, especially white sugar, can damage the liver, while tea with honey does not.

According to an A.R.E. Clinic chart: (1) eighty percent of one's daily food intake should consist of fruits and fruit juices, vegetables, water, and herbal teas; (2) twenty percent should consist of dairy products (including whole milk and butter), whole-grain breads, high-fiber cereals (including granola), honey, soups, fowl, lamb, and fish; (3) one serving about three times per week should suffice for beef, brown rice, oils, potatoes with skin, cheese, eggs, spices, gelatin products, and desserts (e.g., ice cream); and (4) fried foods, alcohol, pasta, white bread, pork, and "processed foods" should be avoided—except "crisp bacon," which may be eaten occasionally.

*Edgar Cayce on Diet and Health* offers the following advice to "normal," healthy people who are not overweight:

- Canned tomatoes are usually preferable to fresh.

- Gelatin enhances glandular activity.

- Certified raw milk is to be preferred, unless it came from cows that eat certain types of weeds or grass growing in January.

- Raw green peppers should not be eaten without other foods.

- One's diet should consist of 80 percent alkaline-producing and 20 percent acid-producing foods.

- Citrus fruits and cereals should not be eaten together.

- No combination whatsoever of white bread, potatoes, and spaghetti should be eaten at the same meal.

- Orange juice and milk should be drunk separately at opposite ends of the day.

- Ideally, lime juice should be added to orange juice, and lemon juice to grapefruit juice (an idea, the authors admitted, "probably new to those working in the science of modern dietetics and food research").

- Neither citrus juices nor tomato juice should be consumed with any starch other than whole-wheat bread.

- It is better to consume meats with sweets than with starches.

- Ice cream is far preferable to pie, which combines starches and sweets.

- Cheese and cream are "good for the system."

- It is "normal" to consume above-ground and below-ground vegetables in a ratio of three to one.

- Squirrel should be stewed or well cooked.

The effect on our society of nonsense as diverse, intricate, and profuse as that of the Edgar Cayce tradition is incalculable. As far as I know, however, no study has been conducted to determine the extent to which Cayce advocates follow his advice or what impact their practices have on their lives. Neither has it been determined whether they seek appropriate medical intervention when it is needed. The A.R.E. dietary philosophy—derived from Cayce's "psychic readings"—is nebulous, internally contradictory, and possibly conducive to chronic confusion.

Actually, unreason permeates all forms of vitalistic "healing."

# 17

# The Multilevel Mirage

### Stephen Barrett, M.D.

Don't be surprised if a friend or acquaintance tries to sell you vitamins, herbs, homeopathic remedies, weight-loss powders, or other health-related products. Millions of Americans have signed up as distributors for companies that market such products from person to person. Often they have tried the products, concluded that they work, and become suppliers to support their habit.

Multilevel marketing (also called network marketing) is a form of direct sales in which independent distributors sell products, usually in their customers' home or by telephone. In theory, distributors can make money not only from their own sales but also from those of the people they recruit.

Becoming a distributor is easy. It usually involves completing a one-page application and spending $25 to $50 for a distributor kit. Kits typically include a sales manual, product literature, order forms, and a subscription to a magazine or newsletter published by the company. Distributors can buy products "wholesale," sell them "retail," and recruit other distributors who can do the same. When enough distributors have been enrolled, the recruiter is eligible to collect a percentage of their sales. Companies suggest that this process provides a great money-making opportunity. However, it is unlikely that people who don't join during the first few months of operation or become one of the early distributors in their community can build enough of a sales pyramid to do well. And many who stock up on products to meet sales goals get stuck with unsold products that cost thousands of dollars.

Most multilevel companies that market health products claim that their products can prevent or cure a wide range of diseases. A few companies merely suggest that people will feel better, look better, or have more energy if they supplement their diet with extra nutrients. When clear-cut therapeutic claims are made in product literature, the company is an easy target for government enforcement action. Some companies run this risk, hoping that the government won't take action until their customer base is well established. Other companies make no claims in their literature but rely on testimonials, encouraging people to try their products and credit them for any improvement that occurs.

Most multilevel companies tell distributors to make no claims for the products except those found in company literature. (That way the company can deny responsibility for what distributors do.) However, many companies hold sales meetings at which people are encouraged to tell their story to the others in attendance. Some companies sponsor telephone conference calls during which leading distributors describe their financial success, give sales tips, and describe their personal experiences with the products. Testimonials may also be published in company magazines, audiotapes, and videotapes. Testimonial claims can trigger enforcement action, but since it is time-consuming to collect evidence of their use, government agencies seldom bother to do so.

Government enforcement action against multilevel companies has not been vigorous. These companies are usually left alone unless their promotions become so conspicuous and their sales volume so great that an agency feels compelled to intervene. Even then, few interventions have substantial impact once a company is well established.

**Typical Promotions**

During the past ten years, I have investigated more than forty multilevel companies marketing health products. Here are some examples:

• Enrich International, Pleasant Grove, Utah, markets more than 150 herbal, homeopathic, and supplement products. Its products have included *Tummy Gum*, for appetite control; *Increase*, claimed to be a homeopathic product that can correct all types of baldness problems; *Cataract*, "to aid . . . any eye and vision problems, cataracts being the most severe"; and *Co-Q10*, claimed to improve angina pectoris, congestive heart failure, high blood pressure, diabetes, and gum disease. Distributors are given *The Mini Herb Guide*, which specifies products for seventy types of health problems. A disclaimer says that the information "should not be used for diagnosing and prescribing" and "is not intended as a substitute for medical care." In 1990, the FDA asked the company to recall nine product information sheets that contained misleading and unapproved therapeutic claims. Subsequently, Woodland Books, Provo, Utah, which publishes books about herbs and "alternative" health-care methods, sent a mailing to distributors with a message on the envelope: "Here are the tools to help sell your Enrich products." Inside were its catalog, a similar message from Enrich's president, and a flyer stating that "Woodland's books help create markets for your products." One book was *The Little Herb Encyclopedia,* by Jack Ritchason, a leading Enrich distributor.

• Light Force, of Santa Cruz, California, markets spirulina products with claims that they can suppress appetite, boost immunity, and increase energy. Company sales materials claim that spirulina is a "superfood" and "works to cleanse and detoxify the body." Its magazine, *The Enlightener,* has carried reports about users who lost weight or recovered from arthritis, cancer, multiple sclerosis, and serious injuries while taking Light Force products.

• Matol Botanical International, a Canadian firm, markets *Km,* a foul-tasting extract of fourteen common herbs. Although company literature states that no therapeutic claims can be made for *Km* in the United States, I have received many reports that distributors are making such claims. A *Km* brochure describes alleged uses of the herbs in centuries past. For example, celery seed is said to contain compounds that "have been found to be gently calming," while passion flower was believed to "quiet and soothe the body and assure peaceful rest." *Km* was originally marketed in Canada as *Matol,* which was claimed effective for ailments ranging from arthritis to cancer, as well as rejuvenation. Canada's Health Protection Branch took action that resulted in an order to advertise only its name, price, and contents. In 1988, the FDA attempted to block importation of *Matol* into the United States, but the company circumvented the ban by adding an ingredient and changing the product's name.

• Nature's Sunshine Products, headquartered in Spanish Fork, Utah, markets more than four hundred herbal products, nutritional supplements, homeopathic remedies, skin and hair-care products, water treatment systems, cooking utensils, and a weight-loss plan. Many of its products are claimed to "nourish" or "support" various body organs. Its distributors, dubbed "Natural Health Counselors," are taught to use iridology, muscle-testing (a type of applied kinesiology), and other dubious methods to convince people that they need the products. The company also markets a weight-loss program based on "glandular body types" not recognized by the scientific community.

• Omnitrition International, Inc., of, Carrollton, Texas, markets supplement products based on formulations by Durk Pearson and Sandy Shaw, authors of *Life Extension.* One product is *WOW!,* "a nutritional alternative to coffee," which contains 80 mg of caffeine and various amounts of vitamins, minerals, and amino acids. Another, *Be Your Best,* is promoted as a bodybuilding aid. Still another is *Omni IV,* a liquid multivitamin/vitamin mineral product for "anyone who is tired of troublesome pills and tablets as a source of nutritional supplementation." (The retail cost is $2.18 per day, about one hundred times the cost of equivalent pills.) Omnitrition's sales manual suggests approaching prospects by offering to show how to double and even triple their current income over the next twelve months. The manual also advises distributors to promote the products by telling how much they like them rather than focusing on ingredients. In 1992, a former distributor filed a class action suit charging that the company was operating an illegal pyramid scheme and exaggerating the financial potential of becoming a distributor.

• Rexall Showcase International (RSI), headquartered in Fort Lauderdale, Florida, markets a weight-loss program, homeopathic remedies, and assorted supplement products. One homeopathic product, *In•Vigor•Ol*, is claimed to be "a natural tonic, "designed for those times when you are troubled with everyday fatigue, general tired feeling and exhaustion." The supplement products include *Workout* ("to aid in your own natural muscular recovery process"), *Energy Essentials* (to "provide the nutrients your body needs to help maximize its natural energy-generating abilities"), and *Essential Bodyguard* (needed because "today's stressful lifestyles can deplete the nutrients your body needs to maintain a healthy immune system").

• Sunrider International, of Torrence, California, markets herbal products with claims that they can help "regenerate" the body. Although some of the ingredients can exert pharmacological effects on the body, there is little evidence they can cure major diseases or that Sunrider distributors are qualified to advise people how to use them properly. During the mid-1980s, the FDA took several regulatory actions to stop false and misleading health claims for several Sunrider products. In 1989, the company signed a consent agreement pledging to pay $175,000 to the state of California and to stop representing that its products have any effect on disease or medical conditions. The company toned down its literature but continued to make therapeutic claims in testimonial tapes included in its distributor kits.

Sunrider products were marketed with an elaborate story that company president Tei Fu Chen had derived the formulas from ancient Chinese manuscripts and was a medical doctor, a "senior research scientist," a licensed pharmacist, and a "world-renowned nutritionist." In 1992, a jury in Arizona found the company guilty of racketeering and awarded $650,000 to Debi A. Boling, who had charged that Sunrider products had discolored her teeth, made her severely nauseous, and caused her to lose large amounts of hair from her head. Testimony during the trial indicated that the story about Chen's background was a complete fabrication. To win her case, Ms. Boling had to persuade the jury that she had been injured by a criminal act done with fraudulent intent for financial gain. After hearing testimony over a three-month period, the jury awarded her $50,000 for actual damages, which were tripled under the state's racketeering law, plus an additional $500,000 for punitive damages.

• United Sciences of America (USA) of Carrollton, Texas, which began marketing early in 1986, used high-tech videotapes to promote its products. Its introductory tape was narrated by William Shatner (Captain Kirk of *Star Trek*) and filled with scenes of laboratories, computers, and prominent medical institutions. Another tape related the ingredients in USA's products—including beta-carotene, fish oils, and fiber—to research on the prevention of cancer, heart disease, and other conditions. The company claimed that these products comprised a "revolutionary" nutrition program designed and endorsed by a scientific advisory board that included two Nobel prize winners and several other medical school professors. Eight months after USA began marketing, the company had over 100,000 distributors and was grossing millions of dollars each month. However, it drew a great deal of unfavorable publicity when several advisors denied endorsing the products and other critics challenged the claims made in the videotapes. The resultant scandal plus action by the FDA and three state attorneys-general quickly drove the company out of business.

## Motivation: Powerful but Misguided

The "success" of network marketing lies in the enthusiasm of its participants. Most people who think they have been helped by an unorthodox method enjoy sharing their success stories with their friends. Those who give such testimonials are usually motivated by a sincere wish to help their fellow humans. Since people tend to believe what others tell them about personal experiences, testimonials can be powerful persuaders.

Perhaps the trickiest misconception about quackery is that personal experience is the best way to tell whether something works. When someone feels better after having used a product or procedure, it is natural to give credit to whatever was done. This is unwise, however. Most ailments are self-limiting, and even incurable conditions can have sufficient day-to-day variation to enable bogus methods to gain large followings. In addition, taking some kind of action often produces temporary relief of symptoms (a placebo effect). For these reasons, scientific experimentation is almost always necessary to establish whether health methods are really effective. Instead of testing their products, multilevel companies urge customers to try them and credit them if they feel better. Some products are popular because they contain caffeine, ephedrine (a stimulant), valerian (a tranquilizer), or other substances that produce mood-altering effects.

Another factor in gaining devotees is the emotional impact of group activities. Imagine, for example, that you have been feeling lonely, bored, depressed, or tired. One day a friend tells you that "improving your nutrition" can help you feel better. After selling you some products, the friend inquires regularly to find out how you are doing. You seem to feel somewhat better. From time to time you are invited to interesting lectures where you meet people like yourself. Then you are asked to become a distributor. This keeps you busy, raises your income, and provides an easy way to approach old friends and make new ones—all in an atmosphere of enthusiasm. Some of your customers express gratitude, giving you a feeling of accomplishment. People who increase their income, their social horizons, or their self-esteem can get a psychological boost that not only can improve their mood but also may alleviate emotionally-based symptoms.

Multilevel companies refer to this process as "sharing" and suggest that everyone involved is a "winner." That simply isn't true. The entire process is built on a foundation of deception. The main winners are the company's owners and the small percentage of distributors who become sales leaders.

Do you think that multilevel participants are qualified to judge whether prospective customers need supplements—or medical care? Even though therapeutic claims are forbidden by the written policies of each company, the sales process encourages customers to experiment with self-treatment. It may promote distrust of legitimate health professionals and their treatment methods. It even may cause some people to become alienated from their family and friends. Some would argue that the apparent benefits of "believing" in the products outweigh the risks involved. Do you think that people need false beliefs in order to feel healthy or succeed in life? Would you like to believe that something can help you when in fact it is worthless? Should our society support an industry that is trying to mislead us? Can't Americans do something better with the billion or more dollars being wasted each year on multilevel "health" products?

**Recommendations**

Consumers would be wise to avoid multilevel products altogether. Those that have nutritional value (such as vitamins and low-cholesterol foods) are invariably overpriced and may be unnecessary as well. Those promoted as remedies are either unproven, bogus, or intended for conditions that are unsuitable for self-medication.

Government agencies should police the multilevel marketplace aggressively, using undercover investigators and filing criminal charges when wrongdoing is detected.

# 18

# Acupuncture:
# Nonsense with Needles

### Arthur Taub, M.D., Ph.D.

Immediately before and after the visit of former President Richard M. Nixon to the People's Republic of China in 1972, reports circulated in the West suggesting that major surgery could be accomplished with acupuncture as the only anesthetic agent. The impression was given that acupuncture was widely used and could be applied in high-risk cases, in children, in the aged, and in veterinary surgery. Perhaps the best-known rumor about "acupuncture anesthesia" was that *The New York Times*'s noted political analyst James Reston had his appendix removed with acupuncture as the anesthetic. Whatever the reasons for the currency of these ideas, they were, every single one of them, untrue.

## Acupuncture as a System of Medicine

Chen-Chiu, or acupuncture-moxibustion, is a technique of medical treatment that began in Stone Age China. It consists of the insertion of needles into the skin, or muscles and tendons beneath, at one or more named points that are said to "represent" various internal organs. These "acupuncture points" are generally located where imaginary horizontal and vertical lines ("meridians") meet on the surface of the body. The organs are also "represented" by points on the surface of the ear or on one finger. Originally there were 365 points, corresponding to the days of the year, but the number identified by proponents has grown to over two thousand, and various charts locate the points differently.

According to classical theory, good health is said to be produced by a harmonious mixture of yin and yang, the fundamental activity characteristics of the universe, which combine to form the life force, *Ch'i* or *Qi*. The

259

disorganization of the flow of *Ch'i* is said to produce illness. The acupuncture needle supposedly can regulate this flow. Moxibustion is a technique in which the herb *Artemesia vulgaris,* or wormwood, is burned at specified points on or near the skin, sometimes to the point of blistering.

Classical Chinese physicians applied these techniques to the entire range of human illness. Surgery as such (save for the operation of castration used to supply eunuchs for the imperial household) was not a part of classical Chinese medicine. The diagnosis of disease was based mainly upon examination of the "pulse." This was not a measurement of the rate and rhythm of the heart, as is done nowadays. Rather, the "pulse" (with six varieties) was related to such things as the "texture" and force of the radial artery at several points of the wrist, while the artery was being compressed lightly or forcefully. Pulse diagnosis supposedly revealed the state of health of the various internal organs. Diagnosis was also based upon the history of the patient's symptoms, the appearance of the patient's tongue, and the state of the weather. Because dissection of the human body was not practiced, internal organs were imagined in rather odd positions and shapes, and some organs were invented. One of these was the "triple warmer," whose precise location baffles even the most astute translator of Chinese acupuncture classics.

Herbal pharmacology has played and continues to play a significant role in classical Chinese medicine. Herbs were generally made into a sort of tea. Some of these herbs (such as ma huang, which is known to contain ephedrine, a drug useful in the treatment of asthma) possess useful therapeutic properties. The majority of such preparations, however, are worthless. In recent years, many classical preparations have been "adulterated" with active agents that have not been listed as ingredients.

Classical Chinese medicine was practiced for thousands of years, maintained by the force of Buddhist and Confucian conservatism. Discerning Chinese were not always content with it, however, particularly when other forms of medical and surgical treatment became known to them.

### Resistance to Acupuncture in China

In the late nineteenth century, efforts by the waning Manchu dynasty toward modernization included an unsuccessful attempt to forbid acupuncture. In the following years, vigorous opposition to acupuncture was mounted by both right- and left-wing intellectuals. Notable among the latter group was Lu Hsun, a major figure in the literature of the People's Republic of China and an author much favored by then Communist party chairman Mao Tse-tung. Lu Hsun ridiculed traditional notions of physiology and indicted Chinese medicine for ineptness, ignorance, and greed.

These indictments were echoed in the 1930s and 1940s by Pa Chin, a revolutionary writer. Many conservative Chinese Nationalist intellectuals shared these authors' feelings of revulsion toward acupuncture and Chinese medicine. Repeated attempts by the Kuomintang (the nationalist people's party) to forbid acupuncture failed primarily because of political pressure. In spite of its low therapeutic value, many party members saw Chinese medicine as a part of the "national essence." Prior to the military unification of Mainland China in 1948–49, the Chinese Communists did not emphasize acupuncture as a medical technique.

Even though the Chinese Communist party made an intensive effort to eliminate traditional modes of thought and to reform social structure, acupuncture was retained as an integral portion of its national medical system. The party realized that the approximately ten thousand Western-trained physicians in China at the time of the Chinese Communist Revolution were too few to carry out the gigantic public health tasks necessary to modernize China. Medical personnel would therefore have to be recruited from among the approximately half a million practitioners of traditional Chinese medicine. It was apparently expected that these practitioners would gradually become more scientific in their work. As Chairman Mao put it: "Traditional Chinese medicine and pharmacology are a great treasure house. Efforts must be made to explore them and raise them to a higher level." Efforts by the Communists to elevate traditional Chinese practitioners, however, were hampered by the party's other political doctrines. As a result, unscientific medical practices remain widespread throughout China.

It appears, however, that acupuncture is not highly regarded within China's scientific community. The great majority of papers in the many journals published by the Chinese Medical Association are about scientific rather than traditional methods. Few articles concern themselves with acupuncture, herbalism, or their variants.

## Acupuncture Quackery

Many claims that acupuncture is effective have been publicly advanced—in China as well as elsewhere—without evidence to back them up. One strategy by which the Chinese promoted this fiction was to use acupuncture therapy together with known effective medication. For example, one Chinese textbook published in the early 1970s states:

Epilepsy is generally caused by rising air and congestion causing the heart to be stuffed and confused. The disease is in the heart, the liver, and the bladder. Treatment should be designed to ease the liver, to stop the rising air, to eliminate congestion, and to open up stuffed circulation.

The text then advocates six kinds of herbal mixtures, three forms of acupuncture, and the injection of vitamins into one of the acupuncture points. However, the effective medications diphenylhydantoin, phenobarbital, and primidone are suggested also. For myasthenia gravis, a disease in which muscles including those of breathing are easily fatigued, vigorous physical training methods including cold baths (which could be dangerous in this disease) are suggested by this same book. Thirteen acupuncture points are discussed, with vitamin injections suggested at some of them. Traditional Chinese herbs are suggested as a "tonic" to improve the "air." Again, however, the effective agents neostigmine, physostigmine, and ephedrine are also advised. A similar approach is used in treating Parkinsonism, for which acupuncture, Chinese herbal medicine, and effective medications such as the belladonna alkaloids are prescribed. There is not the slightest evidence to show that the traditional Chinese medical methods improve the modern treatment of these diseases in any way.

Another strategy used by the Chinese to suggest that acupuncture is effective was to suppress knowledge of the natural course of illnesses that improve spontaneously. Acupuncture was then given credit for curing illnesses that would have improved by themselves.

In 1974, I was a member of the Acupuncture Study Group of the Committee on Scholarly Communication with the People's Republic of China. Our group visited the Acupuncture Research Institute in Peking as well as traditional medical hospitals in the Shanghai region. There I observed one patient receive acupuncture treatment beginning two weeks after a stroke. Patients of this type tend to recover spontaneously and gradually. In fact, this patient, who had received acupuncture for six months, recovered no more and no less quickly than would be expected with no treatment or with a minimum of physical therapy. Several young women I examined had monthly migraine headaches associated with nausea, vomiting, spots before their eyes, and sensitivity to bright light. They told me that monthly acupuncture treatment limited their headaches to several days per month. They apparently did not know that this is the usual state of affairs without treatment.

Another strategy used by the Chinese was to claim benefit from acupuncture where none, in fact, existed. One nearsighted child I saw was given acupuncture treatment before receiving her eyeglasses. I was told that the treatment would enable her problem to be corrected with weaker lenses. This was simply untrue. Other patients with Parkinson's disease, spinal cord damage, and after-effects of head injury were also said to have gotten better, but my examination detected no improvement. Patients were also said to receive treatment for "nerve deafness." However, controlled studies conducted in the United States have failed to show that acupuncture can help nerve deafness.

### "Acupuncture Anesthesia"

Acupuncture is not widely used in China as an "anesthetic." A reasonable estimate of the total use of "acupuncture anesthesia" is approximately 5 to 10 percent. During our visit to China, the Acupuncture Study Group was able to substantiate a number of previous reports that almost all patients operated upon under "acupuncture anesthesia" received other agents in addition. This almost always included phenobarbital (a sedative) and meperidine (a narcotic pain-killer) before and during the operation. Local anesthesia was also used liberally. I personally witnessed operations in which local anesthesia was used from beginning to end, but which were nevertheless classified as done under "acupuncture anesthesia."

Acupuncture needles may be inserted as much as several inches beneath the skin directly into major nerve trunks. These can be stimulated with electric shocks to exhaust their ability to conduct impulses and produce local anesthesia—which is not an acupuncture effect.

"Acupuncture anesthesia" is not generally used for children under twelve because of their inability to cooperate. Elderly patients are generally not operated upon with "acupuncture anesthesia," and it is considered "experimental" in animals. (When it is done with animals, they are strapped tightly to the operating table.) On an occasion that I witnessed, a horse kicked vigorously during the operative procedure, suggesting that anesthesia was not working. The horse also drank with particular eagerness the water that was offered to it, suggesting that it was in surgical shock.

Acupuncture anesthesia is never used for emergency surgery. It is said to be applicable only to "classical" surgery—operations in which no complications are expected. These operations are performed so as to minimize tissue damage and pulling upon muscles or internal organs. To achieve this end, surgical incisions are made small. This means that the operative field is often poorly exposed, increasing the risk that important structures may be damaged. Proper exploration is usually not possible, wasting the opportunity to detect previously undiagnosed disease such as cancer.

The Chinese have stated that general anesthesia is always available as a "backup" procedure in case the patient experiences overwhelming pain when "acupuncture anesthesia" is used alone. In such cases, however, general anesthesia would be started in the midst of an already hazardous surgical situation. The most dangerous time during anesthesia is when the patient is being put to sleep, the time where spasms of the vocal cords or cardiac arrest are most likely to occur. If general anesthesia is delayed until severe pain requires its use, these dangers are increased.

Despite these drawbacks, some major surgical procedures have been performed in China using only small amounts of premedication, little or no local anesthetic, and the insertion of acupuncture needles. Surgical procedures that have been witnessed have gone well, but postoperative studies have not been done. Proper studies should not merely describe what has taken place, but should also consider that Chinese and Western patients may differ in their reactivity to pain and in cultural attitudes toward surgery. Since good statistical studies are not available from the Chinese, "acupuncture anesthesia" should be considered experimental. Doctors who undertake it, and patients who submit to it, should do so only under carefully controlled conditions in established research programs.

Are you wondering what happened to James Reston? Chemical anesthesia was used during the operation to remove his appendix. Acupuncture needles were said to have relieved his postoperative pain on the day following surgery, one hour after they were used. It seems more likely, however, that the relief resulted from the spontaneous return of normal intestinal function.

### Acupuncture "Clinics" and Failed Treatment in the United States

The popularization of acupuncture and its supposed therapeutic results led to rapid development of acupuncture "clinics" and "centers" throughout the United States. Some even provided bus transportation from local shopping centers to their premises. While the majority of these facilities were "supervised" by licensed physicians, acupuncture was performed in the usual manner, and diagnostic investigations were minimal. Previous diagnoses or misdiagnoses were often accepted, with therapy prescribed by ancient rule of thumb. The patients would generally be abandoned to their own devices if acupuncture did not prove successful after a few treatments. As in classical times (and in modern China), treatment was given for disorders in which symptoms vary with the weather and the disposition of the patient, such as generalized osteoarthritis, and for disorders in which remissions are the rule, such as multiple sclerosis.

During this period, I participated in a taped discussion with the director of one clinic who maintained that patients previously unable to walk because of multiple sclerosis had walked out of his facility unaided. The gentleman did not indicate how he had substantiated the diagnosis. Nor could he state what had prevented the patients from walking, whether their legs had been weak, their coordination or balance impaired, or some other reason. Nor could he state how and to what degree these functions had improved as a result of treatment. It should be clear that if a "paralyzed" patient walks unaided after brief treatment, it is certainly more appropriate to question the diagnosis than to praise the treatment!

As the number of acupuncture facilities increased, many patients for whom acupuncture had failed were seen at pain and arthritis clinics. Among those I personally attended were:

- A middle-aged gentleman with sexual impotence and suicidal depression. He had been treated with acupuncture needles placed in the thighs and in the region between the penis and the rectum. Later he required psychiatric treatment.

- A middle-aged woman with pain in the upper teeth who was treated with acupuncture stimulation with needles placed between the second and third toes of her foot. She required extensive dental diagnosis and treatment, as well as psychiatric care to compensate for the intense feelings of frustration that followed the failure of treatment.

- A middle-aged public relations man who was born with a malformed spinal canal. This gentleman had more pain at the end of treatment than when he began.

- Patients with osteoarthritis of the hands who showed minimal relief after the first, but increased pain after the last treatments, and who eventually abandoned them as useless.

- Patients with neuralgic pain following shingles which acupuncture did not help.

A remark characteristic of my patients was made by a middle-aged man with back pain, who said that acupuncture therapy had relieved him only of his money.

## Does Acupuncture Relieve Pain?

It is reasonably clear that acupuncture cannot cure any disease. Does it relieve pain? My clinical experience with acupunctured patients suggests that any pain relief following the procedure is short-lived. Formal studies have shown conflicting results. In most instances, acupuncture produced no better relief than was produced by a placebo. In other studies, acupuncture did produce some degree of difficulty in distinguishing a previously painful stimulus from a nonpainful stimulus, but this relief was minimal, of short duration, and not at all comparable with the degree of relief claimed for conventional acupuncture therapy. In 1990, a trio of Dutch epidemiologists analyzed fifty-one controlled studies of acupuncture for chronic pain and concluded that "the quality of even the better studies proved to be mediocre. . . . The efficacy of acupuncture in the treatment of chronic pain remains doubtful."

"Auriculotherapy" is a variant of acupuncture based on the notion that the body surface and organs are "represented" on the ear in a pattern that resembles an inverted fetus. Proponents claim that pain can be relieved by electrical stimulation of points that "correspond" to the painful area of the body. In 1984, the *Journal of the American Medical Association* published the results of a controlled study of thirty-six patients given auriculotherapy for chronic pain. The researchers found that stimulating locations recommended by auriculotherapy proponents was no more effective than barely touching remote points with or without electrical stimulation. The experiment demonstrated that any relief produced by auriculotherapy would be due to a placebo effect.

## Adverse Effects

Acupuncture has not merely failed to demonstrate significant benefits. In some instances, it has also been very dangerous.

Acupuncture needles are not only inserted into the skin. Needles, up to one foot in length(!), may be inserted deep into the body; serious harm may result when they penetrate vital structures. In one case of back pain and burning around the mouth and vagina, needles were inserted through the skin of the chest. The lung was penetrated and collapsed, filling the chest cavity with almost a pint of blood. The patient required two weeks of hospitalization which was complicated by pneumonia.

Death from puncture of the heart has been reported. Other reports mention puncture of the liver, spleen, bladder, kidneys, and the pregnant uterus. Since classical Chinese medical practice does not recognize that germs cause disease, acupuncture needles might not be sterilized. Lack of sterile technique can, of course, result in bacterial and viral infections. In China, acupuncture needles are stored in alcohol solutions. Since alcohol does not kill the virus that causes infectious hepatitis, contaminated needles can spread this serious infection from patient to patient. Cases of bacterial endocarditis (a life-threatening infection involving a heart valve) have also been reported.

Some acupuncture needles are unusually thin and poorly made. Such needles tend to break. One scientist suffered excruciating pain in an acupuncture experiment when the needle broke off in his foot. An operation was needed to remove the needle.

"Acupuncture anesthesia" may include electrical stimulation of needles placed directly into the sciatic nerve (the main nerve to the leg). If the nerve is stimulated for several hours with high-frequency current, permanent nerve injury is almost guaranteed. The nerve fibers may burn, the nerve sheath may tear, and bleeding into the nerve may occur.

Stimulation of the so-called Ya-men point is recommended for the treatment of nerve deafness in children. Scientific study has demonstrated that this technique is useless. The Ya-men point is located directly above the most sensitive part of the human nervous system, the junction between the spinal cord and the base of the brain. A needle entering this sensitive area can produce instant paralysis of arms and legs, stoppage of breathing, and death.

Textbooks of acupuncture therapeutics advise acupuncture for some conditions that can lead to death or serious disability if not properly diagnosed and treated. Among these conditions are high fever and whooping cough in children, tender breasts in women, and urinary difficulties in men.

While adequate training in medicine or in acupuncture techniques may decrease the incidence of complications, this is no comfort to the victims of these complications.

## Acupuncture Teaching

Acupuncture is not part of the curriculum at most American medical schools, although a few schools offer electives and/or courses accredited for continuing education. Proponents claim that several thousand physicians in the United States and Canada use it in their practices. However, many people who practice acupuncture are not adequately trained either in acupuncture techniques or in medicine.

For what it is worth, in China, formal training in acupuncture requires several years. Some American practitioners, however, have merely attended "quickie" courses, some of which lasted only one or two days. During the early 1970s, a chiropractor who traveled around the country teaching such courses to his colleagues was asked by a reporter how long it would take to acquire a working knowledge of acupuncture. The chiropractor replied, "I can teach you all you have to know in ten minutes." Today he operates a school with more than three hundred hours of courses.

**The Checkered Marketplace**

In the United States today, acupuncture is used mainly for pain relief—particularly in the hands of physicians. However, it is also advertised for "facial rejuvenation" and a myriad of problems including nerve deafness, overweight, paralysis, allergies, impotence, arthritis, and "candidiasis." According to a recent report in *The Wall Street Journal,* veterinary acupuncturists are treating such ailments as listlessness in goldfish, "neuroses" in birds, deafness and back problems in dogs, and aches and pains in horses.

All states permit acupuncture to be performed—some by physicians only, some by lay acupuncturists under medical supervision, and some by unsupervised laypersons. Although lay acupuncture groups advocate standards of training and practice, they have also spawned laws permitting independent practice. In a few states, they actually are lobbying to force physicians who wish to use acupuncture to undergo acupuncture training similar to theirs. An article in the April 1993 *Vegetarian Times* stated that in the United States there are more than fifty acupuncture schools and about 6,500 practicing acupuncturists.

An attempt is being made to set standards through voluntary certification by the National Commission for the Certification of Acupuncturists (NCCA). Several thousand practitioners have become certified, and some states have adopted the NCCA exam as all or part of their criteria for licensing. The credentials used by acupuncturists include C.A. (certified acupuncturist), M.A. (master acupuncturist), D.A. (diplomate of acupuncture), and O.M.D., (Oriental medical doctor). These credentials are not recognized by the scientific community. In 1990, the U.S. Secretary of Education recognized the National Accreditation Commission for Schools and Colleges of Acupuncture and Oriental Medicine as an accrediting agency. However, as with chiropractic and naturopathic schools, such recognition is not based upon the scientific validity of what is taught but upon other criteria.

The FDA believes that acupuncture devices "have not been shown to be safe and effective for any diagnostic and therapeutic use." The National Council Against Health Fraud considers acupuncture an unproven modality that should be restricted to research settings. It also believes that acupuncture licensing should be abolished. I agree. No amount of acupuncture training can enable unsupervised laypersons to safely manage patients who need medical care. Nor is there reason to believe that licensing laws can control acupuncture abuse.

Acupuncture mythology spread rapidly through our country and remains with us. Our best hope is that with time, education, and gradual appreciation of its worthlessness, acupuncture will be resisted by the public. Then it will pass beyond us, as have its sister quackeries: purging, leeching, bleeding, *et cetera.*

# 19

# Nutrition for Athletes: Myths vs. Facts

### Ellington Darden, Ph.D.

For ten years—from 1959 to 1969—I was a firm believer in high-protein supplements, vitamin pills, and other so-called "health foods." I took vitamin $B_{12}$ for endurance, wheat germ oil for energy, garlic for purifying the blood, kelp tablets for muscle definition, and vitamin $B_6$ for strength. At the same time, I avoided white bread, carbonated drinks, ice cream, and most other carbohydrate foods. I was convinced that this dietary program would help me become a superior athlete.

Where did I acquire these beliefs? The majority came from physical fitness and health magazines. According to these publications, most recent champions had followed such a program. I never questioned these concepts until I entered graduate school at Florida State University. In fact, I kept trying to find new ways or more concentrated protein supplements to be certain that I was consuming over 300 grams of protein per day—about four times as much as I actually needed.

During my first postgraduate year, I attended a seminar at which Dr. Harold E. Schendel spoke on the role of nutrition in physical fitness. Dr. Schendel was professor of nutrition at the university, but had spent four years in Africa and elsewhere directing research on problems of protein malnutrition. He had more than seventy published papers to his credit. After our first meeting, we spent many hours discussing how various foods and eating habits might affect athletic performance. To say the least, Dr. Schendel disagreed with most of my nutritional concepts and did not believe that my special eating habits were necessary, beneficial, or even safe. According to him, an athlete did *not* require large amounts of vitamins, proteins, or any special foods.

Nevertheless, Dr. Schendel did not convince me. After all, his knowledge was mostly theoretical, but I was actually eating a special diet and "knew" about its value. I was following the methods of champions and was not about to change my athletic training program because of any university professor or research done on rats! Rather than argue, however, Dr. Schendel suggested that I experiment on myself to determine whether an athlete in hard training could actually use the massive amounts of protein I was eating.

For two months, I kept precise records of my dietary intake, my energy expenditures, and how I felt. My protein intake varied from less than 100 grams per day to more than 380 grams, most of which was obtained from a 90 percent protein powder. All of my urine was collected and analyzed to see whether the protein I ate was being used by my body or merely broken down and excreted in my urine.

The results of this study started me thinking in a different direction. According to the Recommended Dietary Allowances (RDAs), my protein need (for a body weight of 215 pounds) was 77 grams per day. To my surprise, whenever I consumed more than this amount, the excess was excreted. My weight remained relatively constant and I noted no difference in strength regardless of the amount of protein consumed. In fact, when I went off my massive protein diet (relieving my body of the burden of metabolizing the excess protein), I experienced a surge of energy!

Further experimentation made it clear that when I consumed more than the RDA of various vitamins and minerals, excess amounts of these substances were also excreted rather than used by my body. Similar observations had been made by nutrition scientists since the 1930s, but it took a personal experience to undo the brainwashing I had undergone during my early years as an athlete. Today, with a Ph.D. under my belt, I understand why optimum nutrition for athletic performance requires no more than a well-balanced diet composed of foods that are readily available at grocery stores and supermarkets. The only people who benefit from expensive supplements are those who sell them.

When champion athletes attribute their outstanding speed, strength, or endurance to a dietary program, it is perfectly natural for other athletes— or those participating in serious fitness or exercise programs—to pay attention. If a magic food, pill, potion, or dietary regimen might change one overnight into a world champion, why not give it a try? It may be natural, but it is still a mistake. I have yet to meet a single such athlete who had a basic understanding of what happens to his or her favorite foodstuffs after they enter the body. Such athletes obtain their results in spite of their nutritional beliefs and not because of them.

I don't mean to suggest, however, that nutrition is unimportant to athletic performance. While most of the alleged benefits of special diets are myths, correct nutrition can make the difference between having enough stamina and tiring halfway through a game, or between a sense of well-being and a feeling of not being up to par.

Much of what is known today about nutrition and athletic performance can be presented briefly in a fact-fallacy discussion. Since exercise is closely related to nutrition, this chapter also examines some common misconceptions about conditioning activities.

**Protein Foods**

*Fallacy*: Large amounts of protein foods and protein supplements are especially important during intense training.

*Fact*: There is no scientific evidence supporting the popular belief that athletes require massive amounts of protein-rich foods or protein supplements. Surveys show that athletes often consume four to five times their actual requirements. Yet there is absolutely no health or performance benefit from high-protein eating. The following table was developed from the National Research Council's 1989 RDAs:

|  | Age | Average Weight | Multiply Weight by: | Average Protein Need |
|---|---|---|---|---|
| Male | 11–14 | 99 pounds | .45 | 45 grams |
|  | 15–18 | 145 pounds | .41 | 59 grams |
|  | 19–24 | 160 pounds | .36 | 58 grams |
|  | 25–50 | 174 pounds | .36 | 63 grams |
|  | 51+ | 170 pounds | .36 | 62 grams |
| Female | 11–14 | 101 pounds | .45 | 46 grams |
|  | 15–18 | 120 pounds | .36 | 44 grams |
|  | 19–24 | 128 pounds | .36 | 46 grams |
|  | 25–50 | 139 pounds | .36 | 50 grams |
|  | 51+ | 143 pounds | .35 | 50 grams |

These amounts are readily obtainable from a balanced diet.

*Fallacy*: Bodybuilders can get bigger muscles by consuming free-form amino acids.

*Fact*: Amino acids are the building blocks of proteins. Twenty-two of them are important in human nutrition. Some of them can be separated into very pure forms and sold as free-form amino acids. However, there is no advantage to taking free-form amino acids. They will not help build muscle faster.

Nutritionist James J. Kenney, Ph.D., R.D., has noted that "free-form amino acids are anything but free." For example, 100 grams (about 3.5 ounces) of a popular amino acid powder retails for $26.98—which is $122.49 per pound. Similar amounts of free-form amino acids can be obtained from chicken breasts—which can be purchased at a supermarket for one fiftieth of the price. When protein foods are consumed, the body digests them into their component (free-form) amino acids and puts them to work where they are needed.

*Fallacy*: Certain writers and food-supplement manufacturers state that consuming large amounts of arginine and ornithine produce "faster-than-ever-before muscle growth."

*Fact*: Such statements are not correct. Arginine and ornithine are amino acids. There's nothing special about their ability to facilitate the muscle-building process.

A few years ago the Federal Trade Commission entered into a consent agreement with one large manufacturer regarding its advertising for an amino acid supplement. The company can no longer advertise that its free-form amino acid products cause greater or faster muscular development because there is no reliable scientific proof that they do. The manufacturer was also required to offer refunds to people who purchased these products as a result of the misleading advertisements.

Remember that a deficiency of protein or any of the amino acids that make up protein foods will not occur in bodybuilders who eat anything close to a balanced diet. Regardless of what's written in the fitness magazines, don't waste money on expensive free-form amino acids or protein supplements.

*Fallacy*: Protein foods are great for promoting power-packed energy.

*Fact*: The promotion of "power-packed" protein is a sales gimmick. Although proteins can be used as energy sources if necessary, carbohydrates and fats are preferable. They are used more easily by the body and also cost less than protein foods. A diet that is too high in proteins will actually cause fatigue.

*Fallacy*: High-protein diets are a must for fat reduction.

*Fact*: Proteins and carbohydrates both have four calories per gram. Fats have nine calories per gram. Since "high-protein" foods (such as steaks) can contain a high percentage of fat, a "high-protein" reducing diet may actually have 70 percent or more of its calories coming from fat.

Part of the weight loss on a high-protein diet is caused by loss of appetite, which leads to reduced caloric intake. As proteins are broken down, their waste products are flushed out of the body by the kidneys. The resultant water loss, perhaps five to eight pounds in the first week, may mislead the dieter into thinking he or she is losing fat. The water actually comes from muscles, vital organs, and fluid outside of the cells. Any weight lost due to dehydration will be regained as soon as normal eating is resumed.

*Fallacy*: Large amounts of protein cannot hurt the body.
*Fact*: Scientists have found that too much dietary protein can be dangerous. The metabolism and excretion of nonstorable protein can impose serious stress and cause enlargement of the liver, kidneys, and other vital organs.

## Other "Special" Foods

*Fallacy*: Precompetition meals for athletes should consist of special foods.
*Fact*: Although it may give an athlete a feeling of strength and security, food consumed on the day of competition has very little to do with the production of energy for that day. Athletes who compete in nonstop, marathon-type events are an exception to this rule. They can benefit from pre-event meals of carbohydrate-rich foods, as well as several days of carbohydrate loading.

Nutrition scientists have found that it takes from two to fourteen days for the food a person eats to be utilized for energy. The following guidelines should be considered in planning precompetition meals:

- Energy intake should be adequate to ward off any feelings of hunger during competition.

- The necessity for urinary or bowel excretion during competition can be serious or even disabling. For this reason, large amounts of protein foods, bulky foods, or highly spiced foods should be avoided.

- The meal should be eaten at least three hours prior to competition to allow for digestion to take place.

- Fluid intake before, during, and after prolonged competition should guarantee optimal hydration. This can be accomplished with water and various fruit juices.

- The precompetition meal should be food with which the athlete is familiar. Food that provides psychological assurance can strengthen the determination to win.

*Fallacy*: Honey is good for quick energy.
*Fact*: There are no "quick-energy" foods. Nor is there any magic in eating honey. Honey contains glucose and fructose, the same simple sugars that are produced by the digestion of table sugar. Honey contains a higher percentage of fructose, but it is not significantly superior to other common sweets.

Unfortunately, dietary quacks have falsely promoted honey as a sweet that is better tolerated than other sugars.

Taken in large quantities, honey can produce several detrimental effects. Excessive amounts of honey, or other sweets, can draw fluid from other parts of the body into the gastrointestinal tract. This shift in fluids can dehydrate the athlete in long-distance events where sweat loss can affect performance. A concentrated sugar solution may also distend the stomach, causing nausea, cramps, and/or diarrhea. Athletes who are determined to take honey or sugar should do so in small quantities with plenty of water. They should have no more than three tablespoons of the sweets in any one-hour period. This will appease a psychological need, but it will not improve performance.

*Fallacy*: Bee-pollen tablets offer a tremendous breakthrough in helping an athlete run faster and farther.
*Fact*: The athletic world can thank the Finns for publicizing bee pollen. It all started in 1972 when Finland's Lasse Viren won the 5,000 and 10,000-meter runs in Munich and began buzzing the news about pollen tablets. When Viren repeated his success in Montreal in 1976, health-food companies decided to increase the availability of bee pollen—at a cost of up to $45 per pound.

The cost is a result not only of bee pollen's supposed magical properties, but also of the way it is harvested. As bees obtain nectar from flowers, pollen collects on their body. When they return to their hive, the pollen is scraped off by wire brushes that have been placed around the entrances. The very fine-grained powder is then collected and manufactured into tablets.

Promoters call bee pollen "the perfect food" and stress that it contains all of the essential amino acids and many vitamins and minerals. However, none of these nutrients offers any magic, and all can be obtained easily and less expensively in conventional foods.

Research at Louisiana State University has shown that bee pollen has no effect on the performance of runners and swimmers. When confronted with this evidence, an American distributor noted that the LSU study used bee pollen from France, and not the full-potency pollen from England which, naturally, he sold. But he also admitted that bee pollen is unnecessary when the diet is already well-balanced.

Recently, a leading American manufacturer of bee-pollen products was prohibited from making false claims that the products could produce weight loss, alleviate allergies, reverse the aging process, and alleviate sexual dysfunction (see Chapter 27).

*Fallacy*: Large doses of wheat germ oil will improve your stamina.
*Fact*: Wheat germ oil is rich in B vitamins, protein, and vitamin E. Some athletes

drink it straight from the bottle. It is high in calories and more expensive than most foods that contain the same nutrients, but contains no unique ingredients that will improve endurance.

*Fallacy*: Steak is the breakfast of champions.
*Fact*: Thick, juicy steaks were a training table staple for many years, particularly the 1950s and 1960s. Even today, some coaches and trainers believe there is a corollary between red meat and strength and endurance. However, scientific research has shown repeatedly that steak, which contains protein and fat, is not as efficient in supplying energy for athletic performance as food that is rich in carbohydrates. The ideal diet for most athletes should be about 59 percent carbohydrate, 28 percent fat, and 13 percent protein.

## "Forbidden" Foods

*Fallacy*: Table sugar should be avoided.
*Fact*: Although refined sugar is a concentrated form of calories, it does not contain a single harmful substance. Nutritionists would prefer that athletes get most of their carbohydrates from fruits, vegetables, breads, and other foods that also supply vitamins, minerals, and fiber. Table sugar need not be avoided, but should be used in moderation.

*Fallacy*: Fried potatoes are harmful to the digestive tract.
*Fact*: Greasy foods are digested slowly because fat retards the emptying time of the stomach, but this does no harm to a normal digestive tract. Most fats are digested at about the same rate whether they are found in butter, margarine, salad dressing, shortening, or cooking oils used to fry foods such as potatoes. As for potatoes, they are one of the most nutritious vegetables. Fried potatoes are certainly not taboo for athletes, though total fat intake should be kept moderate as a general health measure.

*Fallacy*: Hamburgers should be avoided during training.
*Fact*: There is no good reason why athletes with normal blood cholesterol levels cannot eat hamburgers several times a week if their overall diet is balanced. People who eat regularly at fast-food chains would be wise to make sure that their other meals include enough fruits, vegetables, grains, and dairy products.

*Fallacy*: Bread is a fattening food that athletes should avoid.
*Fact*: Bread is one of the most nutritious foods. It is low in calories— about 60 per slice—and contains ample amounts of niacin, riboflavin, thiamine, iron, protein, carbohydrates, and calcium. The real reason most people associate bread with gaining weight is not the bread itself, but what they put on it.

*Fallacy*: Athletes should avoid white bread and eat only whole-grain bread.
*Fact*: There are only minor differences in the nutrient content of whole-grain and enriched breads. Whole-grain breads are a fair source of fiber, which can be helpful to bowel function. Ample amounts of fiber are also present in other common foods such as oat cereals, apples, carrots, corn, broccoli, pineapples, bananas, and many types of beans.

## Salt and Water

*Fallacy*: Athletes should consume several salt tablets each day during hot weather.
*Fact*: Salt tablets usually do more harm than good. Athletes need more salt during hot weather, but salt tablets often irritate the stomach or pass through the system without being absorbed. Nationally syndicated columnist Lawrence E. Lamb, M.D., recommends that in addition to drinking plenty of water, athletes should drink at least a quart of low-fat milk or fortified skim milk a day, plus two eight-ounce glasses of orange juice. Milk has about the same salt content as the healthy human body, and orange juice contains potassium, which is also important in hot weather. A liberal use of the salt shaker during meals is usually sufficient for extra salt.

*Fallacy*: Drinking water during practice will upset an athlete's stomach.
*Fact*: Prohibiting water on the practice field has no physiological basis. Withholding liquids during hot, humid weather makes an athlete susceptible to heat cramps, heat exhaustion, or the more serious and sometimes fatal heat stroke. Dehydration causes fatigue, which in itself makes an athlete more vulnerable to injury. All coaches, athletes, and even nonathletes should realize the necessity of drinking fluids before, during, and after vigorous activity. Furthermore, the fluids may be iced. The old idea that people warm from exercise should not drink ice water because it causes cramps is completely unfounded.

## Vitamins and Minerals

*Fallacy*: It is a good idea to take a multiple vitamin and mineral supplement every day.
*Fact*: Some television commercials have depicted athletic-looking individuals explaining how they stay healthy—by watching their diet, getting plenty of exercise, and, "just to be sure," taking a daily vitamin-mineral supplement. The ad implies that a balanced diet cannot provide enough nutrients. This is untrue.

All necessary nutrients are easily obtained from a sensible diet of ordinary foods. The sole exception is that some women who have excessively heavy menstrual periods may need to take iron supplements. Other ads have suggested that supplements will provide extra energy. This, too, is untrue. Energy comes from the metabolism of foods.

Another dubious type of vitamin advertising is the result of action by the United States Olympic Committee (USOC). For a sizable contribution, the USOC will award a company the exclusive right to advertise that its product was "selected by" the U.S. Olympic team or that it is "supplier to" or "contributor to" the team. The exact wording depends upon the size of the contribution. Several vitamin companies have donated money and advertised their affiliation without indicating its basis.

Years ago, George V. Mann, M.D., professor of biochemistry at the University of Tennessee called this practice "pure promotional hyping. . . . Of all the people in the world, international class athletes probably need supplementary vitamins the least."

## Conditioning

*Fallacy*: An athlete who wants to gain weight or bulk should resort to a high-calorie diet.

*Fact*: To most athletes and coaches, gaining weight or bulk means getting fatter by eating more calories. But gaining fat will make an athlete slower, less coordinated, less healthy, and more prone to disease in later life.

Unfortunately, "forced" feeding is still done at some college training tables, especially those of football players. Few athletes and coaches realize that such eating does more harm than good. Athletes should be lean and muscular. Their goal should be to gain extra muscle, not extra fat. Muscle is over 70 percent water. It takes only 600 extra calories to build a pound of muscle, but unless the athlete has stimulated muscle growth beforehand, eating extra calories will build fat rather than muscle. Muscular growth is stimulated best by a program of progressive resistance exercises or proper strength training.

*Fallacy*: Strength-training movements should be performed in an explosive manner.

*Fact*: Explosive strength training is of absolutely no value to any athlete except a competitive weightlifter. Yanking an athlete's muscles and tendons does *not* build strength and may produce injuries. Such injuries occur when a force exceeds the structural integrity of the body. All ligaments, tendons, muscles, and bones have breaking points.

During the 1975 National Weightlifting Championships, cinematographic data were collected as a 181-pound athlete ruptured his patellar (kneecap) tendon while attempting to jerk 385 pounds. Kinetic analysis revealed that as the weight was jerked overhead, over three thousand pounds of force were exerted on the patellar tendon! Many Olympic weightlifters suffer permanent damage to the tendons, ligaments, and muscles that surround major joints. This is evidently a risk they are willing to take; it should not, however, be one to which other athletes subject themselves. Competitive sports are dangerous enough without the added jeopardy of explosive weightlifting. Maximum results from strength training will be obtained if each repetition is performed in a slow, smooth manner. The weight should be lifted, not thrown.

*Fallacy*: The stronger the athlete, the more exercise is needed.
*Fact*: The opposite is actually true. Advanced trainees need harder exercises but, in most cases, less exercise. Strength-training sessions should not be performed more than three times a week. Most in-season training should be only twice a week.

*Fallacy*: Women should avoid strength training because they will build large muscles and lose their femininity.
*Fact:* Proper training can strengthen a woman's muscles without significantly increasing their size. Building large muscles requires two factors. First a genetic potential must be present in the muscles themselves—the individual must have long muscle bellies and short tendon attachments. Second, an adequate supply of male hormones, particularly testosterone, must be present in the blood stream. Women very rarely have either of these factors. Heavy exercise is worthwhile for women because it strengthens their muscles, prevents injuries, and turns the respective body parts into trimmer and more solid flesh.

*Fallacy*: Muscles will turn to fat if strength training is discontinued for several months.
*Fact*: If athletes in training do not eat less when they become less active, they will gain weight in the form of body fat. At the same time, their muscle masses will get smaller (atrophy) from lack of use. But these two processes are not directly related. The muscle does not actually turn to fat.

*Fallacy*: Only professional athletes need strong muscles.
*Fact*: Anyone can benefit from stronger muscles. Strengthening of muscles will lead to increased power, speed, efficiency, and productivity. Strong muscles are also less prone to injury.

*Fallacy*: Sit-ups, with or without equipment, can flatten your abdomen.
*Fact*: Despite the spot-reducing exercises and devices promoted on TV and in

the tabloids at the grocery checkout, the scientific literature has never been ambivalent about this subject. There is no such thing as spot-reduction of fat. Feeling "muscle burn" in your abdomen from sit-ups does not mean that belly fat is being incinerated. Heredity determines which fat cells are mobilized and to what degree, and this pecking order cannot be altered.

Studies with people doing hundreds of sit-ups, and one comparing the playing arm to the nonplaying arm of tennis players, have shown that an individual cannot pinpoint the shrinkage of fatty tissue.

But don't give up on exercise. Strengthen all the muscles, particularly the large muscle groups. Each pound of added muscle will burn approximately seventy-five extra calories a day, even at rest. Overfat individuals who create a net calorie deficit through exercise will burn body fat and become leaner.

## Drugs, Real and Imagined

*Fallacy*: Steroid drugs can effectively increase muscular size and strength.
*Fact*: The most popular are androgenic-anabolic steroids. "Androgenic" refers to the production of male body characteristics, while "anabolic" refers to the building processes of the body. Common drugs include *Winstrol, Anavar, Nilevar, Durabolin*, and *Methyltestosterone*. These drugs are synthetic forms of testosterone and other male hormones. They are obtained legally from physicians or illegally on the black market.

In 1977, the American College of Sports Medicine published a position paper stating that anabolic steroids do not significantly improve muscular strength and lean body mass. The organization recognized that gains in muscular size and strength achieved through high-intensity exercise and proper diet can be increased by the use of anabolic steroids in some individuals. However, they still are not safe.

Many athletes who use large doses of steroid drugs do permanent damage to their body, and many more experience temporary complications that last for months after the drug is stopped. The problems include testicular atrophy, pituitary inhibition, prostate enlargement, fluid retention, high blood pressure, kidney damage, acne, fibrosis of the liver, breast enlargement (in both sexes), and unwanted hair growth (in women). Some athletes have even died as a result of steroid use.

*Fallacy*: Many over-the-counter food supplements can help build bigger muscles and enhance athletic performance.
*Fact*: More than a hundred companies are marketing so-called "ergogenic aids." Ads for these products typically contain an endorsement from a cham-

pion athlete or bodybuilder who attributes success to the products. The claims made for the products are mostly nonsense. Many of them are touted as "natural steroids" or "steroid replacements"—which they are not. Their ingredients include chromium picolinate, vanadyl sulfate, ferulic acid, royal jelly, yohimbe bark, branched-chain amino acids, medium-chain triglycerides, hypothalamus, pituitary, orchic, thymus, heart, prostate, liver, sterols, ginseng, Mexican yam, tarrow root, licorice root, dandelion root, grapefruit powder, kelp, cider vinegar, potassium, calcium, zinc, vitamin B$_6$, bromelain, and papain. In lay terms this is a collection of carbohydrates, proteins, fats, herbs, enzymes, some vitamins and minerals, and many nonessential chemicals. None of these ingredients, or any combination of them, has been proven to build bigger muscles and enhance athletic performance any better than the foods in a well-balanced diet.

In 1992, the New York City Department of Consumer Affairs issued "Notices of Violation" to six companies marketing "ergogenic aids" and challenged the FDA to clean up the marketplace nationwide. Investigators from the department reported that manufacturers they contacted for information about their products were unable to provide a single published report from a scientific journal to back the claims that their products did any of these things. Calling the bodybuilding supplement industry "an economic hoax with unhealthy consequences," the department warned consumers to beware of terms like fat burner, fat fighter, fat metabolizer, energy enhancer, performance booster, strength booster, ergogenic aid, anabolic optimizer, and genetic optimizer. The department calculated that a supplement program recommended in the leading bodybuilding magazine (*Muscle & Fitness*) would cost more than $11 per day!

### The Bottom Line

The foremost dream of many athletes is to find a food, exercise, or magic formula that somehow will turn them into champions overnight. This dream is stimulated by the enormous pressure to "win at all costs." While exercise and nutrition gimmicks may sometimes improve performance by increasing self-confidence, they cannot be recommended from the viewpoint of health, safety, or economy. Scientifically based training methods offer much more.

# 20

# Quackery by Mail

## Stephen Barrett, M.D.

Many people believe that advertising claims for health products must be true or somehow would not be "allowed." Many assume that media outlets screen such ads carefully, and some even think that the U.S. Postal Service licenses mail-order advertisers. Each of these beliefs is wrong.

The total amount of money Americans waste on bogus mail-order health products is not known, but probably ranges from $50 to $150 million a year. Most mail-order health schemes attempt to exploit people's fear of being unattractive. Smaller numbers involve products claimed to increase fitness or solve health problems. Misleading claims for mail-order products are made in magazine and newspaper ads, direct mail solicitations, multilevel marketing, television commercials, and telemarketing schemes. Table 20:1 summarizes the typical characteristics of each of these channels.

### Magazine and Newspaper Ads

During the summer of 1977, I headed a Pennsylvania Medical Society Committee on Quackery project that screened more than five hundred nationally circulated magazines. About 25 percent carried display ads for products marketed through the mail with claims that they were effective against disease or could affect the structure or function of the body. The study did not include classified ads or ads for nonprescription drug products sold primarily through pharmacies and supermarkets. Nor did it include ads placed in "health food," fitness, and bodybuilding publications. (We define "health-food magazines" as those whose articles promote vitamins and other supplement products with claims regarded as dubious by the scientific community.)

The products we evaluated fell into two general groups: sex aids, and youth and beauty aids—with about 150 products offered by fifty sellers. Cosmetics, pamphlets, and books were not included in the tabulations.

The sex-aid products included supposed aphrodisiacs, pleasure-

### Table 20:1. The Mail-Order Health Marketplace

| Communication Channel | Typical Products |
|---|---|
| Magazines, astrology | Psychic help with health problems |
| Magazines, fitness/bodybuilding | "Ergogenic aids" |
| Magazines, general audience | Youth and beauty aids |
| Magazines, health | Nonprescription drugs sold through drugstores and supermarkets |
| Magazines, health food | Supplement products sold through health food stores. Misleading claims tend to be made through articles rather than ads. |
| Magazines, pornographic | Sex aids |
| Newspapers, general | Weight-reduction schemes |
| Newspapers, tabloid | Weight-reduction schemes, psychic healing |
| Classified ads | Mostly information and product catalogs rather than specific products |
| Direct mail | Weight reduction schemes, anti-aging products, sex aids |
| Post-it ads | Weight reduction schemes, anti-aging products, pinhole eyeglasses |
| Prizes (mail or phone) | Vitamins, water purifiers |
| Catalogs from mail-order supplement distributors | A multitude of "dietary supplement" products with misleading therapeutic claims |
| Multilevel companies | A multitude of supplement products with illegal claims made through brochures, videotapes, and word-of-mouth |
| Television infomercials | Weight-loss schemes, beauty aids, hair-loss remedies |

enhancers, penis enlargers, and erection aids. The youth and beauty aids included supposed weight-reduction products, breast developers, blemish removers, hair-loss remedies, "spot-reducers," and products claimed to increase longevity. The weight-reduction schemes included promises that you would "melt off fat" while you sleep, "lose five pounds overnight," and lose more than a pound a day without hunger. The "spot-reducers," which included various sorts of belts and wraps, were claimed to trim arms, legs, and abdomen without dieting. The medical society committee concluded that not a single product could live up to its advertised claims.

During the spring and summer of 1990, I obtained one copy each of 463 nationally circulated magazines, either from a local distributor or through direct subscription. The project was funded by a grant from the Dick Goldensohn Fund, a New York City-based foundation interested in promoting economic justice. This time, "health food," fitness, and bodybuilding publications were included, but automobile and computer magazines, which never carry health ads, were not. Mail-order ads for dubious health products appeared in fifty-six out of 423 (13 percent) of the general audience magazines and twenty-three out of forty (58 percent) of the health and fitness magazines (see Table 20:2). In the general magazines, about fifty companies advertised approximately seventy

## Table 20:2. Magazines with Dubious Mail-Order Health Ads*

| Type of Magazine | No. in Category | No. with Dubious Ads |
|---|---|---|
| 1. Fitness/bodybuilding | 14 | 9 (64%) |
| 2. Health | 11 | 4 (36%) |
| 3. Health food | 15 | 10 (67%) |
| 4. General audience | 360 | 33 (9%) |
| 5. Pornographic | 56 | 19 (34%) |
| 6. Astrology/paranormal | 7 | 4 (57%) |
| Total health-related (1-3) | 40 | 23 (58%) |
| Total not health-related (4-6) | 423 | 56 (13%) |
| Overall total | 463 | 79 (18%) |

*These numbers are not exact because a few products were advertised in more than one magazine category. When this occurred, I counted the category in which the ad occurred most often. It is also possible that a few sellers were operating under more than one company name. Some magazines carried ads for products sold at retail outlets as well as through the mail. Such products were counted only if their ads contained claims, price, and ordering information. One product—a device used to reduce sweating—appeared capable of living up to its advertised claims and is not included in this tabulation.

dubious products. In the health food publications, fifteen companies advertised twenty-four dubious products. In the fitness/bodybuilding category, twenty-six companies advertised more than sixty products. Table 20:3 gives examples of the products and the claims made for them.

Fitness and bodybuilding magazines are loaded with ads for "ergogenic aids"—supplement concoctions that contain vitamins, minerals, amino acids, and/or various other substances. These products are primarily sold through stores and fitness centers rather than by mail. They are claimed to increase stamina, endurance, muscle bulk, and/or athletic performance. Some ads make explicit claims, while others do nothing but feature pictures and endorsements of bodybuilding champions and other athletes. All such products are fakes. Table 20:4 gives examples of claims made for them.

Newspaper ads for health products are similar to those in general magazines in both scope and illegitimacy. In 1979, a reporter for the *El Paso Times* recruited volunteers to test forty-six mail-order products whose ads—in newspapers and magazines—looked suspicious. Most were alleged health and

### Table 20:3. Claims from General Audience Magazine Ads

| Product | Dubious Claims |
| --- | --- |
| Aloe Vera Capsules | Real and lasting relief of arthritis; strengthens the immune system. |
| BT-5 Brain Tuner | "May produce a balancing stimulation of brain neuro-transmitters. Sold as an experimental device and no medical claims are made or implied. Investigational areas . . . may include: memory improvements . . . reduced fatigue . . . sound sleep, mood elevation . . . increased vitality." |
| Chinese Exercise Balls | Improves circulation of vital energy throughout the body |
| HPG-C7 | Nutritional supplement for sexier, more beautiful breasts—a secret European formulation |
| Memory Fuel | Memory enhancement, improved neurological functioning |
| Regina Royal Jelly | Helps insomnia, fatigue, asthma; improves immune system |
| Subliminal tapes | Total recall, raise your I.Q., permanent weight loss, powerful immune system, total pain relief, reach any goal, fast healing, flat stomach, etc. |
| Vitacel 7 | An advanced GH-3, beneficial for the relief of degenerative diseases and almost all symptoms of old age: arthritis, Parkinson's, muscular fatigue, poor circulation, varicose veins, depression, and multiple sclerosis |

**Table 20:4. Claims for "Ergogenic Aids"**

| Product | Dubious Claims |
|---|---|
| Gammaplex | Increases testosterone to produce massive gains in strength and size |
| Gorilla Nitro | The most advanced and powerful natural anabolic formula ever. Designed for hard core and serious body builders |
| Hot Stuff | Anabolic activator. Muscle development that would normally take one year or more can be achieved in a matter of months. Increase your muscle mass and thickness by up to 30 percent in just six weeks while decreasing fatty tissue by up to 15 percent |
| Max Amino 2300 | Growth hormone releasers accelerate muscle growth |
| Max Flex Muscle Formula | Doubles rate of muscle growth |
| Metabolic Opti-Max GH | Ultimate results in performance, endurance, and muscular gains |
| Suddenly Slim | Stimulates natural sweating process to remove excess water weight from problem areas |
| Waist Shaper | Lose pounds and inches right where you need it most |

beauty aids, and the rest were household aids. The results were published in a week-long series of articles that covered more than ten full pages. The only product that lived up to its claims was an egg-slicer.

Some bogus ads are submitted to hundreds of newspapers simultaneously with a request that they be accepted without payment in advance. Newspapers that grant credit in this manner often don't get paid. The American Newspaper Publishers Association credit bureau investigates prospective advertisers when asked to do so by its members.

The tabloid newspapers (*Globe, National Examiner, Sun, National Enquirer,* and *Weekly World News*) usually run several misleading health-related ads per issue. Table 20:5 gives examples published during the past few years. My study found that Macfadden Holdings, the parent company of the *National Enquirer, Weekly World News,* and thirteen monthly romance magazines, appeared to publish more dubious ads than any other company in the United States. Six of its magazines, *True Story, True Confessions, Modern Romances, True Experience, True Romance,* and *True Love,* accounted for 23 percent of the dubious ads in the 1990 magazine survey.

### Table 20:5. Ads in the Tabloids

| Product | Dubious Claims |
|---|---|
| Cellulite Control & Scrub | Penetrates skin to dissolve fat and increase circulation. |
| Chinese Vitamins | Youthful vigor due to high energy formulas. give extra energy, reduce fatigue, give extra energy and vitality, help you resist colds and flu, make you feel years younger. |
| Holy Water | Blessed in Lourdes. Guaranteed 100% pure holy healing water. Extraordinary healing power. |
| Magma 700 Pads | Apply the bandaid-like pads to the problem areas and within minutes you'll feel your pains and discomforts disappear. The pads have provided amazing results for sufferers of arthritis, rheumatism, back, neck and shoulder pain, painful legs and feet, sciatica, lumbago, neuralgia, migraine and nervous headaches, poor circulation, high blood pressure, insomnia, cramps, sprains, and countless others. Magnetic therapy can improve blood circulation, increase the blood oxygen level, enhance metabolism and remarkably relieve muscular pain and stiffness. |
| Vigor-X | Increases virility & vigor, increases stamina & energy, increases sexual functions, arousal & sensitivity. |

## Catalog Sales

Most dietary supplement ads appearing in health-food and health-related general-circulation magazines are designed to stimulate the sale of these products through health food stores. Such ads tend to contain few explicit claims that the products are effective against health problems. If they did, the products would be considered "drugs" and be subject to federal regulation. Instead, most manufacturers rely on magazines and books to boost the ingredients of the products. The manufacturers hope that readers will be stimulated to visit stores where retailers can talk to them privately with little or no risk of triggering government regulatory action.

Dietary supplement products also are sold through mail-order catalogs. Some companies market their own lines of products in this manner. Others include a few pages of supplement products in general merchandise catalogs. A few compete with health food stores by carrying the products of many manufacturers at discount prices.

The three largest discounters appear to be Swanson's Health Products, of Fargo, North Dakota; L&H Vitamins, of Long Island City, New York; and The Vitamin Shoppe, of West Bergen, New Jersey. All three offer the products of many manufacturers at discounts of 20 percent or more. Each issues tabloid newspaper or magazine-style catalogs that contain articles promoting products and/or the ingredients they contain. Often the articles are accompanied by display ads for the products to which they pertain. Table 20:6 describes a few of the false claims I have noted in these catalogs.

The largest company selling its own product line by mail is probably

**Table 20:6. Products From Supplement Discounters**

| Product | False Claims |
| --- | --- |
| Diet Systems 2001 (Vitamin Shoppe) | Dissolves cellulite naturally. You can continue eating as much as you want of all your favorite foods. Within minutes your body's fat cells begin shrinking. Letters pour in daily reporting large losses . . . 22 pounds in 7 days. Unlike our competition, you are not bothered with diets, calorie counting, charts, meal cards, food groups, torturous exercise, nervousness, hunger irritability, starvation, discipline, strong will power or plans to follow. |
| Ginkgo biloba (Vitamin Shoppe) | Fights senility. |
| Prolong Sx (Vitamin Shoppe) | Increase muscle strength, endurance, and sexual performance for both men and women. |
| Enduraplex (L&H Vitamins) | The main ingredient, octacosanol, "improves stamina and endurance, reduces heart stress, and quickens reaction time." |
| Sugar Block (L&H Vitamins) | Blocks the absorption of sugar calories. |
| K Complex (L&H Vitamins) | Helps prevent stress from damaging health, enhances body's resistance levels, strengthens organs, increases physical and mental energy, improves the heart and circulation, fights chronic fatigue and weakness. |
| See (Swanson) | Provides eyes with nutrients that may prevent cataracts and macular degeneration. |
| Dilovasic (Swanson) | "Non-drug alternative" for treating high blood pressure, arthritis, impotence or frigidity, memory loss, or stress caused by a circulation problem. |
| Cal-Arrest (Swanson) | "Unique negative calorie energizer that consumes more calories than it contains." |

Nature's Bounty, of Bohemia, New York, doing business as Puritan's Pride. In 1989 the company purchased the mail-order division of General Nutrition Corporation (GNC), which, during 1988, had a total customer base of approximately one million and total sales of $21,775,000. The transaction included the right to use the GNC trademark for two years.

In 1985, GNC had signed consent agreements with the Postal Service to stop making unsubstantiated claims for fourteen products sold through the mail. After acquiring GNC's mail-order division, Puritan's Pride gradually phased out the GNC label but continued to make illegal claims for some GNC products as well as many others under its own label. Its February 1990 catalog, for example, contained at least forty-two product representations that were false, misleading, or unproven. In November 1990, postal officials filed a false representation complaint against Nature's Bounty, charging that at least nineteen of its products were falsely advertised. The products included *Cholesto-Flush, Fatbuster Diet Tea, Kidney Flush, Memory Booster, Prostex,* and *Stress B with 500 mg Vitamin C.* In May 1991, the case was settled with a consent agreement under which Nature's Bounty admitted no wrongdoing but agreed not to make unsubstantiated claims about the efficacy of any product marketed for treating the physical conditions covered in the Postal Services complaint.

After the consent agreement was signed, the number of disease-related claims in Puritan's Pride's catalogs decreased sharply and some of the disputed products were discontinued. But the company began marketing books and booklets that make false claims for vitamins, minerals, and many other substances promoted as dietary supplements. The books included *Prescription for Nutritional Healing,* which recommends long lists of vitamins, minerals, and/or herbs for more than 150 different diseases and conditions. The booklets, which included "Spirulina," "Evening Primrose Oil," and "Beta-Carotene," were published by Keats Publishing Inc., of New Canaan, Connecticut, the health-food industry's leading publisher of unscientific nutrition books. Claims that would be illegal in advertising or on product labels are protected by the doctrine of freedom of the press as long as they are not tied to brand-name products.

## Direct Mail Ads

Some entrepreneurs advertise health products by direct mail, using subscriber lists from publications and other sources. Most of these ads are for weight-reduction schemes, anti-aging products, and beauty aids. The Iowa Attorney General has seen evidence that people who buy one bogus diet product often receive ads for others. One list broker sells names from a database of 280,000 "arthritis/rheumatism sufferers" who have purchased such items as a "sacred Aztec talisman" or a "Chinese miracle weight-loss program."

For only $19.95, "psychic astrologer" Irene Hughes offers to provide a year's worth of instructions for accruing "up to millions" and coping better with personal relationships. "Your name got on my special list," she claimed in a recent mailing. "Right this minute I'm concentrating on you. . . . What my gut feeling tells me is this. You have a serious personal problem. It is eating away at you. . . . You don't know how lucky you are that a truly qualified psychic counseling expert – someone known to be 'right' as a psychic 74 out of 75 times – is now on to your problem." The name to which the letter was addressed belonged to an investigative reporter who uses pseudonyms to inquire about offbeat health matters and get-rich-quick schemes. The reporter gets a steady stream of mail from entrepreneurs who utilize "sucker lists."

Several months later, the reporter heard from "paraspiritual astrologer" Irene M. Morgan. In about a month, her mailing stated, "you will enter . . . a time in which all of your inner energy may channel and act as a catalyst to thrust you toward a life of perhaps unending reward and Instant Wealth. . . . You are lucky, destiny has led me to you in time." Ms. Morgan promised (for $19.95 and completion of a questionnaire) to "guide you to the events that may transpire" and to attempt to disarm a "jealous spirit" that was trying to interfere. A similar offer came from "Metaphysical Super-Natural Advisor" Nicole W. Christoffe, who wrote that "someone who has passed over to the other side just poked me in the ribs that awoke me from a deep sleep and told me to contact [you] as soon as possible."

Some direct mail solicitations for bogus products look like reproductions of newspaper articles or ads, although they probably have not been published. They are accompanied by a handwritten endorsement in the margin or on a Post-it, addressed to the recipient by name or first initial. "Dear Bill," the note might read, "This really works! Try it. S."

## Telemarketing Schemes

Telemarketing schemes typically involve notification by mail or phone that the recipient has won a "valuable" prize. To collect, the recipient must order a large supply of vitamins, a water purifier, or something else that costs hundreds of dollars. If delivery is made, the prize almost always is worthless, the product overpriced, and the "money-back guarantee" not honored. When the product has been ordered by credit card, the buyer can usually prevent loss by asking the credit card company to reverse the payment. But many buyers don't realize this or waste so much time trying to get a refund that the deadline for action through the credit card issuer expires. The National Alliance for Fraud in Telemarketing believes that during the next decade, telephone scams involving arthritis remedies, weight-loss plans, sexual aids, baldness cures, and other health and nutrition products will increase.

## Television Infomercials

The Federal Trade Commission has warned consumers to be aware that some television programs that look like talk shows are actually program-length commercials. Some programs of this type have promoted dubious weight-loss plans, hair-loss products, and food supplements. One tipoff, says the FTC, is that the product promoted during "commercial breaks" is related to the program's content. The FTC has stopped most of the blatantly misleading promotions, but others will undoubtedly take place.

## "Spiritual" Advice

Many "psychics," "astrologers," and "healers" offer to help with life's problems through the mail or by telephone. The purported benefits may include better luck, better health, and/or a financial benefit.

Some of these individuals attempt to persuade respondents to send money repeatedly for their services. During the 1970s, for example, a "spiritual reader" who operating as "Mother McGown," "Mother Luther," and "Mother Alma" guaranteed help within three days for illnesses, loneliness, and other problems. All respondents to her ads received identical mimeographed letters stating: "I have received your letter and found out that I could help you. I have found that you have hoodoo [bad luck] in your home along with sickness and love life problems. As soon as you read this letter, call me immediately."

Those who telephoned were told that their problems would be solved if they sent a specific sum of money, usually $50 (but no personal checks). Follow-up letters would then ask for more money because the problem was worse than it was initially believed to be. The Postal Service took action in response to complaints from victims who had spent money but received no results. It turned out that the perpetrator belonged to a gypsy clan whose female members operated under various names in many states. The scheme was derailed when one of them was prosecuted by the Postal Service and sentenced to three years' probation by a federal judge in Austin, Texas.

## A "Contemporary" Scam

In June 1989, a full-page ad for "Cho Low Tea" was published in the *Washington Post, Los Angeles Times, Forth Worth Star Telegram, Newark Star Ledger, Pittsburgh Press* and one hundred other newspapers. The ad claimed that this tea would reduce blood cholesterol levels while still allowing you to eat whatever you please. The tea was also claimed to add years to your life, make you look and feel better, aid digestion of fatty foods, reduce water retention, and have none of the possible side effects of cholesterol-lowering drugs. The ad contained testimonials from a prominent young television actor, endorsements from seven medical sources, and the logo of the Better Business Bureau.

Fortunately for consumers, James Ralph, vice president of the American Newspaper Publishers Association Credit Bureau, had received inquiries about the advertisers before the ad was published. Ralph, who conducts seminars on how to detect fraudulent ads, is probably the industry leader in trying to persuade newspapers not to publish such ads. On the first day the ad was published, he obtained a copy, concluded the promotion was a scam, and contacted the Council of Better Business Bureaus as well as state and federal law enforcement agencies.

It turned out that the endorsements were fabrications and the marketers did not belong to the Better Business Bureau. They were two Australians who had entered the United States in February 1989. One of them had fled England while awaiting trial for a scheme involving the sale of almost $7 million worth of a Chinese tea that was falsely claimed to cause weight loss. It also turned out that no Cho Low Tea existed. The con men claimed that they had planned to repackage another company's tea but had not yet done so! Three weeks after their ads were published in the United States, both were arrested and jailed in lieu of bail. Early in July, they pleaded "no contest" and received short sentences plus three year's probation. Orders for the tea exceeded $250,000, but the authorities acted so swiftly that all of the money was returned to its senders. Most mail-order victims are not that lucky.

## A Dangerous Product

For several years, *Cal-Ban 3000* was falsely claimed to provide automatic weight loss without dieting or exercise. *Cal-Ban* contained guar gum—claimed by its marketers to decrease appetite and block the absorption of fat. When taken by mouth, guar gum forms a gel within the stomach that may contribute to a feeling of fullness and may block some nutrients so they are not absorbed.

However, there is no proof that either of these effects would be enough to produce weight loss automatically or consistently. For one thing, many overweight people keep eating even when their stomach signals that it is full. For another, if food absorption is decreased, the individual may eat more to compensate. No long-term controlled test of guar gum as a weight-control agent has been reported in the scientific literature.

In 1987, after conducting an investigation, the Postal Service acted quickly to block the sale of *Cal-Ban* through the mail. However, its Florida-based manufacturer continued to solicit orders through a toll-free number, with payment by credit card or COD, and delivery by United Parcel Service. *Cal-Ban* was also marketed through pharmacies and health-food stores. These channels are outside the Postal Service's jurisdiction.

In February 1990, *Cal-Ban*'s marketers signed a consent agreement promising to stop selling it in Iowa and to pay $20,000 to cover the state's cost of taking action against them. The company did not admit wrongdoing, but agreed to notify its 1989 customers that the Iowa Attorney General believed its ads were misleading and that a refund would be sent if requested. The company also agreed to pay restitution for 1987 and 1988, using a formula based on the response to the refund offer. Up to $50,000 would be earmarked for the state's Consumer Education Fund, while any excess would be given to an appropriate nonprofit organization. Subsequently, 80 percent of the 1989 customers asked for a refund, triggering total restitution of $320,000. Iowa officials estimated, however, that total U.S. sales of *Cal-Ban* had exceeded $20 million in 1989.

A few months later, spurred by evidence of danger, more regulatory actions were taken. Early in July, postal authorities, working with the U.S. Attorney in Tampa, Florida, obtained a temporary injunction prohibiting sales and directing telephone companies to disconnect the company's toll-free lines. During the same week, the Hillsborough County (Florida) Sheriff filed charges of fraud against three company officials. In mid-July, the Florida Department of Health and Rehabilitative Services ordered Florida retailers to remove *Cal-Ban* from their shelves and to stop selling it immediately. The department said it had acted after reviewing complaints involving more than one hundred people, at least fifty of whom required some type of medical intervention. The complaints included esophageal obstruction, gastric obstruction, upper and lower intestinal obstruction, nausea, and vomiting.

One week later, the FDA issued a regulatory letter stating that *Cal-Ban* was an unapproved new drug and was misbranded and asking that it be recalled immediately. The FDA also announced that it had collected reports of at least seventeen cases of esophageal obstruction. Hospital stays were required by ten of these people, one of whom died. Shortly afterward, the California

Department of Health Services warned consumers not to use *Cal-Ban* and warned retailers not to sell it. California authorities also embargoed more than twenty million tablets and capsules at a warehouse and manufacturing plant in Anaheim, California.

In August the Florida civil case was settled with payment of a $1.3 million penalty, and the criminal case was settled with a plea bargain in which *Cal-Ban's* marketers pled guilty to one count of organized scheme to defraud, paid a $5,000 fine, and pledged never to sell guar gum or *Cal-Ban* again in the United States. The federal case was settled with a similar consent agreement plus a penalty of $25,000. In addition, if company officials ever promote another weight-loss aid, the promotional material must make it clear that any weight loss will result from increasing exercise and/or consuming fewer calories. Some civil suits have been filed by people who believe they were harmed by using *Cal-Ban.*

Since the weight-reduction claims made for *Cal-Ban* made it a drug under federal law, the FDA could have ordered the manufacturer to stop making these claims. A simple regulatory letter might well have stopped the company dead in its tracks during its first year of operation.

## Advertising Standards

The Postal Service has a very active program to detect and stop the sale of bogus health products through the mails. Even so, many mail-order thieves operate long enough to make a profit—as do media outlets that collect money for running the ads. Each year buyers of these products lose small amounts of money individually, but tens of millions of dollars collectively. At the same time, taxpayers have to pay for government enforcement actions that would be unnecessary if media outlets had uniformly higher standards.

When questioned about standards, advertising managers typically respond that it is impossible, too difficult, or even legally risky to check every ad that comes their way. Some also respond that it should not be their responsibility to judge health claims. At the same time, they feel entitled to complete freedom to decide for themselves which ads to print. The net result is that they, too, profit from deceiving the public.

During 1984 the FDA and the Council of Better Business Bureaus sent information packets to the advertising managers of 9,500 newspapers and magazines as well as to 10,000 television and radio stations. The mailing included tips on checking ad copy as well as the marketer's credentials. Armed with this information, advertising departments could weed out the vast majority of fraudulent health ads with little effort—if they wanted to do so. In addition, if they really care about public protection, they could notify the Postal Service whenever they receive a *proposal* for an obviously fraudulent ad.

A few periodicals—most notably *The New York Times,* the *St. Petersburg Times,* and *Good Housekeeping*—have published standards and do an effective job of following them. Many others rarely run ads for bogus mail-order health products but occasionally slip up. The major television networks screen ads fairly carefully, but rarely publicize the procedures they use. No large study has tabulated how media outlets screen their ads. James Ralph believes that almost all of them make an effort to detect frauds and do reject many that are submitted. But it is clear from the Cho Low Tea incident alone that something is radically wrong.

### Advice to Consumers

Be very skeptical of advertising claims for mail-order "health" products. Almost all such products are misrepresented. Don't be misled by the promise of a "money-back guarantee." There is no reason to believe that such a guarantee is any better than the product. Remember:

- No product can "melt away fat" or cause effortless weight loss.
- No mail-order product can erase scars, wrinkles, or "cellulite."
- No device can selectively reduce one part of your body.
- No mail-order product can increase bust or penis size.
- No mail-order product can prevent or cure hair loss.
- No mail-order nutrient product can increase stamina or endurance, or increase strength or muscle mass.
- No nutrient product can "prevent aging" or prolong life.
- No nutrient product can prevent senility or increase memory.
- No pill can increase sexual stimulation or pleasure.
- Musical tapes with "subliminal" messages can't do anything more for physical or mental well-being than listening to ordinary music.

In fact, so few mail-order health products work as advertised that you should never buy one without competent medical advice.

# 21

# The Tooth Robbers

**Bob Sprague**
**Mary Bernhardt**

More than two thousand American communities have decided the matter of fluoridation at the voting booth. In thousands of others, the decision to fluoridate has been made by city councils. In recent years, however, many voters have rejected fluoridation. In fact, according to the U.S. Centers for Disease Control and Prevention, fluoridation lost in 83 out of 123 referendums held from 1980 through 1986. During the same period, 162 out of 215 city councils and other governing bodies that considered the measure approved it.

Although this trend is discouraging, it does not surprise public health leaders. As long ago as 1951, Dr. Frank A. Bull, Director of Dental Education for the Wisconsin State Board of Health, summed up the problem quite well in a speech to the Fourth Annual Conference of State Dental Directors:

> I don't believe that you can win approval of any public health program where there is organized opposition. I mean clever, well thought-up opposition. I think it is possible to beat almost anything.

In the years since this statement was made, antifluoridationists have developed clever political tactics that can play on the fears of ordinary citizens. Increasingly, these tactics have been employed to defeat fluoridation proposals. The sad fact is that people can easily be frightened by things they do not understand and can readily be confused by contradictory arguments.

## Fluoridation's Credentials

There should be no mystery about what fluoridation is. Fluoride is a mineral that occurs naturally in most water supplies. Fluoridation is the adjustment of the natural fluoride concentration to about one part of fluoride to one million parts of water. Thousands of scientific studies attest to fluoridation's safety and effectiveness in preventing tooth decay.

The history of fluoridation in the United States underlines its unique standing as a public health measure copied from a natural phenomenon. In the early 1900s, Dr. Frederick S. McKay began an almost thirty-year search for the cause of the staining of teeth that was prevalent in Colorado, where he practiced dentistry. In his investigation, McKay found the condition common in other states, including Texas, where it was known as "Texas teeth." In 1928, he concluded that such teeth, although stained, showed "a singular absence of decay," and that both the staining and the decay resistance were caused by something in the water. In 1931, the "something" was identified as fluoride.

The Public Health Service then took over to determine precisely what amount of fluoride in the water would prevent decay without causing staining. Years of "shoeleather epidemiology" by Dr. H. Trendley Dean traced the dental status of seven thousand children who drank naturally fluoridated water in twenty-one cities in four states. In 1943, he reported that the ideal amount of fluoride was one part per million parts of water. This concentration was demonstrated to result in healthy, attractive teeth that had one-third as many cavities as might otherwise be expected—and no staining. Dean, later known as the "father of fluoridation," thus paved the way for public health application of this natural phenomenon.

The next step was to determine whether water engineering could copy nature's amazing dental health benefit. At several test sites, the fluoride concentration of the public water supply was adjusted to one part per million.

One such test was conducted in the neighboring cities of Newburgh and Kingston, New York. First, the children in both cities were examined by dentists and physicians; then fluoride was added to Newburgh's water supply. After ten years, the children of Newburgh had 58 percent fewer decayed teeth than those of nonfluoridated Kingston. The greatest benefits were obtained by children who had drunk the fluoridated water since birth. Other studies showed that teeth made stronger by fluoride during childhood would remain permanently resistant to decay. As the evidence supporting fluoridation accrued, thousands of communities acted to obtain its benefits.

Too much fluoride can cause dental fluorosis, which, in its mildest form, causes small, white, virtually invisible opaque areas on teeth. In severe form, fluorosis results in brownish mottling. However, dental fluorosis is not caused by artificial fluoridation, because the levels are kept low enough to avoid this effect.

Recent data have shown that fluoridation has been reducing the incidence of cavities 20 to 40 percent in children and 15 to 35 percent in adults. The reduction is less than it used to be, probably due to improved dental hygiene and widespread use of fluoride toothpaste. Currently, more than 135 million Americans live in fluoridated communities. But eighty million others receive public water supplies that are not fluoridated—thanks largely to the efforts of poisonmongers.

## Opposition to Fluoridation

From the beginning, fluoridation has encountered opposition from scattered groups and individuals. Many of them have been associated with the "health food" industry—which views antifluoridation claims as aligned with its general propaganda that our food supply is "poisoned" (see Chapters 2 and 5). Chiropractors have opposed fluoridation as interfering with "free choice of health care." Christian Scientists have regarded it as "forced medication," and the John Birch Society has seen it as a "Communist plot."

The early efforts of the antifluoridationists ("antis") were assisted by the caution and conservatism of many physicians, dentists, and other scientists who felt that not enough research had been done for them to take a positive stand. As time went on and data piled up, however, the overwhelming majority of health scientists concluded that fluoridation is safe and effective.

But while scientists were refining and publishing their experiments, the antis were refining and publishing their battle plans. In the mid-1960s, the National Health Federation published "An Action Guide ... On How to Fight Fluoridation in Your Area." Sold for 25¢, this four-page leaflet detailed a strategy that can be used in any community where fluoridation is considered.

## "Neutralizing" Politicians

Once fluoridation proponents are known to be active, the leaflet said, antis should immediately send a letter to each member of governing bodies. The letter should emphasize "the most recent evidence" that fluoridation is harmful. Most important, it should urge the officials to "remain absolutely neutral" by putting the matter to public vote. "When this is done," the leaflet stated, "whatever political figures may be concerned are relieved of any and all responsibility in the matter."

This opening blast is designed to neutralize politicians and to raise doubt about the safety of fluoridation. It also offers an easy excuse for delaying favorable action—while the antis begin their hatchet job on public opinion.

## How Poisonmongers Work

The antis' basic technique is *the big lie*. Made infamous by Hitler, it is simple to use, yet surprisingly effective. It consists of claiming that fluoridation causes cancer, heart and kidney disease, and other serious ailments that people fear. The fact that there is no supporting evidence for such claims does not matter. The trick is to keep repeating them—because if something is said often enough, people tend to think there must be some truth to it.

A variation of the big lie is the *laundry list*. List enough "evils," and even if proponents can reply to some of them, they will never be able to cover the entire list. This technique is most effective in debates, letters to the editor, and television news reports. Another variation is the simple statement that fluoridation doesn't work. Although recent studies show less difference than there used to be in decay rates between fluoridated and nonfluoridated communities, the benefit is still substantial. In fact, the Public Health Service estimates that every dollar spent for community fluoridation saves about fifty dollars in dental bills.

A key factor in any anti campaign is the use of printed matter. Because of this, antis are very eager to have their views printed. Scientific journals will rarely publish them, but most local newspapers are willing to express minority viewpoints regardless of whether facts support them. A few editors even welcome the controversy the antis generate—expecting that it will increase readership.

The aim of anti "documents" is to create the illusion of scientific controversy. Often they quote statements that are *out of date* or *out of context*. Quotes from obscure or hard-to-locate journals are particularly effective. Another favored tactic is to *misquote* a profluoridation scientist, knowing that even if the scientist protests, the reply will not reach all those who read the original misquote.

*Half-truths* are commonly used. For example, saying that fluoride is a rat poison ignores the fact that poison is a matter of dose. Large amounts of many substances—even pure water—can poison people. But the trace amount of fluoride contained in fluoridated water will not harm anyone.

*"Experts"* are commonly quoted. It is possible to find someone with scientific credentials who is against just about anything. Most "experts" who speak out against fluoridation, however, are not experts on the subject. There are, of course, a few dentists and physicians who oppose fluoridation. Some of them object to fluoridation as a form of government intrusion, even though they

know it is safe and effective. Curiously, even when anti experts change their mind in favor of fluoridation, they sometimes find that the antis keep on quoting their earlier positions.

*Innuendo is* a technique that has broad appeal because it can be used in a seemingly unemotional pitch. Some antis admit that fluoridation has been found safe "so far," but claim that its long-range effects have "not yet" been fully explored. *The waiting game is* a related gambit in which antis suggest that waiting a bit longer will help to resolve "doubt" about fluoridation's safety. No doubt, some antis will continue to use this argument for a few hundred more years.

The *bogus reward* is a fascinating technique. Some antis have offered large rewards to anyone who would prove that fluoridation is safe. If an offer's wording is not extremely careful, however, the pros can actually collect. In 1965, a California chiropractor offered $1,000 to anyone who could produce an expert from California who had done any conclusive research or who could produce documentary evidence that fluoridation is safe. A local dental group assembled a barrage of experts and more than one hundred research reports testifying to fluoridation's safety and effectiveness. When the chiropractor refused to pay, the dental group filed suit and later settled out of court for $500.

A $100,000 reward offer survived for a longer time—but a close look will show why. In order to collect, pros had to post a bond "to cover any costs which the offerers of the reward might incur if the proof is deemed invalid." The offer did not state who would judge the evidence, but it is safe to assume that the antis themselves would have appointed the judges. If a suit had been filed to collect the reward, the court might have ruled that the offer was a gambling bet that should not be enforced by a court. Such a suit would have required at least $25,000 for the bond and legal fees. Even if it had been won, however, there was no assurance that the money would have been recovered from the individuals who sponsored the reward. Most of them were elderly and scattered widely throughout the United States and Canada.

Since the scientific community is so solidly in favor of fluoridation, antis try to discredit it entirely by use of the *conspiracy gambit.* The beauty of the conspiracy charge is that it can be leveled at anyone and there is absolutely no way to disprove it. After all, how does one prove that something is not taking place secretly? Favorite "conspirators" are the U.S. Public Health Service, the American Dental Association, the American Medical Association, the Communist Party, and the aluminum industry. Apparently, in the minds of the antis, these groups could all be working together to "poison" the American people!

Local promoters are often accused of being in the employ of "vested interests." An individual is rarely accused directly since that could trigger a lawsuit for defamation of character. Instead, a question is asked: "Could it be that Dr. So-and-so is really working for the aluminum industry?" Years ago, conspiracy claims would work primarily with the very paranoid. But modern-day government scandals may make them seem realistic to a wider audience.

*"This is only the beginning!"* is a related gambit. "First *they* will add fluoride, then vitamin pills, and the next thing you know it will be birth control pills!" Who *"they"* are not need be specified.

*Scare words* will add zip to any anti campaign. Not only the more obvious ones like "cancer" and "heart disease," but also more specialized terms like "mongoloid births" and "sickle-cell anemia." *Ecology words* are also useful. Calling fluoride a "chemical" (rather than a nutrient) can strike fear in the minds of many Americans who fear we are already too "chemicalized." The fact that water itself is a chemical and the fact that responsible use of chemicals is extremely helpful to our society will not reassure everyone. Fluoride is also called "artificial" and "a pollutant," which is "against nature." Faced with the fact that fluoridation merely copies a natural phenomenon, the antis reply that "natural" fluoride differs from "artificial" fluoride—a "fact" as yet undiscovered by scientists.

Suggesting *alternatives* is a common tactic. Here the antis propose that the community distribute free fluoride tablets to parents who wish to give them to their children. The suggested program sounds "democratic," but it will not be effective from a public health standpoint. Most parents are not motivated to administer the 4,000+ doses needed from birth through age twelve. The plea for alternatives is often made by a "neutral" individual who sounds like he will support an alternative program if water fluoridation is defeated. Don't bet on it. Such advocacy is almost always a propaganda ploy.

Profluoridationists can sometimes turn the tables on the "alternatives" argument by suggesting that nonfluoridated water remain available at a special tap for residents who want it. Despite the antis' professed fears, however, such taps get little use. After one was installed in 1979 in Lawrence, Kansas, for example, fewer than ten people out of 64,000 used it regularly.

Once fluoridation has begun in a community, antis can resort to the *"cause-of-all-evil"* gambit—blaming fluoridation for everything that occurred after it started. An example of this tactic, one that backfired on opponents, took place in Cleveland on June 1, 1956—when fluorides were to be added to the city's water supply. That day, the phone calls began: "My goldfish have died." "My African violets are wilting." "I can't make a decent cup of coffee." "My dog is constipated." Although the basis of such complaints is emotional rather than physical, this time fluoridation's innocence was beyond question. Last-minute problems had delayed its start until July!

**"Let the People Decide"**

The antis' most persuasive argument, both to legislators and to the general public, is to call for a public vote. On the surface, this appears to be the democratic way to settle the issue. But the antis are dealing from a stacked deck. First, the people who need fluoridation the most—the children—do not vote. Second, it is not difficult to confuse voters by flooding the community with scare propaganda. Average citizens do not have the educational background to sort out claim and counterclaim or to judge which "authorities" to believe. To turn against fluoridation, they don't need to accept *all* the anti arguments—*only one*. The sheer bulk of the controversy is itself likely to arouse doubt in the minds of most voters.

Occasionally, a brave profluoridation group will attempt a referendum as a last resort to overcome the resistance of its local government. But make no mistake about it—the referendum is *primarily* an antifluoridation device. Antis who say, "Let the people decide," may sound as if they wish to use a democratic process to make the decision, but experience in many cities has shown otherwise. If fluoridation wins a referendum, the usual anti response is to work for another one. In some communities that allow repeated referendums on the same subject, fluoridation has been in and out, and in and out again. When this happens, not only do children suffer, but taxpayers are saddled with the cost of the referendums.

Curiously, studies have shown that referendums can lose even in communities where public opinion favors fluoridation. People will usually go to the polls to vote against what they *don't* like. So the crucial factor in many referendums is the ability of proponents to mobilize the supporters.

The value of getting out the vote was never more strikingly demonstrated than in the 1973 referendum in Seattle, Washington. The vote was 115,000 for fluoridation and 49,000 opposed. The key to victory was an unprecedented move by Sheldon Rovin, D.D.S., who was then dean of the University of Washington School of Dentistry. Two weeks before the vote, Dr. Rovin excused students and faculty members from class so that they could participate in a door-to-door campaign. In all, five hundred doorbell-ringers saturated the city with pleas to residents. Person-to-person contact just before the vote worked in Seattle just as it might for any political candidate anywhere—by instructing voters on how to cast the ballots and by giving them a brief opportunity to share their concerns. One homeowner agreed to vote for fluoridation if the canvassers would help him move his television set to the basement.

The Seattle fluoridation forces were extremely well organized and were very sophisticated politically. They had a broad base of support from community organizations such as unions, the PTA and the Chamber of Commerce. But they also had no sizable opposition.

## The Devout Anti

Most people who power local and national antifluoridation movements see themselves as saviors of their fellow humans. Some of them make opposing fluoridation their single great mission in life; others include fluoridation among a variety of health-related causes. Staunch antifluoridationists have worked against mental health programs, compulsory immunization, and the use of animals in research.

Fluoridation's cause is damaged most by the few antis who are physicians, dentists, or others who presumably should be able to judge fluoridation on its merits. Some of them are simply misinformed. Others are alienated for reasons unconnected with fluoridation, but use this cause to get back at the scientific community which they feel has "slighted" them.

What makes a devout anti tick? Three prominent psychiatrists suggested an answer in "Psychodynamics of Group Opposition to Public Health Programs," an article that appeared in 1960 in the *American Journal of Orthopsychiatry*. Some are motivated, they wrote, by factors of personal power, prestige, or gain. Some are driven by great anxieties or hostilities, the sources of which are unconscious. Antis commonly perceive certain health measures as a threat to their "sense of wholeness," and must passionately defend themselves against the "forcible entry" of any "foreign body" or "foreign agents"—whether this be a vaccination, an interracial contact, or a wave of immigrants from overseas. Any of these is apt to be felt as a threat to their "whole way of life."

It is important to realize that a devout anti cannot be dissuaded by facts.

## NHF's Cancer Scare

The most active anti in America today is John Yiamouyiannis, Ph.D., whose background is in biochemistry. In 1974, the National Health Federation (NHF) hired him as "Science Director" and announced that he would "break the back of promoters' efforts to fluoridate more American cities." In the ensuing years, Yiamouyiannis has written several reports and has traveled around the country to give speeches, testify at hearings, and meet with legislators. Often he was accompanied by Dean Burk, Ph.D., a retired employee of the National Cancer Institute who was also a major promoter of laetrile.

In the mid-1970s, Yiamouyiannis and Burk issued several reports claiming that fluoridation causes cancer. Experts concluded that these reports were based on a *misinterpretation* of government statistics. In true anti fashion, Yiamouyiannis and Burk had compared cancer death rates in fluoridated and nonfluoridated cities but failed to consider various factors in each city (such as industrial pollution) that are known to raise the cancer death rate. By 1977, independent investigations by eight of the leading medical and scientific organizations in the English-speaking world had refuted the cancer claims.

Meanwhile, NHF concealed information about a study it had commissioned. In 1972, it granted $16,000 to the Center for Science in the Public Interest (CSPI), a group founded by former associates of Ralph Nader. While CSPI's study was under way, NHF proudly announced that it would "put the fluoride controversy into proper perspective." When the report came out *favorable* to fluoridation, however, NHF suddenly became silent about it.

During 1978, *Consumer Reports* published a two-part series on fluoridation that criticized Yiamouyiannis's work and concluded:

> The simple truth is that there's no "scientific controversy" over the safety of fluoridation. The practice is safe, economical, and beneficial. The survival of this fake controversy represents, in Consumers Union's opinion, one of the major triumphs of quackery over science in our generation.

A few months later, Yiamouyiannis filed suit for libel, charging that he had been defamed by Consumers Union's report. After a lower court dismissed the suit, Yiamouyiannis appealed to the United States Court of Appeals for the Second Circuit, which upheld the dismissal. The appeals court's ruling, issued in 1980, stated:

> It is clear that [Consumers Union] ... made a thorough investigation of the facts. Scientific writings and authorities in the field were consulted; authoritative scientific bodies speaking for substantial segments of the medical and scientific community were investigated. The unquestioned methodology of the preparation of the article exemplifies the very highest order of responsible journalism: the entire article was checked and rechecked across a spectrum of knowledge and, where necessary, changes were made in the interests of accuracy.

At about this time, Yiamouyiannis had a falling out with other NHF officials, left NHF, and started a group of his own. Without NHF's financial backing, however, his antifluoridation activities became much less effective.

In 1985, a prestigious group appointed by the British Department of Health and Social Security issued yet another review of the Yiamouyiannis/

Burk data plus more recent studies from a dozen countries. Agreeing that fluoridation does not cause cancer, the group said, "The only contrary conclusions are in our view attributable to errors in data, errors in analytical technique, and errors in scientific logic."

During the same year, Yiamouyiannis's credibility was attacked further when a team of public health experts from the Ohio Department of Health published a book analyzing his eight-page pamphlet, "A Lifesaver's Guide to Fluoridation." This pamphlet, which was invariably distributed wherever community fluoridation was considered, cited 250 references that supposedly backed up Yiamouyiannis's claims that fluoridation is ineffective and dangerous. However, when the Ohio team traced the references, they found that almost half had no relevance to community water fluoridation and many others actually supported fluoridation but were selectively quoted and misrepresented.

Without Yiamouyiannis, NHF's antifluoridation activity has slowed to a trickle. Though its magazine still blasts fluoridation occasionally, its political priorities are elsewhere. These events, in addition to the deaths of Burk and several other leading opponents, should enable communities interested in fluoridation to have a much easier time achieving it.


**Another Cancer Scare**

Early in 1990, the cancer charge was raised again—spurred by an article in *Newsweek* magazine. The magazine's story was triggered by an unauthorized release of data from an experiment in which rats and mice were exposed to high dosages of fluoride.

The experiment had been conducted by the National Toxicology Program, a branch of the National Institute of Environmental Health Sciences. More than one thousand rats and mice drank water containing 0, 11, 45, or 79 ppm (parts per million) of fluoride. No mice showed any signs of cancer, but one male rat in the 45 ppm group and four males in the 79 ppm group developed bone cancer. In addition, one male rat in the 45 ppm group, three female rats in the 79 ppm group, and one female rat in the control group developed tumors of the mouth. These dosages, of course, are enormously higher than those in fluoridated water.

Before conclusions are drawn, data normally go through extensive peer review by a panel of pathologists and epidemiologists at the agency. But in this case, raw data had been leaked to the press before the review took place. The final report concluded that there was no evidence of cancer-causing activity in female rats or in male and female mice and only "equivocal evidence" in male rats. Subsequent review by a U.S. Public Health Service expert panel concluded that the data were insignificant and that fluoridation posed no risk of cancer or any other disease. Although experts believe that the experiment has no practical significance for humans, it has furnished ammunition for antifluoridation propaganda. In the March/April 1990 issue of *Nutrition Forum,* Dr. Stephen Barrett stated:

> I believe that *Newsweek*'s article is the most irresponsible analysis of a public health topic ever published by a major national news outlet. How sad it is that a magazine which has ignored the *real* dangers of cigarette smoking is willing to devote two pages to attacking a nonexistent danger.

**Don't Be Misled**

As a public health measure, fluoridation is unusual in several ways. It is a copy of a naturally occurring phenomenon. It is supported by libraries full of articles that document its safety and effectiveness—more so than any other public health measure. It is supported by a variety of health, scientific, and civic groups that could hardly be expected to agree on any other single measure. But most significant, it is the only health measure that is often put to public vote.

If you live in a community with fluoridated water, consider yourself lucky. If you do not, don't let the poisonmongers scare you. Fluoridation is still a modern health miracle.

# 22

# Dubious Dental Care

John E. Dodes, D.D.S.
William T. Jarvis, Ph.D.

Dental problems are among the most common ailments in the United States, with a total annual cost of more than $30 billion for prevention and treatment. The majority of dentists work in the privacy of their own offices, where they are usually not subject to review by knowledgeable colleagues. This situation, plus the fact that the consequences of poor dental care may not become apparent for many years, makes it difficult for consumers to evaluate the quality of the treatment they receive. Although reliable dentistry has made great strides in recent years, quackery experts believe that over a billion dollars a year is spent annually on dubious dentistry.

## Dubious Credentials

The American Dental Association (ADA) recognizes eight dental specialties: endodontics (root-canal therapy), oral and maxillofacial surgery, oral pathology, orthodontics, pediatric dentistry, periodontics (treatment of gum disorders), prosthodontics, and public health dentistry. Some dentists who have not completed specialty training but who limit their practice or emphasize an aspect of their practice refer to themselves as specialists. Many such dentists practice in a scientific manner and do high-quality work. However, some claim to be specialists in fields that are either unrecognized, unscientific, or both. These include "cosmetic dentistry," "TMJ disorders," "holistic dentistry," "bonding," "implants," and "amalgam detoxification." A few dentists base their claim of specialization on attendance at a weekend seminar.

Now let's look at some questionable practices.

**Suboptimal Care**

This section covers six areas of dental practice that involve considerable controversy. The first is a root canal treatment that may work but is less predictable than standard endodontic treatment. The second is an approach to gum disease that has been discredited but is still used. The third is the "no-man's-land" of "TMJ therapy," in which some practitioners act responsibly while others make extravagant claims and prescribe expensive treatment that is ineffective. The remaining three treatments—implants, bonding, and tooth bleaching—are legitimate and useful when properly administered by a dentist. However, some dentists who are doing implants are not qualified to do so. Bonding is sometimes promoted with exaggerated claims. Do-it-yourself bleaching has not been proven safe and effective.

• *Sargenti root canal therapy.* The root canal is the hollow area within each tooth that normally encloses the pulp, the central part of the tooth that contains nerves and blood vessels. If the pulp becomes badly diseased or injured, root canal therapy may be able to save the tooth. During root canal therapy, the pulp is removed and the space is filled with a substitute material. Ideally, the filling material should be inert and easy to handle. The most common and scientifically accepted material is gutta percha, the coagulated sap of certain tropical trees.

In the early 1950s, a Swiss dentist named Angelo Sargenti developed a root canal filling he called N2. Its active ingredient is paraformaldehyde, which, in contact with water, forms formaldehyde, a toxic substance used in embalming fluid. Paraformaldehyde pastes have not been proven safe and have caused painful injuries to surrounding tissues.

Injecting N2 paste into the root canal is easier and faster than placing gutta percha, but the pressure needed to get the paste to the tip of the root can force the toxic mixture into the area beneath the tooth. In 1990, Laurie Ann Shoop of Pompano Beach, Florida, received a $1 million settlement from the malpractice insurance company of a dentist who had used the Sargenti technique. The N2 injured the left side of her jawbone, necessitating its removal and requiring more than forty surgical procedures to partially correct the deformity. Dr. Stephen Cohen, a root canal specialist from San Francisco who gave a pretrial statement, said he had testified in eighty cases involving N2 and that its use today is inexcusable. "If a dentist makes an error with the Sargenti paste, the consequences are dire," he said in a newspaper report on the settlement.

The American Endodontic Society (AES), an organization formed by proponents of the Sargenti method, dismisses this apparent danger and states that thirty thousand dentists in the United States and Canada use N2 or a similar paste-filler. Although AES provides its members with an impressive-looking certificate, this credential has no standing within the scientific dental community. The officially recognized endodontic specialty group is the American Association of Endodontists.

• *Keyes gum disease treatment.* In the late 1970s, an oral hygiene program called the Keyes technique was widely promoted as a nonsurgical alternative for treating advanced periodontal disease (pyorrhea). The technique includes microscopic examination of the bacterial film covering the teeth (plaque) and cleaning the teeth and gums with a mixture of salt, baking soda, and peroxide. Although studies have shown that these agents have some effectiveness against harmful bacteria in laboratory tests, this does not mean they are effective in people. A study by proponents of the Keyes method found some effectiveness in humans, but the study lacked a control group. In addition, the participants received antibiotics, so it wasn't possible to tell whether the benefits they experienced were actually due to the baking soda regimen. Despite the dearth of research, the Keyes method became popular with patients, who were happy to avoid periodontal surgery; and with dentists, who found it both profitable and an excellent marketing tool.

By 1983, at least three long-term studies had found that surgical treatment was more effective than nonsurgical treatment for advanced periodontal disease. More recently, researchers at the University of Minnesota conducted a four-year controlled study of 171 adults with moderate periodontal disease. The researchers concluded that while the baking soda mixture did help in maintaining oral health, it was no more effective than ordinary toothpaste. They also found that those using the baking soda regimen were three times as likely to stop their program because it was inconvenient. Thus it seems unlikely that the Keyes technique can contribute more toward healthy gums than brushing with ordinary toothpaste and using dental floss.

• *Inappropriate TMJ therapy.* A confusing muddle of diseases and conditions have been lumped under the term "TMJ" disorders. The most common symptom of "TMJ" is chronic facial pain, often accompanied by difficulty in fully opening the mouth. "TMJ" is actually the abbreviation for "temporomandibular joint," the hinge joint that connects the lower jaw to the skull. Since the joint itself may not be the source of the symptoms, the term temporomandibular disorders (TMD) is more accurate.

TMJ disorders have been described as dentistry's "hottest" area of unorthodoxy and out-and-out quackery. Pains in the face, head, neck, and even remote parts of the body have been erroneously diagnosed as TMJ problems. Some practitioners also claim that a "bad bite" causes ailments ranging from menstrual cramps, impotence, and scoliosis, to a host of systemic diseases.

The correction of a "bad bite" can involve irreversible treatments such as grinding down the teeth or building them up with dental restorations. The most widespread unscientific treatment involves placing a plastic appliance between the teeth. These devices, called mandibular orthopedic repositioning appliances (MORAs), typically cover only some of the teeth and are worn continuously for many months or even years. When worn too much, MORAs can cause the patient's teeth to move so far out of proper position that orthodontics or facial reconstructive surgery is needed to correct the deformity. TMJ expert Charles S. Greene, D.D.S., of Northwestern University Dental School, cautions that plastic appliances should be used only when necessary, for limited periods of time, and never while eating.

Plastic appliances are sometimes misprescribed when a patient's jaw joint makes a clicking or grinding noise, even when there are no other symptoms. Research shows that joint sounds without pain or restricted or irregular jaw movement do not indicate any disease process and that no treatment should be undertaken in these circumstances.

Some dentists use electronic instruments to diagnose and treat TMJ disorders. The diagnostic procedures include: surface electromyography (EMG), jaw tracking, silent period durations, thermography, sonography, and Doppler ultrasound. Use of these procedures for diagnosing TMJ is not supported by scientific evidence. Similarly, treatment with ultrasound or TENS (transcutaneous electrical nerve stimulation in which a low-voltage, low-amperage current is applied to painful body areas) has not been proven effective. Some dentists obtain TMJ x-ray films as part of their routine dental examination. These films should be obtained only when there is a history of trauma or progressive worsening of symptoms, but not as a *routine* screening procedure.

Some "TMJ specialists" are soliciting personal injury attorneys by offering to certify accident victims as having accident-related TMJ injuries—including "mandibular whiplash," a diagnosis not recognized by the scientific community. Attorneys have even been invited to free medicolegal seminars with a brochure stating that a patient "was awarded a settlement of over $100,000 for TMJ injuries *alone* ... based on ... emotional and physical distress resulting from the TMJ injury." Ultimately the insured public has to pay for such abuse.

There is considerable evidence that for patients with real TMJ problems, safe, simple, inexpensive treatments (such as warm moist compresses, simple jaw exercises, and a soft diet) will produce high rates of improvement similar to those of risky, complex, irreversible, expensive treatments. Surgery should be considered only for tumors, "frozen jaws," or other definitively diagnosable problems that can only be resolved through surgery. Other alternatives should be exhausted first. If surgery is recommended, it is prudent to obtain a second opinion, preferably from the oral surgery department of a dental school.

• *Improper implants.* Implants are artificial root substitutes that are placed within the jaw bone to anchor artificial teeth. They are usually made of metal, especially titanium. Today there are implant systems that provide a good chance of success with little danger of serious complications. However, some implants are being placed by dentists whose training has consisted of a short course (sometimes only one day) or simply viewing a videotape. For this reason, consumers should carefully investigate the experience of any dentist they consult about implants. An oral surgeon or periodontist is likely to have the best surgical skills in placing the implants, but some general dentists have undergone sufficient training to do the surgery properly. Consumers should request complete information about the type of implant and possible complications.

• *Inappropriate bonding.* Bonding is a safe and useful technique for repairing broken, chipped, or discolored front teeth. However, it does have limitations. The teeth to be bonded should be supported by healthy bone and gums. Patients may have to adjust some of their eating habits, and should be aware that bonding materials are not as durable as silver, gold, or porcelain. Despite its limitations, bonding is being promoted by some dentists as a substitute for more durable repairs (crowns) and as an alternative to orthodontics. Although bonding is an excellent way of eliminating a simple (cosmetic) gap between a patient's front teeth, it is not appropriate for complicated cases in which the teeth are so poorly positioned that they don't function properly. It is also being promoted as a treatment for loose teeth (a symptom of periodontal disease)—which it is not.

• *Do-it-yourself bleaching.* Bleaching of the teeth by dentists is a legitimate procedure that requires care to ensure that the patient is not injured by the caustic bleaching agent. In recent years there has been a flurry of advertising for tooth-bleaching agents for home use. None of these products has been proven safe and effective by well-designed studies. Experts warn that these home-use products may not be effective and might even be dangerous.

**Nutritional Pseudoscience**

Many dentists are promoting unscientific "nutritional" methods that can be quite lucrative. A 1985 article in a dental trade journal stated: "Are you interested in doubling your net practice income? We almost did it last year.... We used nutritional counseling as the vehicle."

The increased income is produced by selling dietary supplements that are unnecessary and overpriced. The "counseling" may be based on discredited diagnostic methods such as hair analysis, lingual vitamin C testing, or dubious tests for "food allergies." Some dentists are distributors for multilevel companies that market supplements and herbal preparations with suggestions that everyone should use them.

• *"Balancing body chemistry"* is based on the notion that dietary practices can prevent a wide variety of "degenerative" diseases. Its advocates use various laboratory tests to determine the biochemical state of the patient and recommend special diets and expensive food supplements to achieve "balance." Supporters of these methods greatly exaggerate what nutrition can do. Their patients acquire false hopes and waste money on lab tests and food supplements.

• *Hair analysis.* Closely connected to balancing body chemistry is the technique known as hair analysis. Here a sample of hair is sent to a laboratory for spectrographic analysis. The laboratory report states which components are "deficient" and recommends specific supplements—often the lab's own brand. The practitioner then sells the product to the patient. As explained in Chapter 2, this is not legitimate practice. If you encounter it in a dental office, switch to another dentist.

• *Computer analysis.* Some dentists use computers to analyze the diets of their patients and recommend supplement concoctions, usually by brand name. While computer analysis of diet can be valuable when done properly, use as a basis for recommending supplements is not valid.

• *"Holistic dentistry."* As noted in Chapter 26, promoters of "holistic" approaches typically claim that disease can be prevented by maintaining "optimum" health, or "wellness." "Wellness" is something for which quacks can get paid when there is nothing wrong with the patient. In the dental office, these schemes usually involve the purchase of expensive dietary supplements or a plastic bite appliance.

## Other Bizarre Practices

Some dentists use pendulums to test for "food compatibility." Some perform dental procedures under pyramid-shaped structures that they believe will reduce the incidence of infection. Some dentists employ what they call Chinese medicine—including herbalism, acupuncture, vitamin therapy, and whatever else they wish to throw in. Others are dabbling with iridology, reflexology, body "auras," Kirlian photography, black box devices, and other occult practices.

• *"Applied kinesiology"* is a pseudoscience involving the notion that many health problems can be diagnosed by testing muscles while various substances are in contact with the body (see Chapter 26). Practitioners of "dental kinesiology" may consider muscle testing useful in locating diseased teeth, determining sensitivity to tooth filling materials, restricting orthodontic treatment, constructing oral devices, and more. Typically they test muscle strength by pushing or pulling the patient's arm before and after vitamins or other substances are placed under the patient's tongue. "Treatment" then consists of expensive vitamin supplements or a special diet.

• *Cranial osteopathy.* Although the bones of the skull are fused, dentists who practice "cranial osteopathy" claim that they can be manipulated. This, say proponents, causes "the energy of life" to flow and can cure or prevent a wide variety of health problems ranging from headache and visual impairment to an "imbalance" in leg lengths. The "manipulation" is accomplished by pushing hard on the face and skull. The only demonstrable results of this therapy are loss of money and extensive bruising of the patient's face.

• *Auriculotherapy.* Auriculotherapy (acupuncture of the ear) is based on the notion that the body and organs are represented on the surface of the ear. Auriculotherapy is claimed to be effective against facial pain and ailments throughout the body. Its practitioners twirl needles or administer small electrical currents at points on the ear that supposedly represent diseased organs. Courses on auriculotherapy are popular among holistic dentists. Although complications from unsterilized and broken needles have been reported, this bizarre practice is touted as "quick, easy, inexpensive, effective, and completely reversible."

## Anti-Sugar Crusaders

Dentists generally say that sugar is bad for your teeth. But research shows that the physical nature of foods and frequency of intake are even more important in producing tooth decay than the amount of sugar that is consumed. Length of contact with the tooth's surface is the key factor. For this reason, honey, dried fruits, pastries, and cereals—which can stick in the pits and fissures of teeth—are the foods most likely to produce cavities. Soda pop, a major sugar-containing product, doesn't have as great a decay-producing effect because it generally doesn't stay in contact with the tooth surface for very long.

The dental profession has long sought to teach people not to eat sweets as snacks—especially sticky, gooey sweets. But some dentists seem to have an obsession about refined (white) sugar and attack it with the fervor of evangelists. Many of these anti-sugar warriors have been influenced by the writings of Weston Price, an early twentieth-century dentist who imagined that sugar causes not only tooth decay but physical, mental, moral, and social decay as well. During a whirlwind tour of areas where primitive people could be viewed, Price examined them superficially and jumped to fantastic conclusions. While extolling their health, he overlooked their short life expectancy, high infant mortality, endemic diseases, and malnutrition. While praising their diets for not producing cavities, he ignored the fact that malnourished people don't usually get many cavities.

Price noted correctly that primitive people who had few cavities when they ate native food developed dental troubles when exposed to civilization. But he did not realize why. Most primitive people are used to "feast or famine" eating. When large amounts of sweets are suddenly made available, they overindulge themselves! Not knowing the value of balancing their diets, they also ingest too much salt and fatty foods.

Price also noted that exposure to civilization had led to an increased incidence of other diseases. But this increase was not caused simply by exposure to the food supply of the civilized world, as Price imagined. Although diet was a factor, it was a matter not merely of eating "civilized" food but of *abusing* it. Price overlooked other factors that were important in increasing the disease rate. One was exposure to unfamiliar germs, to which the natives were not resistant. Another was the drastic change in their way of life as they gave up strenuous physical activities such as hunting. Alcohol abuse was also a factor.

Today's anti-sugar warriors are highly philosophical in their approach. Many of them believe that dental problems are not caused by local factors in the mouth but are due to problems of the body as a whole. They are often the same dentists who make public statements against the proven benefits of fluoridation—suggesting instead that elimination of refined sugar from the diet is all that is needed to prevent cavities. Removing refined sugar from the diet is not a realistic suggestion. Even if this could be done, tooth decay would not be eliminated. All fermentable carbohydrates can contribute to the decay process.

The anti-sugar warriors often endorse "natural" sweets as safe for teeth, but scientific studies of snack foods do not support this recommendation. Years ago, for example, it was found that an All Natural Carob Proteen Energy Bar was twice as cavity-producing as a Milky Way bar. Unsweetened grape juice proved slightly worse than a Coke, and a Natural Honey Sesame Bar was more than twice as cariogenic as a Hershey bar.

### "Silver-Amalgam Toxicity"

One of the simplest ways to bilk people is to tell them something they have is no good and sell them something else. During the past decade, a small but vocal group of dentists, physicians, and various other "holistic" advocates have been doing exactly that—by claiming that mercury-amalgam ("silver") fillings are a health hazard and should be replaced.

"Silver" fillings are an alloy of silver, tin, copper, zinc, and mercury. While the vast majority of dentists recognize that silver fillings are safe, some blame a large number of diseases—such as multiple sclerosis, immune deficiency diseases, and emotional conditions—on leakage of mercury from the fillings.

Anti-amalgam dentists typically use a mercury vapor analyzer to convince patients that "detoxification," is needed. To use the device, the dentist asks the patient to chew vigorously for ten minutes, which causes tiny amounts of mercury to be released from the fillings. Although this exposure lasts for just a few seconds and most of the mercury will be exhaled rather than absorbed by the body, the machines give a high readout, which the anti-amalgamist interprets as dangerous. The most commonly used device, the Jerome mercury tester, is an industrial device that multiplies the amount of mercury it detects by a factor of 8,000. This gives a reading for a cubic meter, a volume far larger than the human mouth. The proper way to determine mercury exposure is to measure blood or urine levels, which indicate how much has been absorbed by the body. Scientific testing has shown that the amount of mercury absorbed from fillings is insignificant.

Anti-amalgamists may also use a galvanometer to measure tiny differences in the electrical conductivity of the teeth. One such device—the "Amalgameter"—was investigated by the FDA because literature accompanying the device alleged that it could be used to recommend the removal of dental fillings. In a 1985 regulatory letter, the agency said "there is no scientific basis for the removal of dental amalgams for the purpose of replacing them with other materials as described in your leaflet. . . . We consider your device as being directly associated with. . . . a process that may have adverse health consequences when used for the purposes for which it was intended." Although the dentist who manufactured this product has stopped production, these and similar devices are still in use.

There is overwhelming evidence that mercury-amalgam fillings are safe. Although billions of amalgam fillings have been used successfully, fewer than fifty cases of allergy have been reported in the scientific literature since 1905. Yet anti-amalgam dentists often recommend that they be replaced with either plastic or gold; a profitable recommendation for the dentist involved, but one that can lead to serious complications for the patient.

In 1985, a $100,000 settlement was awarded to a fifty-five-year-old California woman whose dentist removed her silver fillings after testing them with a Dermatron, a device said to measure "energy flow" through "acupuncture meridians." The dentist claimed that the fillings were a "liability" to the patient's large intestine. In removing the fillings from five teeth, the dentist caused severe nerve damage necessitating root canal therapy for two teeth and extraction of two others.

The false diagnosis of mercury-amalgam toxicity is potentially very harmful and reflects extremely poor judgment on the part of the practitioner. We believe that dentists who engage in this practice should have their license revoked.

The leading advocate of "balancing body chemistry" and "mercury-amalgam toxicity" is Hal A. Huggins, D.D.S., a dentist from Colorado Springs, Colorado. Huggins is also crusading against root canal therapy, which he claims can make people susceptible to arthritis, multiple sclerosis, amyotrophic lateral sclerosis, and other autoimmune diseases. As is the case with mercury-amalgam fillings, there is no scientific evidence that teeth treated with root canal therapy produce any adverse effect on the immune system or any other part of the body.

### The Spread of Misinformation

Not all techniques used by dentists are learned at dental schools. New ideas and techniques are constantly being developed. Unfortunately, the dental profession has not yet developed a system to evaluate the validity of new methods promoted through seminars conducted by other practitioners. Too often, a questionable practice must become a major issue before a scientific body like the American Dental Association Council on Dental Research is prompted to issue a guiding statement. By that time, its promoters may have a following of dentists who continue their practices despite recommendations to the contrary.

Information can also spread by word of mouth. Consider the experience of a dentist who had been in practice for nine years when he bumped into an old schoolmate. "Vitamin E seems to help the gums," his friend said. "Just have your patients chew up a capsule, swish the remains around their mouth, and floss them between their teeth." When the dentist tried it, he thought he could see an improvement, and his patients thought so, too. He would ask them such questions as, "Have you noticed that your gums aren't as red as they used to be?" "Do your gums bleed less now?" and "Have you noticed less soreness?"

Some tricky things can happen when a clinician looks for something as subtle and subjective as changes in color and pain. Both patient and doctor tend to see what they hope to find. More important, when improvement does occur, people tend to credit the treatment even though a natural healing process may be responsible. There was a time in medical history when conclusions based upon simple observation were accepted because doctors didn't know better. Clinical observations are still a source of research leads, but they are not a substitute for scientifically designed studies.

True scientists base their beliefs on objective reviews of measurable data. Their commitment should not be to current beliefs but to the pursuit of truth; if they receive better evidence, they should be able to change their position. But some people arrive at beliefs that are *delusional* and held so rigidly that new knowledge is either altered to fit their notions or rejected as false. While genuine scientists change their theories to bring them in line with new facts, deluded investigators will alter facts to fit their theories!

Unfortunately, deluded or misguided dentists don't wear signs around their neck proclaiming themselves to be unorthodox. Let's illustrate with a fictitious example: Steve Warmheart has been a dentist for fifteen years. He likes what he is but feels that most people do not appreciate dentistry's true worth. He firmly believes that the mouth is the barometer of total body health and that problems in the mouth are not just local but involve the patient's entire system. Steve relates everything he learns about health to this basic principle. No one can change his mind because he is so sure that his fundamental belief is correct. Unhappily, it is exactly that—resistance to change—which makes Steve untrustworthy as a practitioner.

Many people believe that the actions of quacks are so preposterous that any thinking person (which we all regard ourselves to be) can spot them easily. This is a fallacy. Dubious dentists tend to be extremely self-confident and to do an exceptional job of selling themselves to patients.

Several factors may have contributed to quackery's prevalence among dentists. These include: increased competition, advertising; higher costs for education and for opening a practice, lower incidence of tooth decay due to fluoridation and better oral hygiene, diminished dental education in the methods of science, and the failure of organized dentistry to develop guidelines and policies for combatting quackery. Some dentists with an entrepreneurial bent seem willing to embrace virtually any dubious practice that has profit-making potential.

Many dental quacks actually believe in the techniques they promote. The instruction of dental students may be partially to blame. Little about the scientific method, scientific reasoning, or statistics is included in dental education. Some dental schools are largely authoritarian—with an emphasis on memorizing facts rather than understanding their scientific basis. These factors leave many students willing to accept the views of a perceived authority figure without checking whether they are scientifically supportable.

Although most teachings at the postgraduate level are valid, courses on unproven and disproven topics are more common than they should be. Many schools and dental organizations permit the delivery of pseudoscientific ideas through their continuing education programs and publications. For example, Boston's Goldman School of Dentistry has sponsored a course "Adventures in Dental Hygiene," presented by a self-styled holistic dentist who is a leading crusader against amalgam fillings. Although the course included reflexology and acupressure, it was accredited by the Academy of General Dentistry and the ADA. Georgetown University School of Dentistry has offered a five-day postgraduate course on cranial osteopathy which cost $1,250. At the 1989 Greater New York Dental Meeting (the largest dental convention in the world), a course was given by a physician who is a proponent of clinical ecology, a disreputable form of "allergy" treatment. During his talk he called silver-amalgams fillings "toxic time bombs." And at the 1993 Greater Long Island Dental Meeting, a chiropractor shared his views on distinguishing between "TMJ" and "cervical syndrome," which he said was a misalignment ("subluxation") of the neck that mimics TMJ pain. If the patient's legs have equal length, he said, the problem is dental. If one leg is shorter, however, spinal realignment is needed, with periodic check-ups to make sure the problem does not recur.

When a prestigious dental school or reputable professional group sponsors a course eligible for continuing education credit, it is easy to mistakenly conclude that the course is scientifically valid. ADA officials have expressed concern about dubious seminars but are afraid that aggressive actions (such as "blacklisting" speakers) could trigger expensive lawsuits. Another factor perpetuating these seminars is that they can be very profitable for their sponsors. In 1993, the ADA began a voluntary Continuing Education Recognition Program (CERP) for sponsors of continuing education courses. To achieve recognition, sponsors are supposed to ensure that the courses they accredit have a sound scientific basis. However, CERP's published standards contain no guidelines on topic or speaker selection. Thus it remains to be seen how effective the CERP program will be.

The media often promote quackery by not investigating thoroughly. In one case, on CBS TV's "New York Nightly News," a dentist with a degree in nutrition from a nonaccredited diploma mill was allowed to terrorize the public with false allegations of the toxic effects of "mercury" fillings. A recent article in *Newsweek* greatly distorted the significance of several studies on amalgam fillings. And a piece on the CBS newsmagazine "60 Minutes," which included the same distortions, has caused countless patients to seek removal of their mercury fillings.

The "60 Minutes" story was one of the most irresponsible programs ever aired on a health topic. The program featured a woman who said that her severe symptoms of multiple sclerosis had disappeared the day after her mercury-amalgam fillings were removed. Even if the mercury in fillings could cause multiple sclerosis, the woman's claim was still preposterous. Drilling out the fillings causes small amounts of mercury vapor to be inhaled, producing a temporary *increase* in body mercury load, not an overnight decrease!

## Greater Protection Is Needed

We hope this chapter will help consumers to recognize current situations in which their health or pocketbook may be in jeopardy. We also hope that dentists who read this will become more wary of certain dental promoters. Recognizing quackery in all its forms is a formidable task. Its methods may seem honorable, its promoters convincing. Sometimes the only dividing line between quackery and an innovative idea lies not in what is done, but in how much is promised by the doer.

If the profession of dentistry is to remain reputable, it must find a way to control the spread of dubious methods. Steps should also be taken to stop the spread of misinformation to dentists through accredited courses. This can be accomplished by enforcing standards for the sponsors of courses and guidelines for the selection of speakers. It would also help if dental education included more instruction on the scientific method and the detection of quackery. Indeed, courses on consumer health strategy should be included in everyone's education.

# 23

# The Gadgeteers

### Wallace F. Janssen

There was dead silence in the courtroom. The tense little man in the witness chair leaned forward and shook his finger at the jury.

*"I had fits all my life till Dr. Ghadiali cured me!"* he shouted. *"His Spectrochrome stopped my fits and now I feel grand!"*

Suddenly the witness paled, stiffened in his chair, and frothed at the mouth. As he began to convulse, a government physician and courtroom attendants stepped forward, placed something in his mouth, and carried him away.

This shocking moment was but one of several dramatic episodes that marked the trial of Dinshah P. Ghadiali, "seventh son of a seventh son" and organizer of a nationwide healing cult that became a religion to his followers.

Ghadiali was a "gadget quack," inventor of the "Spectrochrome," a machine that resembled a theatrical spotlight. Spectrochrome, he claimed, would cure all diseases by projection of colored light. Not ordinary light, of course, but rays from a 1,000-watt bulb passed through a glass tank of water and focused by a crude lens through colored glass slides. Spectrochrome offered something special—"no diagnosis, no drugs, no manipulation, no surgery"— simply "attuned color waves." The light boxes bore labels stating they were "for the measurement and restoration of the human radioactive and radio-emanative equilibrium."

Directions for the treatment were spelled out in Ghadiali's textbook, *Spectrochrometry*. Combinations of light colors were specific for body areas and diseases being treated. Time of treatment was determined by the phases of the moon and the dictates of astrology. Latitude and longitude of the place of treatment were determined according to "solar, lunar, and terrestrial gravitation." The patient had to be nude, with his body facing north.

A three-volume *Ghadiali Encyclopedia* defined the technical language of Spectrochrometry and contained case histories of people who were supposedly helped by it. "For legal protection," the *Encyclopedia* suggested that words like "imbalance" be used for "disease" and "normalate" for "cure."

Appropriately for an astrological society, followers of the cult were organized in local congregations called "planets." Each planet was headed by a "Normalator" who gave treatments and instructed the faithful. Spectrochrome was more than colored-light seances—it was a way of life to its followers! They were to eat no meat and to use no alcohol, tea, coffee, or tobacco. Honey and eggs were likewise taboo. Membership cost $90. Most amazing was the growth of the cult: At the time of the trial, Ghadiali had some nine thousand followers who paid dues and many others who took "treatments."

Pathos and tragedy marked the trial in federal court at Camden, New Jersey, where victims of the fraud and survivors of other victims told their stories. The saddest testimony concerned people who had abandoned rational medical treatment and then succumbed to their diseases while depending on Spectrochrome.

The "case histories" Ghadiali had published in his *Encyclopedia* were pathetic. The Government spotlighted five of these cases in court and proved that the allegedly successful results were false. Three of the victims had died from the conditions Ghadiali claimed to have cured—two from tuberculosis, and a third from complications following severe burns. In the third case, the *Encyclopedia* contained photographs purporting to show the stages in the healing of burns that covered a little girl's body. The mother testified that scars and open sores had continued until the girl died. The fourth case was that of a girl whose sight Ghadiali claimed to have "restored," but who in fact was still totally blind. The fifth victim, a spastic girl completely paralyzed from the waist down, was carried to the witness chair. She had been photographed standing alone and reported to walk unaided. She testified that she had been supported by others except at the moment the picture was snapped.

Most dramatic was the testimony of the son of a man who died from diabetes. Pointing at the defendant, he charged: *"You told my father to stop insulin. You told him to eat plenty of brown sugar and starches. You said he would recover with Spectrochrome!"*

The evidence showed that Ghadiali himself did not believe in Spectrochrome. Certainly he was aware of the importance of suitable "qualifications" and had obtained a false M.D. degree from a diploma mill at a cost of $133.33. Other "degrees" were secured in a similar manner. One institution he did attend was the Atlanta Penitentiary, where he "matriculated" in 1925 after a conviction for violating the Mann Act, a federal law prohibiting transportation of women across state lines for immoral purposes. (He said he had been "framed" by the Ku Klux Klan.) Testifying in the 1930s against the passage of the Federal Food, Drug, and Cosmetic Act, Ghadiali claimed to have a million-dollar business.

The forty-two-day trial was the longest in the history of the FDA up to that time. Ghadiali had 112 witnesses who testified they had used Spectrochrome successfully, making a total of 216 persons whose cases figured in the trial. Government witnesses included experts on cancer, diabetes, tuberculosis, heart disease, blood pressure, and nervous and mental disorders. The Government had to prove beyond a reasonable doubt that Spectrochrome was a fraud and Ghadiali its perpetrator.

On January 7, 1947, the jury brought in a verdict of guilty on all twelve counts in the case. The sentence, by Federal Judge Philip Forman, was carefully designed to avoid making a martyr of Ghadiali and to put a stop to his gigantic swindle. This was accomplished through a $20,000 total fine, probation for five years, and a three-year prison term to be served if the defendant resumed his illegal activities.

On the very day his probation ended, Dinshah Ghadiali announced his intention to found a new "Institute." Changing the name slightly, he built more machines and resumed leadership of the local branches, renamed "studios." New literature was issued bearing substantially the same unwarranted claims as before. The FDA requested an injunction which became permanent in July 1958, finally ending the operations of this "colorful" cult.

## An Endless Variety of Gadgets

The Spectrochrome was but one of hundreds of contraptions and gadgets that the FDA has dealt with since it obtained legal powers over "therapeutic devices" in 1938. The extraordinary variety of these health fakes is in itself significant. They range from seemingly complex electronic instruments to disarmingly simple articles of everyday use.

One of the most amusing I can recall was the Chiropra Therapeutic Comb, invented by Herr Dr. Theo. Schwarz, of Mannheim, Germany. Imports were spotted by U.S. Customs and turned over to the FDA. Herr Schwarz theorized that the act of scratching is beneficial, a well-known fact that he extended to extraordinary lengths. The Chiropra Comb, a soft rubber article with curved teeth, came with a thirty-six-page illustrated manual of instructions on how to

324    *The Health Robbers*

scratch—for the treatment of virtually all diseases. Charts showed the proper scratching patterns for men, women, and children. For high blood pressure, for example, the instructions called for scratching the back of the trunk and the back of the lower legs. For arthritis deformans, criss-cross scratching of the lower back and the back of the left leg was prescribed.

The Chiropra system was promoted in Germany by the "Chiropra Institute" of Heidelberg. The FDA detained the imports on the basis of false claims that scratching would benefit such conditions as cancer, multiple sclerosis, asthma, heart and circulatory diseases, insomnia, constipation, lumbago, arthritis, stomach ache, fallen arches, and cold feet.

The variety of gadgets to cure anything and everything never ceases to amaze! But even more amazing is the uncritical capacity of so many people to believe that any one thing can do so much. About the same time I heard of the Chiropra Comb (the mid-1950s), the FDA seized a little device called "Babylon's Zone Therapy Roller." This was simply a single large ball-bearing mounted on a block of wood—resembling a furniture caster. The general idea was that massaging the feet on the ball-bearing could benefit many different conditions. After all, are not the feet connected to the rest of the body, and do they not affect the way you feel? So why not treat the whole body through the soles of the feet?

Dr. Scott's Electric Hair Brush for the Bald—a turn-of-the-century marvel—was warranted to cure nervous headache, bilious headache, and neuralgia in five minutes! Over half a century later, it took a hard-fought court case to stop a dentist's claims that regular use of his toothbrush kit was the best way to prevent heart disease, cancer, and birth defects in one's offspring.

A seemingly harmless device can turn out to be inherently dangerous. Consider the "Relax-A-Cisor," an electrical contraption for the overweight— designed to provoke muscle spasms through mild electrical shocks. This was promoted as "passive exercise," a pleasant and effortless way to reduce. It took years of investigation and a five-month court battle to put this profitable gismo out of business. Forty witnesses testified about the injuries they had received from its use. Medical experts explained the hazards of treatment with such a machine. Federal Judge William P. Gray concluded that the Relax-A-Cisor would be hazardous in a wide range of conditions including gastrointestinal, orthopedic, muscular, neurological, vascular, skin, kidney, and female disorders. He found it could cause miscarriages and could aggravate such pre-existing problems as epilepsy, hernia, ulcers, and varicose veins.

More than 400,000 Americans fell for this major health hoax of the late 1960s. Obviously, to round up all these machines from all their users would have been practically impossible. Accordingly, the FDA issued a public warning and arranged for public notices to be displayed in U.S. Post Offices throughout the country.

Much gadget quackery is designed for use by health practitioners, especially chiropractors. During the 1950s and early 1960s, more than five thousand "Micro-Dynameters" were sold. Chiropractors purchased most of them at prices of up to $875. This machine was represented as capable of diagnosing and treating virtually all diseases (a sure sign of quackery). It consisted of a highly sensitive galvanometer fitted with various electrodes that were applied to different areas of the patient's body. Actually, the only condition it could detect was perspiration! Because of its uselessness, the Court of Appeals found the device unsafe even in the hands of a licensed practitioner.

Announcing a nationwide campaign to round up all Micro-Dynameters in use, the FDA Commissioner called the machine "a peril to public health because it cannot correctly diagnose any disease." Thousands of people, he said, had been hoodwinked into believing they had diseases they did not have, or had failed to get proper treatment for diseases they did have.

In 1972, the FDA began conducting a nationwide round-up of "Diapulse" devices. This machine was represented as an effective means of diathermy (deep heat) treatment. But FDA tests showed it produced an insignificant amount of heat—not enough for any therapeutic effect. Promoted mainly to M.D.s, Diapulse was backed by pseudomedical literature based on uncontrolled experiments. Many sales were made at seminars for doctors. During 1973 alone, more than one thousand of the machines were seized or voluntarily turned over to the FDA.

In recent years, the FDA has taken action against several bogus devices that involve galvanometers connected to a voltmeter or a computer (see Chapters 13 and 27). These devices, used mainly by homeopathic physicians, are said to detect and balance "electromagnetic energy" emanating from bodily organs.

The cost to patients of diagnosis or treatment with ineffective machines far exceeds the cost of the equipment. A conservative estimate would be $100 million annually.

## From Witchcraft to Science Fiction

Since much gadget quackery is absurd, why do people fall for it?

Gadget quackery had its beginnings thousands of years ago when people first used charms and fetishes to ward off evil spirits and cure disease. Belief in magic is still a major factor in the success of health fads and cults. At the same time, the miracles of science have made it easy to believe in science fiction.

When Benjamin Franklin published his now famous discoveries on electricity, he also helped open the door to two of the most famous frauds in medical history. The idea that this mysterious force might have medical applications was widely popular. Franklin himself had worked with a physician who attempted to use electric shock in treating a woman for convulsions.

In 1784, while representing the United States in France, Franklin was appointed to a royal commission to investigate the hypnotist Antoine Mesmer, whose treatments had become the rage of Paris. Mesmer, clad in a lilac suit, carrying a metal wand, and playing a harmonica, healed by what he called "animal magnetism." Patients sat around a huge vat or "battery," holding iron rods that were immersed in a solution. The treatments went on for hours, accompanied by shouts, hysterical laughter, and convulsions. The Franklin commission included the noted chemist Lavoisier ("The Father of Modern Chemistry") and a physician named Guillotin (inventor of the device for execution by beheading). After performing some experiments, they reported finding no electricity in Mesmer's tub. Nor did they detect the current known as "animal magnetism." A royal decree banned further treatments, but Mesmer was allowed to take his winnings to England.

Ten years later, Elisha Perkins, a mule trader turned physician, secured a patent for "Perkins Tractors." Franklin was dead, but popular interest in electricity was still great. The tractors, two pointed rods about three inches long, one gold-colored, the other silver, were simply drawn downward across the afflicted part of the anatomy, in a sort of scratching motion. This, it was theorized, would draw off the "noxious fluid" (electricity) that was alleged to cause disease. "Tractoration," of course, was universal therapy—good for everything. For a time, the Perkins treatment enjoyed amazing popularity, with ministers, college professors, and Congressmen giving enthusiastic endorsement. The Chief Justice of the Supreme Court bought a pair, and President Washington was a customer and wrote letters recommending the treatment. The medical profession was initially impressed; but in 1796 the Connecticut Medical Society condemned the treatment as "gleaned from the miserable remains of animal magnetism." In the following year the Society expelled Dr. Perkins from membership. In 1799, he voluntarily served in a yellow fever epidemic in New York, caught the disease, and died. Tractoration soon died out as well.

But electrical health gadgetry marched on—through the nineteenth century and into the twentieth. Electric belts, peddled by pitchmen at county fairs, seemed credible because the magic of magnetism was demonstrated in such marvels as the telegraph, the dynamo, and the telephone. Then came the x-ray and radio, with accompanying waves of electronic quackery.

In the 1920s, Albert Abrams, M.D., invented the system of diagnosis and healing he called "Radionics." Soon more than three thousand local practitioners, mainly chiropractors, were sending dried blood specimens from patients to be inserted in Abrams' "Radioscope." The diagnosis would come back on a postcard, with recommended dial settings for treatment with other Abrams machines.

Abrams left his lucrative business to the College of Electronic Medicine, which he reportedly endowed with some $3 million to carry on his medical theories. The "college" was succeeded by the Electronic Medical Foundation. When FDA agents investigated this business in the early 1950s, they looked first into the blood-spot system of diagnosis. Inspectors arranged to send blood from an amputee and got back a report of arthritis in the right foot and ankle, which the man had lost several years before. The blood of a dead man brought back a diagnosis of colitis, and that of an eleven-week-old rooster resulted in a report of sinus infection and bad teeth!

Investigating the thirteen different treatment machines, the FDA found just two basic types. The Depolaray and six other units simply produced magnetism from circuits like that of an electric doorbell. The Oscilloclast and five similar machines had short-wave radio circuits resembling a taxicab transmitter. None could heal anything.

Officials of the Electronic Medical Foundation consented to a Federal court injunction in 1954, agreeing to stop all further promotion of the diagnostic system and devices. Shortly thereafter, they established the National Health Federation, an organization that would crusade against any government interference with quackery (see Chapter 28).

What made "radionics" seem sensible to its victims? Certainly one factor was the experience of millions of Americans who had built homemade radios with crystal detectors and heard music in their earphones. Why couldn't blood crystals function like the crystal in the radio and reveal a person's diseases? Besides, hadn't their own trusted doctor taken the blood specimen and sent it away for analysis?

## Treatment by Remote Control

Albert Abrams had many imitators, among them Ruth Drown, a Los Angeles chiropractor. One of her many nonsensical inventions was the Drown Radio-therapeutic Instrument. With this little black box and two blood spots, Mrs.

Drown claimed to be able to "tune in" specific organs of the body and treat a patient by remote control anywhere in the world! When she was prosecuted by the FDA, one of the defense witnesses testified how she had been cured of pneumonia, from Hollywood, while attending a convention of the National Education Association in Atlantic City. When reporters later identified this witness as chairman of the Los Angeles Board of Education, there was an immediate reaction. How could someone so uninformed and gullible be in charge of the education of 400,000 children and responsible for hiring science teachers, organizing health education programs, and the like? A resignation followed. Even persons who are well-educated in some areas may be extremely naive in health matters.

Dr. Drown claimed that the only current used in her treatments was "the patient's own body energy." She alleged that tuning in on the "radio frequency" of the disease would automatically cause the disease cells to "fall away." Her followers were taught to conserve their "body magnetism." At the trial, one witness enthusiastically endorsed the Drown warning against shower baths. Since water was a conductor, his body magnetism and energy would go down the drain if he showered. In a tub bath, he was careful not to pull the stopper until he had climbed out, and to clean the tub with a long-handled brush!

The trial also had its tragic side. The Government's principal case history was that of a woman treated for breast cancer with the Drown device until her cancer became too advanced for successful surgery. Mrs. Drown was convicted and received what was then the maximum fine of $1,000.

## A Force Unknown to Science

"Unknown forces," as well as those familiar to science, have been exploited by the gadgeteers. William R. Ferguson combined both approaches in promoting his "Zerret Applicator."

More than five thousand of these gadgets were sold to desperate, hopeful people throughout the Midwest in the late 1940s. Made of two blue and white plastic globes that had been joined together (originally components of a baby rattle), the device was nicknamed the "plastic dumbbell." Inside were two plastic tubes containing "Zerret Water." Ferguson said this produced the "Z-ray, a force unknown to science." To have his diseases cured, a patient had only to sit holding the dumbbell, one ball in each hand, for at least thirty minutes at a time. The energy from the Z-rays would flow through the body and "expand all the atoms of your being." Directions warned not to cross the legs during treatment, since this could cause a "short circuit."

All this seems so ridiculous that one wonders why anyone would spend $50 for such a gadget. The reason seems to have been the timing of the promotion. The public was being informed about the wonders and possibilities of atomic energy. The *Chicago Tribune* had carried a series on the experiments at the University of Chicago, involving plutonium and "heavy water," which led to the atom bomb. As in the time of Franklin and Perkins' tractors, people were hearing of possible health applications of a new kind of energy. The medical uses of x-rays were long established. Why shouldn't there be a Z-ray which could cure by its effects on the atoms of the body? Maybe it sounded silly, but why not give it a try? *It might work!* What did they have to lose? Only $50.

The medical con man Ferguson was sentenced to two years in federal prison, while a female associate, Mary Stanakis, received a one-year sentence. During the trial, chemists proved that Zerret water was chemically identical to Chicago tap water.

During the same month, the Chicago Federal Court sentenced George Erickson and Robert Nelson to a year in prison for promoting the "Vrilium Tube" for radiation therapy. They recommended it for cancer, diabetes, leukemia, thyroid disturbances, ulcers, arthritis, and other serious conditions. This gadget was a brass tube two inches long, about as thick as a pencil, with a safety pin for attaching it to clothing. Inside was a tiny glass tube filled with barium chloride, a chemical worth about 1/2000 of a cent. The contraption sold for $306 (tax included).

Having to prove "beyond a reasonable doubt" that the Vrilium Tube was a fraud, the Government called some thirty-five witnesses, including distinguished atomic scientists, who established that the device was not radioactive and was worthless for any medical use. The most effective witness, however, was a man who described the death of his diabetic son, who had abandoned insulin and pinned his faith on the "Magic Spike."

When pronouncing sentence, Federal Judge Walter LaBuy told the defendants:

> The sale of the device constitutes a gross fraud on the public. . . . You have imposed on the poor sick who in their anxiety for relief would try anything at any price. You have fooled the trusting, the credulous, and the gullible. The quackery you have employed is the more despicable because those who were deceived into believing in your fake remedy failed to pursue the treatment proven by medical science to be effective in preventing and curing diseases. This credulous belief in the efficacy of a useless product is the greatest danger inherent in quackery. It discourages and prevents those who use it from seeking proper medical treatment, and the results of such neglect are often fatal.

## The Orgone Energy of Wilhelm Reich

Wilhelm Reich, M.D., one-time pupil of psychiatrist Sigmund Freud, claimed to have discovered "orgone energy," the most powerful force in the universe, and wrote extensively of its manifestations. Physical scientists, however, were unable to find the slightest evidence in Reich's data or elsewhere that such a thing as orgone exists.

Soon after immigrating to the United States in 1934, Reich designed and built "orgone accumulators." Most of them were boxes of wood, metal, and insulation board about the size of a telephone booth. Disease, he claimed, could be cured simply by sitting inside the box and absorbing the orgone. Hundreds of the boxes were sold or leased to practitioners and laypersons for treatment of all kinds of diseases, including cancer. Rentals were around $250 per month. When the FDA sued in 1954 for an injunction to stop the hoax, Reich told the court that neither it nor the FDA would be capable of understanding his orgone science, and therefore he would not offer a defense. The injunction was then issued on the basis of the Government's evidence. When Reich continued to promote the box for treating the sick, he was prosecuted for contempt of court. Found guilty, he was sent to prison, where he died in 1956.

From the outset of his difficulties with the Government, Dr. Reich attempted to pose as a martyr and to make his case a *cause célèbre.* His family and followers have continued this effort. Destruction (by court order) of seized labeling material on the accumulator devices has produced accusations of "book burning." Actually, Reich's books have continued to be available. There has been no destruction of any of his publications other than those that accompanied the seized devices. The American College of Orgonomy and the *Journal of Orgonomy,* founded during the late 1960s by disciples, remain active. Orgone accumulators, blankets, vests, belts, mitts, and wands are available from a company in California that makes no medical claims for them in its catalog.

## Scientology and Its E-Meter

Twenty years after the Spectrochrome trial, the FDA became involved with Scientology, another group that used a supposed healing device in its rituals. The device, a form of galvanometer, is called the Hubbard Electropsychometer (or "E-Meter"). Its inventor, and the founder of Scientology, was a science fiction writer named Lafayette Ronald Hubbard. Hubbard has reportedly said: "If a man really wanted to make a million dollars, the best way would be to start his own religion."

An article by Hubbard in the May 1950 issue of *Astounding Science Fiction* was such a hit that he dashed off a book-length version—*Dianetics: The Modern Science of Mental Healing*. Dianetics quickly became popular, and a Dianetic Research Foundation was established at Elizabeth, New Jersey. Practitioners trained by the Foundation set up offices in Hollywood, on New York City's Park Avenue, and on Chicago's "Gold Coast." The practitioners were called "auditors" and patients were interviewed while they reclined on couches. After a few years, dianetics declined in popularity, but the invention of the E-Meter and the incorporation of Scientology as a church, revived it. Disarmingly simple, the early version of the E-Meter used small soup cans for its hand-held electrodes.

FDA's involvement with Scientology began in 1958 when it learned that the Distribution Center of the organization was selling a drug called "Dianazine." This product was promoted for "radiation sickness," a condition widely feared at that time as a potential consequence of "fallout" from atomic weapons testing. Dianazine, a vitamin mixture in tablet form, was seized and condemned by the court as misbranded.

A follow-up inspection led to an investigation of the E-Meter. Action against the device began when more than one hundred E-Meters were seized by U.S. marshals at the headquarters of the "Founding Church of Scientology" in Washington, D.C. The court papers charged that the devices were misbranded by false claims that they effectively treated some 70 percent of all physical and mental illness. It was also charged that the devices did not bear adequate directions for treating the conditions for which they were recommended in Scientology literature.

A jury trial resulted in a verdict that the E-Meter was misbranded by the Scientology literature—hence both the device and its "labeling" were subject to condemnation. The court rejected as irrelevant in this case the defense that the literature was exempt from legal action because it was issued by a "religious" organization. The Court of Appeals, however, reversed the verdict on the basis that the government had done nothing to rebut Scientology's claim that it was a religion. A new trial was ordered, at the close of which Judge Gerhardt A. Gesell issued a fourteen-page opinion. Regarding the practice of auditing, the judge stated:

> Hubbard and his fellow Scientologists developed the notion of using an E-Meter to aid auditing. Substantial fees were charged for the meter and for auditing sessions using the meter. They repeatedly and explicitly represented that such auditing effectuated cures of many physical and mental illnesses. An individual processed with the aid of the E-Meter was said to reach the intended goal of 'clear' and was led

to believe that there was reliable scientific proof that once cleared many, indeed most, illnesses would successfully be cured. Auditing was guaranteed to be successful. All this was and is false.

Upholding FDA's charges that the E-Meter was misbranded, Judge Gesell ordered that use of the E-Meter be confined to "bona fide religious counseling" and that the device be prominently labeled with the warning notice:

> The E-Meter is not medically or scientifically useful for the diagnosis, treatment or prevention of any disease. It is not medically or scientifically capable of improving the health or bodily functions of anyone.

After eight years of litigation, with two complete trials and three rulings of the Court of Appeals, the E-Meters and literature were returned to the Scientology headquarters. Was anything accomplished? Most definitely. The courts saw the necessity to uphold the food and drug law even in a situation that involved the First Amendment. The court upheld the right of believers to believe—even in science fiction—provided that they do not violate the laws that protect the public health.

## A Chiropractic Device

The Toftness Radiation Detector (TRD) is a hand-held instrument claimed to detect low levels of electromagnetic radiation from the human body and focus it so that a chiropractor can detect conditions that require chiropractic treatment. The device, patented in 1971, consists of a plastic cylinder containing a series of plastic lenses. Its inventor, chiropractor Irwing N. Toftness, claimed that energy with a frequency of 69.5 gigahertz emanates from the human body, most strongly from areas of neurological disturbance. Holding the device close to the patient, the practitioner supposedly would feel resistance to movement while rubbing his fingers on the detection plate. The purported disturbances were then treated by spinal "adjustments." About seven hundred chiropractors leased the device, which cost $700 for the first year and $100 for each of the next fourteen years.

Experts consulted by the FDA noted that even if a diseased organ radiated the tiny amount of energy claimed by Toftness, the radiation would be absorbed by surrounding tissues and would not be detectable at or above the body's surface. Between 1962 and 1975, the agency seized TRDs from chiropractors in several states, charging that the devices were misbranded by "failure to carry adequate directions for use." (Of course, adequate directions cannot be written for a worthless device.) After a jury sided with the FDA, the chiropractors appealed, claiming that the device was used for research only. In 1982, a United States District Judge upheld the jury verdict and permanently prohibited use of the Toftness Radiation Detector. In 1984, after higher courts concurred, the Justice Department ordered chiropractors who still possessed a TRD to return it.

## Consumer Protection Laws

Before 1938, the only federal control over medical devices was through enforcement of the postal laws against device fakes sold by mail. Device quackery became so rampant that the 1938 Federal Food, Drug, and Cosmetic Act included specific provisions to combat dangerous or misbranded devices.

Through court procedures under the 1938 law, hundreds of misbranded devices were taken off the market or had their labels changed to eliminate deception. At the same time, the FDA began to regulate "legitimate" medical devices—testing the accuracy of clinical thermometers, insuring sterility of bandages and sutures, and seizing defective condoms, to mention but a few of its activities.

Unlike new drugs, new devices did not have to be proven safe before being put on the market. To act against a device, the FDA had to learn about it and then be able to prove it was dangerous or misrepresented. Unless a device was clearly dangerous, it could usually continue to be sold until all court proceedings ended. The more profitable the business, the longer the promoters were likely to stretch out the litigation.

The weaknesses of the 1938 Food, Drug, and Cosmetic Act with respect to devices were recognized from the beginning, and corrective legislation was introduced year after year. Meanwhile, great changes were taking place in medical technology. New materials and the development of electronics were bringing about a tremendous increase in the number and complexity of medical devices. Pins and plates to repair bones were followed by replacements for entire joints, artificial arteries and valves were developed, and electronic pacemakers were devised to keep the human engine running. As these products became more commonplace, the need for standards and more specialized regulation became increasingly obvious. Since the government could stop sales only by proving actual harm or deception, a manufacturer could, in effect, test a device on the public and wait for the FDA to take action if something went wrong. Finally, after many years of deliberation, Congress enacted the Medical Device Amendments of 1976.

Taking into account the great variety of regulated products, this law required devices to be classified so that the strongest controls would be applied to the riskiest devices. Thus, premarket approval was required for implanted or life-support devices. Other devices presenting a substantial and unreasonable risk could be ordered off the market. All device manufacturers are now required to register their products with the FDA, but few manufacturers of quack devices bother to do so.

The 1976 law also required that adverse effects observed during research or clinical use be reported to the FDA—but the agency received few such reports. To overcome this problem, Congress passed the Safe Medical Devices Act of 1990, which added hospitals, nursing homes, and outpatient facilities (except physicians' offices) to the reporting network. Unfortunately, the exemption for physicians' offices is a loophole for doctors who use quack devices. The FDA does not regulate the healing arts, a function reserved for the states.

The 1990 law added additional reporting requirements for life-support devices and enables the FDA to order an immediate recall of a device it deems unsafe. Manufacturers can also be assessed civil penalties of $15,000 for each violation of the law and a maximum of $1,000,000 for each proceeding in an FDA civil case before an administrative judge.

The quality of consumer protection against device quackery will depend upon the enforcement priority given to it by the FDA. False claims for devices usually can be stopped by warning letters, but the agency continues to bring court actions when it cannot get compliance by other means.

## Don't Be Fooled!

How can you avoid being cheated by the gadgeteers and their gadgets? For they are still around in great variety in spite of legal efforts to combat them.

- First and foremost, don't believe anyone who says that *one* kind of diagnosis or *one* kind of treatment is effective for a *wide range of diseases.* The ancient Greeks had a word for this kind of oversimplification: "panacea," meaning good for curing everything. All panaceas are quackery. Many of the devices discussed in this chapter belong in this category.

- Beware of all gadgetry claimed to aid in weight or girth reduction. All "passive" or "effortless" exercise machines are fakes. The same is true of massagers or suction devices that are represented as capable of "spot reducing." No device can "reproportion" one's figure without dieting and proper exercise. That includes all so-called "body wraps," "sauna belts," "sauna suits," and other sweat-inducing garments.

• Vibrator devices are marketed in great variety. Essentially for massage, they are often useful for temporary relief of muscular stiffness, aches, and pains. Excessive claims are often made for them, however. Vibrators are not effective for curing arthritis, rheumatism, nervous disorders, heart conditions, and other serious diseases. Nor are they effective for reducing.

• Youth, beauty, and sex are constantly exploited by the gadgeteers, as well as by other quacks. Many externally applied devices to enlarge and develop the female breast have been marketed. Most have been plastic cups that connect to a vacuum pump or water faucet to produce a massage effect. Dozens have been taken off the market by government action. They are not merely ineffective; if cancer cells are present, breast massagers can help them spread. The FDA has collaborated with the U.S. Postal service to stop bust developers sold through the mail.

• "Air purifiers" are sometimes promoted with excessive claims. Even ordinary household vacuum cleaners have been advertised as helpful in preventing allergies, hay fever, and respiratory diseases. Although equipment does exist that can effectively remove dust and pollen, the small units sold by many firms are not able to do so. Nor can the air purifiers marketed for home use help to prevent viral or bacterial diseases such as colds, flu, or pneumonia. "Negative ion generators" have no value in preventing or treating disease.

• No machine can be used to diagnose or treat the full range of disease by applying electrical contacts to the body, turning knobs, and reading dials. Such devices are fakes.

• Beware of gadgetry used by faith healers or promoted by crusading groups of laypersons.

• Don't fall for "science fiction." The miracles of legitimate medicine are much more wonderful and deserving of confidence.

• Last, don't assume that because an article is marketed, advertised, sent through the mail, or used or prescribed by a health practitioner, that it must be legitimate. If you suspect that a gadget is being misrepresented, don't hesitate to contact your nearest FDA office.

# 24

# The Miracle Merchants

### Rev. Lester Kinsolving
### Stephen Barrett, M.D.

Mary Vonderscher of Burbank, California, thought faith healing worked. She felt cured of cancer of the spine, she said, even though doctors had thought her case was hopeless. Appearing on an Oral Roberts TV spectacular in mid-1955, Mrs. Vonderscher gave a glowing testimonial. In January, 1956, relatives of hers in Indiana saw a re-run of this program—just three days before traveling to California for her funeral.

Wanda Beach, another believer, was a thirty-seven-year-old diabetic from Detroit. In 1959, after telephoning her mother that Roberts had "completely cured" her, she threw away her insulin. And died.

## From "Healer" to "Educator"

Though the faith of these two ladies did nothing to heal them, it is not difficult to understand its appeal. Sick people are prone to reach desperately for hope—especially when it is presented in a convincing way. And Oral Roberts could be quite convincing. When he rolled his mighty baritone into overdrive and howled, *"HEAL LORD!"* neither the Almighty nor the ailing appeared able to resist him. *"DO YOU FEEL HEALED?"* he would bellow—as if anyone submitting to such a scenario would dare to say no!

Roberts' enthusiasm for his work was unbounded. He moved into the big time with the skilled coaching of J.L. White, the same publicity expert who launched ultra-right wing anti-Communist Christian crusader Billy James Hargis.

The Jesuit magazine *America,* in a critique of Roberts titled *Faith Healing over T.V.,* noted:

> There is certainly a reasonable doubt that these programs are in the public interest. Of their very nature, they play on the hopes and fears of the credulous and ignorant. There is no positive proof that some of the "cures" are not rigged. At any rate, standard medical treatment seems to be flouted. We can wonder how many, viewing such programs in their homes, are impelled to neglect ordinary medical treatment.

In 1966, Roberts began a rather spectacular transition from Pentecostal Holiness to Methodist—leaving behind the faithful who had launched his healing ministry with many thousands of their dollars. He stopped broadcasting in 1967 and joined the Boston Avenue Methodist Church in Tulsa, Oklahoma, in 1968. Although he had previously been quoted as saying: "I consider Hollywood and all its works unclean," in 1969 he reappeared on TV—in Hollywood. These programs were straight evangelism—a Sunday series plus quarterly prime time specials—all broadcast from the same unclean Hollywood.

Roberts founded and is president of Oral Roberts University, whose five hundred-acre campus is located in Tulsa, Oklahoma. He has been supported by several million "prayer partners" who receive computer-printed "personal" letters approximately once a month from the Oral Roberts Evangelistic Association in Tulsa. He promotes the idea that money donated to him (which he calls "seed-faith") can bring to its donors rich rewards from God. Prayer partners are invited to inform Roberts of their spiritual and health needs to that he can pray for them in a special prayer tower at ORU.

According to Roberts, God told him to build ORU in order to "take His healing power to people all over the world." Another construction project "ordered directly by God" was the City of Faith medical center, opened debt-free in 1981, just south of the ORU campus. Visitors to this $250-million complex could enter by walking between sixty-foot bronze castings of hands joined in prayer. The facilities included a sixty-story-high clinic; a twenty-story research facility; and a thirty-story, 777-bed hospital. Stating that God had told Roberts "not to let the City of Faith get into the hands of the money lenders," the Oral Roberts Evangelical Association asked his faithful flock to pay for it.

"From the beginning," said Roberts in a fundraising letter, "the devil has violently opposed the City of Faith. He doesn't want prayer and medicine joined under [His] loving care"—a reference, perhaps, to the Tulsa Hospital Council's lawsuit that attempted to block opening of the hospital because the community's facilities already had too many unfilled beds. God also directed him, Roberts added, to offer his prayer partners a swatch of cloth "to touch and hold where they need a miracle." For added effectiveness, other solicitations offered an anointing oil, a prayer plaque, a prayer rope, and a Christmas Star. "It seems God never gives me much money in advance to pay for the construction," Roberts explained in another letter.

In 1983, Roberts announced, "God has called this ministry to declare war on cancer and dread diseases. . . . We must believe that a cure for cancer can be found through a supernatural manifestation from God and medical research." In 1987, Roberts told his followers that God had ordered him to raise $8 million for scholarships at Oral Roberts Medical School and would "call him home" unless he did so. He obtained the money, but the appeal set off a storm of protest from television executives and religious leaders. Roberts had envisioned that his center would attract large numbers of devout Christians from across the country. But in 1989 he announced that unfilled beds—a problem from the beginning—had forced him to close the school and shut down his hospital. At its peak, the 777-bed facility had only 148 inpatients.

## Kathryn The Great

After Roberts shifted from the healing circuit to Hollywood, his place was immediately taken by Kathryn ("The Great") Kuhlman, a spectacular successor to the late Aimee Semple McPherson. Kathryn seemed absolutely tireless and had an iron will and positively hypnotic charm. She would skip onto the stage with her golden sheath dress, red hair, pearly teeth, and blue eyes all glistening in the spotlights.

For five hours— without a break—this dynamic woman would preach, pray, lead hymns, lay on her hands, and cheer, for God as well as every one of the hundreds who would announce that they had been healed. As the faithful came forward (healing often presumably took place en route from seat to platform), Kathryn would walk with them or direct them: "Bend down, honey (and prove your arthritis has vanished)," or, "Run down the aisle and show everybody you're healed!" Loudly thanking the Holy Spirit, Kathryn would clutch each miracle recipient—and then would push so that the individual fell into the arms of a ready (and agile) assistant.

When the pace of miracles slackened, Kathryn would give The Spirit a nudge. Beaming those beautiful eyes heavenward, she would become psychic: "Someone in the balcony has just been cured of asthma!" or, "There is someone who has just recovered his hearing!" At this point, one or more elderly men might jump up, wave their earphones madly, and shout that they were no longer deaf.

Kathryn was advertised as "an ordained Baptist minister." But during an interview, she admitted having no theological education prior to receiving "honorary recognition" from something called "Evangelical Church Alliance, Inc.," of Joliet, Illinois. Her formal education ended after two years of high school in Missouri, when her father died. At age sixteen, and looking better than Susan Hayward, Kathryn persuaded a group of Baptist deacons in Twin Falls, Idaho, to let her fill a vacant pulpit. One of the deacons was sufficiently sophisticated to call the local press photographer. Her first scheduled sermon jammed the church to overflowing.

While much of her oratorical style and humor was pure corn-on-the-cob, Kathryn was much smarter than most faith healers. Instead of ignoring or attacking the medical profession, she used it—knowing that there were fundamentalist physicians who would "certify" miracles without checking up on them afterward. One such doctor was Martin Biery, M.D., a retired surgeon from Garden Grove, California. During nine years of regular attendance on Kathryn's platform, Dr. Biery saw dozens of "miracles" that he did not bother to research.

In 1974, Kathryn's certification gimmick was debunked by the book *Healing: A Doctor in Search of A Miracle,* by William Nolen, M.D., a Minnesota surgeon. After recording the names of twenty-five people who has been "miraculously healed" at a service in Minneapolis, Nolen was able to perform follow-up interviews and examinations. Among other things, he discovered that one woman who had been announced as cured of "lung cancer" actually had Hodgkin's disease—which was unaffected by the experience. Another woman with cancer of the spine had discarded her brace and followed Kathryn's enthusiastic command to run across the stage. The following day her backbone collapsed, and four months later she died. Overall, not one person with organic disease had been helped.

In December 1975, Kathryn underwent open-heart surgery at a hospital in Tulsa, Oklahoma. She survived the operation but died two months later.

**The "Science of Prayer"**

Some religious sects favor prayer over medical care. Christian Science is probably the best known of these groups and is the only form of faith healing covered by many insurance policies and deductible as a medical expense for federal income tax purposes.

Christian Science was developed by Mary Baker Glover Patterson Eddy (1821–1910), a New Hampshire native who adopted much of her philosophy from that of Phineas Parkhurst Quimby, a faith healer and "metaphysician" from Maine. Her first husband, Gilbert Glover, died of fever. Left pregnant, penniless, and very sick, she married her dentist, Daniel Patterson, whom she later divorced on charges of desertion. Finally she married Asa Gilbert Eddy, ten years her junior, a mild-mannered man who served her devotedly as she expanded the movement that she called "Christian Science."

In 1882, husband Asa Eddy died of valvular heart disease—but Mrs. Eddy called in the press to announce that he had been "murdered by arsenic mentally administered by malicious mental practitioners," whom she identified as three of her alienated pupils.

Mrs. Eddy taught that dead individuals continue to live "even though unseen by persons on our planes of existence." She also taught that prayer could heal, even at considerable distances. Christian Science contends that illness is an illusion caused by faulty beliefs, and that prayer heals by replacing bad thoughts with good ones. "You can Heal," a pamphlet of the Christian Science Publishing Society, states that "every student of Christian Science has the God-given ability to heal the sick."

Christian Science practitioners work by trying to argue "sick thoughts" out of the afflicted person's mind. Consultations can take place in person, by telephone, or even by mail. Individuals may also attain "correct beliefs" by themselves through prayer or mental concentration. The training of practitioners, which takes two weeks, is based on questions and answers from *Science and Health,* one of Mrs. Eddy's books. After three years of full-time practice, a practitioner may apply for six more days of instruction to qualify as a teacher. The February 1991 *Christian Science Journal* listed 1,450 U.S. churches and about 2,200 practitioners and teachers who were licensed by the Mother Church (of Boston) to perform healing.

The weekly magazine *Christian Science Sentinel* publishes "testimonies" in each issue. To be considered for publication, an account must be "verified" by three individuals who "can vouch for the integrity of the testifier or know of the healing." In recent issues, believers have claimed that prayer has brought about recovery from anemia, arthritis, blood poisoning, corns, deafness, defective speech, multiple sclerosis, skin rashes, total body paralysis, visual difficulties, and various injuries. Most of these accounts contain little detail, and many of the diagnoses were made without medical consultation.

Two studies suggest that devout Christian Scientists, who rarely consult doctors, pay a high price for avoiding medical care. The studies were carried out by William F. Simpson, Ph.D., an assistant professor of mathematics and computer science at Emporia State University. In the first study, published in the September 22, 1989 *Journal of the American Medical Association,* Dr. Simpson compared alumni records from Principia College, a Christian Science school in Elsah, Illinois, with records from the University of Kansas in Lawrence, Kansas. Even though Christian Science tenets forbid the use of alcohol and tobacco, the death rates among those who had graduated from Principia between 1934 and 1948 were higher than those of their University of Kansas counterparts (26.2 percent versus 20.9 percent in men, and 11.3 percent versus 9.9 percent in women). The second study, published in 1991, compared the mortality of Principia alumni with that of Loma Linda University alumni. Most students at Loma Linda are Seventh-day Adventists, for whom use of tobacco and alcoholic beverages is likewise proscribed. However, Seventh-day Adventists also tend to consume little or no meat. This time, the Principia alumni fared even worse in the mortality-rate comparison.

Rita and Douglas Swan, whose sixteen-month-old son Matthew died of meningitis under the care of two Christian Science practitioners in 1977, are not surprised by these statistics. Angered by their experience and determined to help others avoid the needless death of their children, they founded Children's Healthcare Is a Legal Duty (CHILD), Inc., to work for legal reforms that can protect children from inappropriate treatment by faith healers. So far, CHILD has collected 140 cases of children who died in this manner.

During an appearance on the "Donahue" show the Swans were asked why Matthew's illness had not been reported to state health authorities as required by law in Michigan. They replied that no one had made the diagnosis. Devout believers, they did not want to face possible abandonment by the church if they sought a medical opinion. The broadcast triggered many responses, including this one from forty-three-year-old Paul Michener of Waynesville, Ohio:

> At age nine, my left leg was burned in a gasoline fire (1st to 3rd degree). Although the area burned was not too large, from the ankle to just above the knee, it became a lengthy trauma. . . . I was fifteen years old before the injury had grown closed with scar tissue. In the meantime, the knee became stiff and the pain was beyond description. I was bedridden for about two years and walked on crutches for another two and a half years. Today I walk with a four-inch limp, a curved spine, and some recurring back and hip pain. . . . I have undergone three surgical operations in the last four years trying to patch up the damage done by this insidious philosophy. I find it neither Christian nor a science. . . . Today when I look at our nine-year-old daughter, I ask how could any "loving" and "religious" parent put his child through such an experience.

The Christian Science Church does not disclose its membership figures. However, it appears to be declining because its doctrines have little appeal to modern youth. During the past fifteen years, the number of practitioners listed in *The Christian Science Journal* has almost halved and the number of churches has decreased by more than three hundred.

## No Documented Benefit

Is there any evidence that faith healing works? The first step in approaching this question is to specify what should be considered proof that an ailment has been healed by a supernatural method. In our opinion, three criteria must be met: (1) the ailment must be one that normally doesn't recover without treatment (2) there must not have been any medical treatment that would be expected to influence the ailment, and (3) both diagnosis and recovery must be demonstrable by detailed medical evidence.

Louis Rose, a British psychiatrist, investigated hundreds of alleged faith healing cures. As his interest became well known, he received communications from healers and patients throughout the world. He sent each correspondent a questionnaire and sought corroborating information from physicians. In *Faith Healing* (1971), Dr. Rose concluded:

> I have been unsuccessful. After nearly twenty years of work I have yet to find one "miracle cure"; and without that (or, alternatively, massive statistics which others must provide) I cannot be convinced of the efficacy of what is commonly termed faith healing.

C. Eugene Emery, Jr., a science writer for the *Providence Journal,* has looked closely at the work of Reverend Ralph DiOrio, a Roman Catholic priest whose healing services throughout the United States attract people by the thousands. In 1987, Emery attended one of DiOrio's services and recorded the names of nine people who had been blessed during the service and nine others who had been proclaimed cured. DiOrio's organization provided ten more cases that supposedly provided irrefutable proof of the priest's ability to cure. During a six-month investigation, however, Emery found no evidence that any of these individuals had been helped.

Has any "faith healer" ever sent for the medical records of a client? Or had a client examined by a doctor before and after healing is administered? Or inquired about a client's health months or years after the healing? Or even kept statistics to indicate what percentage of people with various ailments appear to have been helped? Or compiled data that an independent investigator could verify? As far as we know, no "faith healer" has done any of these things. Thus, as far as we are concerned, there is no reason to believe that faith healing has ever cured anyone of an organic disease—that is, disease that changes the structure of parts of the body.

What about functional ailments—in which the symptoms are bodily reactions to tension? Whether a healer believes in himself (as most do) or is an outright faker, many people will appear to get symptomatic relief from his attention. Many diseases are *functional,* wherein emotions play a large part in causing symptoms. Functional ailments can sometimes be relieved by the ministrations of a faith healer—or for that matter by the reassurance of a medical doctor or psychiatrist. But any benefit of this type should be weighed against the fact that people who are not relieved may conclude that they are "unworthy" and become depressed as a result. Believers who are not helped may blame themselves. They may become sicker or severely depressed by such thoughts as: *"Faith always heals. I'm not healed. I'm being punished! What have I done wrong? What's wrong with me?"*

The biggest problem with faith healers of all types is that they do not know their limitations. Untrained in medical diagnosis, they rarely even try to distinguish between cases they may be able to help and those that are beyond their ability. Many cases have been documented in which people with serious disease have died as a result of abandoning effective medical care after being "healed." Money spent for a fruitless experience with a healer is another negative factor.

## Documented Fraud

When Dr. William Nolen looked closely at the work of Filipino "psychic surgeons," he found that all used sleight-of-hand to create an illusion that surgery was being performed. Animal parts or cotton wads soaked in betel nut juice (a red dye) were palmed and then exhibited as "diseased organs" that had been removed from the patient's body.

In *The Faith Healers*, James Randi describes how several of the leading evangelistic healers have enriched themselves with the help of deception and fraud. Some of his evidence came from former associates of the evangelists who got disgusted with what they had observed.

Randi's most noteworthy account concerned the unmasking of Peter Popoff, an evangelist who would call out the names of people in the audience and describe their ailments. Popoff said he received this information from God, but it was actually obtained by confederates who mingled with the audience before each performance. Pertinent data would be given to Popoff's wife, who would broadcast it from backstage to a tiny receiver in Popoff's ear. In 1986, after having recorded one of Mrs. Popoff's radio transmissions, Randi exposed the deception on the Johnny Carson Show. First Randi played a videotape showing Popoff interacting with someone in the audience. Then he replayed the tape with Mrs. Popoff's voice audible to illustrate how Popoff used the information.

Randi also exposed the techniques used by W.V. Grant, another evangelist who often calls out people in the audience by name and describes their ailments. Grant obtains this information from letters people send him and by mingling with the audience before his show. To help his memory, he uses crib sheets and gets hand signals from associates who also use crib sheets. After one performance, Randi was able to retrieve a complete set from the trash Grant left behind! Following another performance, Randi found that some members of the audience had given false information about themselves, their ailments, and their medical care. For example, after "Dr. Jesus" had "put a new heart" into a man supposedly awaiting open-heart surgery, Randi found that the details (including the doctor and hospital named by Grant) could not be corroborated.

Grant's subjects typically are "slain in the spirit" and fall backward into the arms of his assistants. In 1986, one of us (SB) observed what happened when Grant encountered an elderly woman who did not wish to fall backward when he touched her forehead. Grant pushed his fingers into her neck so hard that she could not remain standing. He also "lengthened" the leg of a man who limped up to the stage, supposedly because one of his legs was shorter than the other. The man—who was one of Grant's assistants—walked normally before the show began.

### Recommendations

Can anything be done about faith healing? Believers don't see it as a problem, while most nonbelievers don't see it as a priority issue and have little sympathy for its victims. But a few things might help lower faith healing's toll on our society:

- Laws should be passed and enforced to protect children from medical neglect in the name of healing. States that allow religious exemptions from medical neglect should revoke these exemptions.

- Treating minors with faith healing should be made illegal.

- Faith healing should no longer be deductible as a medical expense or reimbursable by health insurance policies.

- Journalists should do more follow-up studies of people acclaimed to have been "healed."

- "Healers" who use trickery to raise large sums of money should be prosecuted for grand larceny.

# 25

# The Eye Exorcisors

**Russell S. Worrall, O.D.**
**Jacob Nevyas, Ph.D., Sc.D.**

Since ancient times, many people have held the mistaken belief that poor eyesight can be cured by special eye exercises. More than a century ago, the textbook *Sight and Hearing,* written by a New York physician named Henry Clark, stated:

> It would appear as if the eye was the organ peculiarly selected by quacks in relation to which they display their ingenuity in extorting money. The suffering patient is so desirous of relief, that he easily believes, and as sight, from his point of view, is of such inestimable value, he cheerfully and liberally pays. I shall mention as a sample, one more of the recent humbugs which have obtained currency, and made money for many pretenders, in consequence of public credulity. An ingenious and enterprising man believed that exercises and application of pressure to the eyeball gradually changed its form, enabling the individual to do without glasses. He afterwards opened an office in New York, and advertised himself as a doctor, declaring his ability to cure all diseases of the eye, and to relieve everybody from the encumbrance of spectacles. Of course multitudes flocked thither.

This commentary on eye-exercise schemes is as appropriate today as it was in 1856!

## The Bates Method

The belief in eye exercises was brought to its highest state of fruition by a one-time reputable physician, William Horatio Bates, M.D., who in 1920 published

347

*The Cure of Imperfect Eyesight by Treatment Without Glasses.* Most of the following account is based on a book by the late Dr. Philip Pollack, a prominent optometrist of New York City. Titled *The Truth About Eye Exercises,* it was published in 1957 and is now out of print.

Pollack considered Bates to have been a sincere individual with an impressive record. Born in Newark, New Jersey, in 1860, Bates graduated from Cornell University in 1881 and from Columbia University's College of Physicians and Surgeons in 1885. For the next seven years, he practiced in New York City as an ethical physician, specializing in eye, ear, nose, and throat diseases and working in a number of prominent hospitals. In 1902, however, Bates fell victim to amnesia and disappeared from view. His wife found him seven weeks later working as a doctor's assistant at the Charing Cross Hospital in London, England. Two days later he vanished again and was missing for eight years, during which time his wife died. In 1910, Bates was found practicing medicine in Grand Forks, North Dakota, and was persuaded to return to New York, where he resumed practice and married again.

Early in his career, Bates displayed an interest in problems of vision. In 1891, he published an article in a medical journal on the cure of nearsightedness by eye exercises. In his office, he taught patients to stare into the sun and to relax their eyes by covering them with their palms. He soon became obsessed with his peculiar theories of vision.

In 1917, Bates teamed up with Bernarr Macfadden, a nationally known food faddist who published the magazine *Physical Culture.* Together they offered a course in the Bates System of Eye Exercises for a fee that included a subscription to the magazine. This venture met with considerable success and led many people to believe in the Bates System. However, the big impact of Bates's work materialized after publication of his book. This book attracted large numbers of charlatans, quacks, and gullible followers who then published scores of unscientific books and articles of their own on the subject of vision. Extolling the Bates System, these authors urged readers to "throw away" their glasses. Some of these writers even established schools.

Contrary to scientific fact, Bates taught that the dimensions of the eyeball and the state of the crystalline lens have nothing to do with poor eyesight. All defects in vision, he said, were caused by eyestrain and nervous tension; to achieve perfect vision, just relax the eyes completely. Bates warned that eyeglasses cause the vision to deteriorate; he also deplored the use of sunglasses. Bates claimed his exercises could correct nearsightedness, farsightedness, astigmatism, and presbyopia (the inability of older people to focus their eyes on nearby objects). They could also cure such diseases as cataracts, eye infections, glaucoma, and macular degeneration. His exercises were as follows:

- *Palming:* This is the principal procedure of the Bates System. The patient must first look intently at a black object, then close his eyes and recall to mind its blackness. This procedure supposedly relaxes the eyes, relieves eyestrain, corrects vision to normal, and eliminates pain during surgery.

- *Shifting:* This is the opposite of staring. By shifting his gaze continually from object to object, the patient will improve his vision.

- *Sun gazing:* Staring directly into the sun, the patient will benefit from the "warmth of light."

It should be obvious that these exercises cannot influence eyesight disorders as Bates claimed. Nearsightedness, farsightedness, astigmatism, and presbyopia result from inborn and acquired characteristics of the lens and the eyeball—which no exercise can change. As for eye diseases, the only thing the exercises can do is delay proper medical or surgical treatment and result in permanent impairment of vision. All reputable eye doctors caution patients against looking directly into the sun. Such a practice can cause permanent damage to the macula, the most sensitive and important area of the retina.

After Bates died in 1931, his office and teaching practices were taken over very successfully by his wife Emily with the help of Dr. Harold M. Peppard. Mrs. Bates had worked with her husband for a number of years, and Peppard was an ardent advocate of the Bates System. An edited version of Dr. Bates's book was published in 1940 as *Better Eyesight Without Glasses.* The book was revised several times and is still in print. Current versions don't advise looking directly at the sun; they say to let the sun shine first on closed eyes and then on the sclera (white portion of the eye) while looking downward. But they also say, "One cannot get too much sun treatment."

Other dubious promoters followed Bates's path. One of the best known was Gayelord Hauser, popular food faddist and Hollywood favorite, who in 1932 published *Keener Sight Without Glasses.* By combining eye exercise and diet theories, Hauser furthered the sale of his own dietary products.

One convert to the Bates System deserves special notice because he had no financial interest in it. This was the well-known British novelist Aldous Huxley. In 1942, Huxley wrote *The Art of Seeing,* claiming that he personally had been helped by the system. He had been a patient of Mrs. Margaret Dorst Corbett, who had written about the system and operated two schools for teaching it to patients and other practitioners. In 1941, Corbett was charged with violating the Medical Practice Act of California by treating eyes without a license. Her defense was that she taught only eye-relaxation exercises and did not impinge upon the practice of medicine or optometry. Corbett's subsequent acquittal was greeted with a large wave of popular approval. A similar case was that of Miss Clara A. Hackett who operated schools in Los Angeles, San Diego, and Seattle. Indicted in New York in 1951, she, too, was acquitted of practicing medicine and optometry without a license.

Several other authors have reached large audiences with their books on the Bates System. Most prominent among them were Bernarr Macfadden *(Strengthening Your Eyes,* 1924); Cecil S. Price *(The Improvement of Sight,* 1934); and Ralph J. Mac Fayden *(See Without Glasses,* 1948). Macfadden's book described how his interest in eye-strengthening had been aroused by "an experience that came near to being tragical." After a period of particularly hard work, he found that his vision became so bad that printed newspaper pages "appeared like solid black." Macfadden's vision improved greatly after a vacation and one-week fast, the book said, and recovered completely through experiments with eye exercises, eye baths, and massage of the areas surrounding his eyes.

It is difficult to understand the widespread popularity of the Bates System unless one considers that its followers make up what is essentially a cult. Its practitioners are *faith healers* who appeal to the gullible, the neurotic, the highly emotional, and the psychosomatic. Even the author Mac Fayden admitted that the System's results are 90 percent "mental," a view shared by Professor Elwin Marg of the University of California, Berkeley, who feels that subjects learn to interpret "blurs" without a demonstrable improvement in clarity of vision. Professor Marg's definitive study of the Bates technique, published in 1952, showed that "perfect sight without glasses" is an empty promise.

We know of a nearsighted woman who, many years ago, traveled from Philadelphia to New York City once a week to see a Bates practitioner. She expected that his treatment would eliminate her need for thick glasses. Each trip cost her a day's lost wages plus train fare, lunch, and the practitioner's fee. For several months a reputable optometrist tried to convince this woman that she was wasting her time and money. He finally persuaded her to ask the practitioner what progress she was making and how long it would take before she could change her glasses. At the same time, the optometrist gave her a sealed envelope to open at the end of her next visit to New York.

When questioned by the woman, the practitioner replied, "I was just about to tell you. We have decided that we can improve you no further. You should return to your optometrist for further care." Opening the envelope, the woman saw that the optometrist had predicted the Bates practitioner's reply almost word for word! She finally saw the light.

This woman was lucky. In another case we know about, a man confronted his Bates practitioner about the lack of improvement in his vision. Somehow the practitioner convinced him that the fact that his vision had not worsened indicated that the costly treatment was working. He also made the patient feel guilty about the lack of improvement by saying that he lacked the "willingness and commitment" to produce change—a ploy used by many types of quacks. The patient didn't become disillusioned until the practitioner said the treatment might take eight years.

The Bates method still has many advocates today. Some cling to traditional Bates techniques, while others use expensive computerized biofeedback machines. Their promotion is not limited to books and magazine articles but includes direct-mail campaigns with glossy brochures and toll-free numbers, pitching similar programs with new gadgets and mail-order videos. Beware of "Institutes" using well-known college towns in their names or "doctors" with dubious credentials, such as one we encountered recently with a degree from the "University in California" (not the University *of* California).

## Vision Therapy

"Vision therapists" claim to strengthen eyesight through a series of exercises and the use of eyeglasses. Their training sessions may take place several times a week and amount to thousands of dollars for a series. In contrast to Bates's use of relaxation, vision therapists promote active exercises. They emphasize exercising hand-eye coordination, watching a series of blinking lights, focusing on a string of objects, and even sleeping in a certain position. Often they prescribe bifocal and prism glasses for nearsightedness. They claim that these methods can improve school and athletic performance, increase I.Q., help overcome learning disabilities, and help prevent juvenile delinquency. However, there is no scientific evidence to support these claims.

Vision therapists who refer to themselves as "developmental" or "behavioral" optometrists adhere to the belief that most vision disorders are the result of learned or environmental factors and can be corrected through training. Often they prescribe low-power glasses ("learning lenses") with bifocals to children. The initials C.O.V.D. after a practitioner's name refers to the College of Optometrists in Vision Development, which is a national organization that provides training, promotional, and referral services for its members. Another proponent group is the Optometric Extension Program (O.E.P.), which organization began as the Oklahoma Extension Program in the 1920s and has contributed greatly to advancing the optometric profession by provide practicing optometrists with postgraduate continuing education. In recent years, however, its programs have emphasized vision therapy. Even though there is no scientific evidence that vision therapy can improve academic performance, the public relations activities of these two organizations have persuaded many teachers and counselors to refer children with dyslexia to a behavioral or developmental optometrist.

Dyslexia, a term that is often misunderstood, simply refers to severe reading problems in an otherwise normal person. Because reading involves sight, teachers and parents often incorrectly assume that vision problems are the cause of reading problems. Vision and eye-coordination problems, however, are not the cause of dyslexia. Glasses will be helpful if a child has trouble focusing on words, but they are often prescribed unnecessarily. Muscle-strengthening exercises (orthoptics) may help if a mild strabismus ("crossed eyes") due to muscle imbalance interferes with focusing, but exercises to improve "coordination" are not helpful for dyslexia. Reading experts have identified many causes of dyslexia, with the majority related to the brain's ability to interpret the sound of spoken words or (rarely) to process visual information.

The preponderance of studies have found that vision-related training has no effect or even a negative effect on reading skill. For example, a study by Dr. J. David Grisham, an optometrist at the University of California, compared three groups of seventh-grade remedial reading students. One group received vision training, another was tutored in reading, and the third group played computer games. Over a ten-week period, the vision training group improved their eye-coordination skills, but all three groups progressed equally in reading.

Recently, a vision training program was promoted in supermarkets with "tear-off" advertisements targeted to unsuspecting parents. The practitioner, boasting that vision training is a low-cost, high-profit specialty, claims he generated close to $950,000 in new billings during the first twelve months of the supermarket campaign. There also are many self-help books aimed at people who want to improve their eyes "naturally" without glasses. Two that are popular at grocery checkout stands are *Dr. Friedman's Vision Training Program* and Lisette Scholl's *Visionetics: The Holistic Way to Better Eyesight.*

An optometrist in Wisconsin offers to teach colleagues how to increase their practice's net "an average of $50,000 to $100,00 in one year." The cost of the "turn-key program" is 10 percent of the "increase in therapy collections" for four years. A recent mailing describes how the system is based on "two simple concepts dentists and chiropractors use . . . all the time. . . . (1) the magic of multiple visits, and (2) how to use staff to generate a lot more of your income." The mailing states that a few days of training can "take a person who has no idea what an optometrist does and, by the following week have that person performing therapy" in the optometrist's office. The recommended charge for the "high-intensity vision therapy program" is $80 per session for thirty sessions ("covered by most major medical insurance companies"), with about two hours of involvement by the optometrist. The mailing also notes:

> A chiropractor will get patients that come back regularly over an extended period. The only problem is that he has to do all of the work himself. With vision therapy, you truly have the best of both worlds: the patient will come back <u>multiple</u> times, but yet the <u>staff members</u> are the ones generating most of the income.

The mailing promises that part of the $4,500 deposit will be refunded if the optometrist cannot generate at least $30,000 in therapy fees.


**Other Unproved Methods**

Pressing on the eyes or surrounding bones has been a perennial favorite for all manner of eye disease. John Quincy Adams once wrote a paper claiming this method could return the "convexity of youth" and eliminate the need for reading glasses. Small "eye-stones" placed under the lids were popular until the early 1900s. Chiropractors who use "craniopathy" or "neural organization technique" claim that vision and eye coordination can be improved by manipulating ("adjusting") the eyes and skull. Current devices include the "Natural Eye Normalizer" for massaging the eyelids, and a pneumatic bag for placement over the head to cure all visual problems.

The use of color to treat various ailments, including those affecting the eye, has been promoted for many years. Edwin Babbit popularized the use of colored light with his book *The Principles of Light and Color: The Healing Power of Color* published in 1878. Today's practice of "syntonics"—also called "photoretinology"—evolved from these theories. Its practitioners use expensive machines to direct various pulsating colored lights into the eyes, claiming to cure optical errors, eye coordination problems, and even general health problems! There is no scientific evidence to support these claims.

Another approach involving color has been popularized by Helen Irlen, a psychologist who has appeared on CBS-TV's "60 Minutes" and franchised more than two thousand individuals and clinics nationwide. She claims that "scotopic sensitivity syndrome" is a leading cause of dyslexia and other school problems, and can be remedied by treatment with colored eyeglasses. Her recommended treatment costs more than $500. As is typical with extraordinary claims, neither Irlen or her supporters offer any scientific evidence that it can improve reading or any other visual skill.

Several entrepreneurs have marketed "pyramid" or "pinhole" glasses consisting of opaque material with multiple slits or perforations. The "technology" involved has been known for centuries and was used before glass lenses were invented. Light passing through a small hole (or holes) is restricted to rays coming straight from the viewed object; these rays do not need focusing to bring them to a point. Modern promoters claim their products are better than conventional lenses. Actually, both reduce the focus effort needed to read, but pinhole glasses are much less useful because they restrict contrast, brightness, and the field of view. Worn as sunglasses, they can even be harmful because the holes allow damaging ultraviolet rays to reach the eye.

In 1992, the Missouri Attorney General obtained a consent injunction and penalties totaling $20,000 against a New York company that sold "aerobic glasses." These glasses, which sold for $19.95 plus postage and handling, had black plastic lenses with tiny holes. The company's ads had falsely claimed that its "Aerobic Training Eyeglass System exercises and relaxes the eye muscles through use of scientifically designed and spaced 'pin dot' openings that change the way light enters the eye." The company had also advertised that continued wear and exercises should enable eyeglass wearers to change to weaker prescription lenses and reduce the need for bifocals or trifocals.

### Stick with Proven Treatment!

There is one rational method of eye training and eye exercises—orthoptics—carried out under competent optometric and medical supervision to correct coordination or binocular vision problems such as "crossed eyes" and amblyopic or "lazy" eyes. If the muscles that control eye movements are out of balance, the function of one eye may be suppressed to avoid double vision. (The suppressed eye is called an "amblyopic" eye.) Covering the good eye can often stimulate the amblyopic eye to work again to provide binocular vision for the patient. Orthoptics, surgery, or a combination of the two often can improve problems in pointing and focusing the eyes due to poor eye-muscle control.

Remember—no type of eye exercise can improve a refractive error or cure any ailment within the eyeball or in any remote part of the body. If you are considering a vision training program, request a written report detailing the problem, the proposed treatment plan, an estimate of the time and costs involved, and the prognosis. If the plan is not targeted toward a specific visual problem (such as amblyopia), or if it includes a broad promise such as improving I.Q., forget about it. If you are not sure what to do, invest in a second opinion, preferably from a university-affiliated practitioner.

# 26

# The "Holistic" Hodgepodge

## Wallace I. Sampson, M.D.

The word "holistic" was coined in 1926 by Jan Christiaan Smuts, philosopher and first prime minister of South Africa, in his book *Holism and Evolution.* Smuts observed that objects have properties that cannot be predicted from mere knowledge of their parts. An automobile, for example, would not be recognizable if its components were assembled randomly instead of by design. In addition, the full nature of automobiles cannot be appreciated without considering their role in modern life—as both transportation and sources of pollution.

Promoters of "holistic medicine" (also called "wholistic medicine") believe that illnesses should not be studied apart from the people who have them and their social and environmental situations. Medical attention should therefore not be limited to current physical problems but should also be directed toward emotional factors and lifestyles. Good physicians have always tried to understand their patients as whole beings. But the holistic movement is promoted *as something new* by unorthodox practitioners, crusading laypersons, and a few hundred physicians. The promotion rests on an elaborate but loosely defined philosophy that refers to scientific concepts. However, a close look will show that much of it is irrational.

## Holistic Philosophy

A good way to begin our inquiry is to examine some prominent "holistic" publications. *Wholistic Dimensions in Healing—A Resource Guide*, compiled by the Berkeley (California) Holistic Health Center and published in 1978, describes about fifty types of healing approaches and lists 1,146 sources of holistic treatment and/or information. According to its editor, Leslie Kaslof, "The ultimate responsibility for health maintenance lies within each of us. By being in contact with our own healing processes, we take the first step beyond the need for the tools of healing—beyond the need for therapy and technique." After noting that a listing in his guidebook "in no way constitutes an endorsement or a recommendation," Kaslof adds that "since many of the terms used in the fields included do not have generally agreed upon meanings," the book contains no glossary of terms.

The general introduction to *Wholistic Dimensions in Healing* was written by Rick J. Carlson, J.D., an attorney who was Assistant Adjunct Professor of Medicine, Boston Medical School, and Senior Research Associate of the Institute of Medicine, National Academy of Sciences. He stated:

> The public should know what the options are in regard to their health. The day is past when we could confidently turn to modern medicine for all or even many of our health needs. By most estimates ... medicine influences most indices of health only to about 10 percent. The remaining 90 percent is dependent on environmental, social, and cultural factors over which doctors and hospitals have little, if any, control. . . . People are now, to an unprecedented degree, looking for alternatives to what some perceive as a dinosaur—the modern medical system.

But Carlson also noted that "many practitioners of new wholistic approaches . . . in their attempt to create a market for their wares, put the money-motivated physicians to shame. . . . As in all areas, the buyer must beware."

In 1985, the Berkeley center produced *The New Holistic Health Handbook,* with more than a hundred topics. Like its predecessor, it lists sources of holistic treatment and/or information, accompanied by a warning: "These organizations were included on the basis of unsolicited promotional materials sent to our office. . . . THERE ARE NO STANDARDS OF PRACTICE FOR THESE FACILITIES." In an introductory chapter, center board member Richard J. Miles states:

> The holistic-health system consists essentially of enabling good health to emerge from within the person who recognizes and acts on life's stresses, and undertakes a commitment to maintain self-expression in an environment of good will. Disease is seen as an important feedback message. . . . The holistic assumption is that the body knows how to heal itself, is a natural "healing" system intent on good health, and that we must learn how to get our stresses and misunderstandings out of the way.

The above passages contain at least five themes that appear central to the philosophy of holistic medicine:

1. Individuals have primary responsibility for their health. Physicians don't treat patients as much as teach them how to remain healthy.

2. General measures, such as "reducing stress" and "correcting imbalances," can make people far less susceptible to disease.

3. Medicine is too rigid and impersonal.

4. Medicine is just one healing system among many.

5. "Alternative" approaches, though indefinable, unendorsable, and unproven, should be promoted vigorously.

Each of these themes involves misconceptions.

## Something Extra?

It is well known to health scientists that cigarette smoking causes cancer, that overeating and excessive alcohol intake are dangerous, that exercise is good for people, and that use of safety belts can reduce the incidence of serious automobile injuries. To the extent that holistic promoters persuade their followers to adopt better health practices, the movement will accomplish some good. As far as I can see, however, holistic promoters offer no useful addition to what good physicians have been doing quietly all along.

Many holistic practitioners see disease as primarily caused by stresses and "imbalances." Although stress is a factor in many ailments, it is by no means clear that stress-reduction techniques advocated in the name of holism are actually effective in preventing disease. The concept of "imbalances" is even more fanciful. Acupuncturists claim to balance "life forces"; chiropractors claim to balance spines; some unorthodox dentists claim to balance "body chemistry"; applied kinesiologists claim to balance muscles; and various other healers claim to balance people's spiritual, mental, and physical "systems" to bring them "into harmony with nature."

Curiously, although these concepts appear to have little in common, their proponents rarely if ever criticize each other. As noted by Douglas Stalker, Ph.D., and Clark Glymour, Ph.D., in *Examining Holistic Medicine*:

> Chiropractors, iridologists, reflexologists, tongue diagnosers, zone therapists, and many others all claim to treat or diagnose the whole from some anatomical part. Of course, they differ about which part, but that does not seem to bother either them or the editors of holistic books.

Holistic promoters tend to view nature as harmonious and benign. They depict primitive humans as living in a utopian state which can be ours if we return to "natural" living. A common goal is a state of optimal health or "wellness" that goes beyond the mere absence of disease. The idea that disease itself may be "natural" is not considered.

Many people do feel negatively toward our health care system, but this is a very curious phenomenon. Polls show that most people *are* satisfied with their own medical care. Their antagonism is toward the "system"—which they view as overpriced or too self-serving. It is also true that more people are turning toward "alternative" methods. However, disillusionment with medicine is by no means the main reason for this (any more than dissatisfaction with astronomy is the primary cause of astrology's popularity). Many people have hopes that cannot possibly be fulfilled by science.

Holistic proponents make a serious error by pretending that all of medical science is one system and then listing various others as separate but equal systems. They may call modern medicine "Western medicine" to distinguish it from "Eastern medicine." Or they may call it "allopathic medicine," a term coined almost two centuries ago by Samuel Hahnemann, the founder of homeopathy. In Hahnemann's day, allopathy included cupping, bloodletting, and many other primitive methods then considered orthodox. These methods were abandoned long ago as medical scientists learned how to determine what works and what doesn't. Scientific medicine now includes all methods of treatment that are sensible, reliable, and reproducible from one practitioner to another. Holistic advocates attempt to reduce its significance by defining it as "one approach." A wide variety of other approaches are then promoted as "alternatives." Here's a brief look at some of them.

## Chinese Medicine

*Acupuncture* defines the body according to systems with functions that have no similarity to what is actually known about body physiology. These systems are said to be affected by color, weather, emotion, and other factors. Meridians and acupuncture points on the surface of the body, which supposedly refer to internal organ functions, cannot actually be seen or measured. They are part of the ancient Chinese way of looking at the body, health, disease, and nature. It is claimed that stimulation of acupuncture points can benefit organ systems and return their functions to normal. The same claims are made for *acupressure,* but no needles are used.

Research during the past twenty years has failed to demonstrate that acupuncture is effective in altering the course of any disease. Controlled experiments have been done to test acupuncture's effectiveness against chronic pain, cigarette addiction, drug abuse, and various other problems. Expert reviewers have concluded that very few such studies have been well designed, and that the better the design, the less the actual effect. Any *perceived* effects are probably due to a combination of expectation, suggestion, counter-irritation, operant conditioning, and other psychological mechanisms.

Dr. William Jarvis believes that acupuncture might be useful as a "psychological aid" that reinforces desired behavior or diverts attention away from unhealthy behavior patterns. "Learning to manipulate psychological reinforcement in a scientific manner might turn out to be much more fruitful than attempting to prove that acupuncture has true therapeutic effect," he said recently.

*Herbalism* involves the use of thousands of substances whose pharmacology may not be known to the herbalists who prescribe them. Herbs are promoted with the mystique of being "natural" and of possibly containing useful substances as yet undiscovered by science. Such promotion ignores the fact that drug companies routinely test large numbers of naturally occurring substances and are quick to investigate new rumors about folk remedies. Many herbal remedies exert no pharmacological effect upon the body; others contain potent drugs, some of which can be toxic.

## Meditation

Most meditation techniques are derived from ancient Oriental efforts to obtain transcendent states of consciousness. Highly trained mystics can alter their heart rate, blood pressure, body temperature, and other functions that are not ordinarily subject to much conscious control. This has encouraged hopes that medical benefits can result from learning these techniques. Indeed, there have been some benefits from yoga and meditation. Serious practitioners can reduce their blood pressures a little—about 10 mm systolic and 5 mm diastolic—while using these techniques on a regular basis. However, expectations of doing without medication and medical care by meditating are unrealistic.

"Psychic healers" claim that health can be maintained by "cleaning out your energy body" each day. Their recommended methods include breath and rhythm exercises, visualization, color channeling, and "unconditional love." There is no way to measure the "energy" flow they postulate.

O. Carl Simonton, M.D., who now operates a retreat for cancer patients, believes that cancers may be affected by meditation. He theorizes that the brain can stimulate endocrine glands to inspire the immune system to attack cancer cells. While training to become a radiation therapist, Simonton noted that some cancer patients who had "positive attitudes" seemed to recover more quickly and live longer than those who seemed less motivated for treatment. Based on this observation, Simonton and his associates developed a system for motivating "positive attitudes" by having patients meditate and "visualize" their cancers degenerating under treatment (see Chapter 6). Some imagine the killing effects of their immune system on the cancers. Although this method may appear harmless, it may also encourage patients to abandon effective care.

Hundreds of published studies have explored the influence of the mind on cancer and vice-versa. So far no clear relationship has been shown between emotions, personality factors, stresses, and cancer. If stress were a major cause of cancer, every great tragedy (such as war) would be followed by an outbreak of cancer. In all of recorded history, no such observation has been made.

Other aspects of "mind-over-matter" were popularized by Norman Cousins, former editor of the *Saturday Review of Literature.* In a 1976 article in *The New England Journal of Medicine,* he claimed that a combination of laughter, high doses of intravenous vitamin C, and other self-chosen remedies had cured him of ankylosing spondylitis (a form of arthritis of the spine). Cousins said he had been given a 1-in-500 chance of recovery from this disease. The fact is, however, that flareups of ankylosing spondylitis *usually* are followed by periods of remission so that, with proper treatment, most patients have minimal or no disability and are able to lead a full productive life. Although Cousins' story made no medical sense whatsoever, it propelled him into a career as a professor in the department of psychiatry and behavioral sciences at the UCLA School of Medicine and inspired him to write several books about the influence of emotions over disease.

## Homeopathy

Homeopathy is a system of treatment that uses a wide variety of herbs, drugs, and other substances in infinitesimal doses. It is based on the theory that if a substance can produce symptoms of an illness in healthy persons, a tiny amount of the substance can cure that illness in a sick person. When substances are so dilute that they could not possibly be effective against anything, homeopathic practitioners may still claim that an "essence" of the active ingredient persists even though the substance itself is no longer present. Homeopathy enjoyed some success during the nineteenth century when its methods (the equivalent of doing nothing) were less dangerous than some of the other treatments of that period. Today its use is utter nonsense (see Chapter 13).

### "Separate and Distinct" Healing Arts

*Chiropractic* is based on the theory that most ailments are caused by spinal problems that can be corrected by spinal manipulation. Its scope is therefore unlimited. Some chiropractors, called "straights," limit their treatment to manipulation. Others, called "mixers," use nutritional approaches and a variety of physical therapy methods in addition to manipulation.

*Naturopathy* is a system of healing said to rely solely on "nature." Naturopaths believe that the basic cause of disease is the violation of nature's laws. They view diseases as the body's effort to purify itself, and cures result from "increasing the patient's vital force by ridding the body of toxins." Naturopathic treatment modalities include "natural food" diets, vitamins, herbs, tissue minerals, cell salts, manipulation, massage, remedial exercise, diathermy, and colonic enemas. Radiation may be used for diagnosis but not for treatment. Drugs are forbidden except for compounds that are components of body tissues. Like chiropractors, naturopaths believe that virtually all diseases are within the scope of their practice. They are licensed in a few states and the District of Columbia. There are also chiropractors who practice naturopathy.

*Iridology* is a system of diagnosis devised more than a century ago by Ignatz von Peczely, a Hungarian physician. It is based on the premise that each area of the body is represented by a corresponding area in the iris of the eye (the colored area surrounding the pupil). Iridologists claim that states of health and disease can thus be diagnosed according to the color, texture, and location of various pigment flecks in the eye. Iridology practitioners also claim to diagnose "imbalances" that can be treated with vitamins, minerals, herbs, and similar products.

Bernard Jensen, D.C., the leading American iridologist, states: "Nature has provided us with a miniature television screen showing the most remote portions of the body by way of nerve reflex responses." He even claims that iridology can locate "toxic material" that has accumulated in body organs and detect "potential problems that will contribute to senility." In 1979, however, Jensen and two other iridologists flunked a scientific test in which they examined photographs of the eyes of 143 persons in an attempt to determine which ones had kidney disease. (Forty-eight had been medically diagnosed as impaired using creatinine clearance tests, while the rest had normal kidney function.) The iridologists scored no better than chance.

The AMA Council on Scientific Affairs has noted that iridology charts are similar in concept to those used years ago in "phrenology," the pseudoscience that related protuberances of the skull to the mental faculties and character of the individual. Another critic of iridology has collected twenty iridology charts that show differences in the location and interpretation of their iris signs.

*Applied kinesiology is* a system of diagnosis and treatment based on the theory that every organ dysfunction is accompanied by a weakness of a specific muscle group. Practitioners also claim that nutritional deficiencies, allergies, and other adverse reactions to food substances can be detected by testing muscles after placing substances in the patient's mouth so that salivation occurs. "Good" substances will lead to increased strength in specific muscles, whereas "bad" substances will cause specific weaknesses. Treatment may then include special diets, food supplements, acupressure, and/or spinal manipulation. Although the notions of applied kinesiology are so far removed from scientific reality that testing them seems to be a waste of time, several investigators have subjected the muscle-testing procedures to controlled tests. One found no difference in muscle response from one substance to another, while others found no difference between the results with test substances and with placebos.

*Reflexology* (also called "zone therapy") is based on the idea that pressure on a hand or foot can relieve the symptoms and remove the underlying cause of disease in other parts of the body. Proponents claim that the body is divided into ten zones that begin or end in the hands and feet, and that each organ or part of the body is represented on the hands and feet. They also claim that abnormalities can be diagnosed by feeling the feet and that massaging or pressing each area can stimulate the flow of energy, blood, nutrients, and nerve impulses to the corresponding body zone.

Most proponents believe that foot reflexology is more effective than hand reflexology. "Perhaps," says one, "it is because the total body weight passes through the feet, and they are weighed down by gravity. Thus the feet have a reciprocal connection with the earth, and they may be imagined as two poles, responsible for the equalization of Man's electromagnetic field."

Most reflexologists claim that foot massage can relieve stress—which undoubtedly is correct but does not require the services of a "certified reflexologist" for $35 to $100 per session. Other claims are equally immodest. One prominent author claims that foot reflexology can cleanse the body of toxins, increase circulation, assist in weight loss, and improve the health of organs throughout the body. Others have reported success with earaches, anemia, bedwetting, bronchitis, convulsions in an infant, hemorrhoids, hiccups, deafness, hair loss, emphysema, prostate trouble, heart disease, overactive thyroid gland, kidney stones, liver trouble, rectal prolapse, undescended testicles, intestinal paralysis, cataracts, and hydrocephalus (a condition in which an excess of fluids surrounding the brain can cause pressure that damages the brain). One practitioner even claims he has lengthened a leg that was an inch shorter than the other.

*Polarity therapy* supposedly "coordinates diet, exercise, and techniques of body manipulation to increase and balance the flow of vital energy for the physical, emotional and mental well-being of the individual." According to Pierre Pannetier, director of the Polarity Center in Orange, California, "Love and understanding are the chief qualifications for applying the art. . . . Teachers are the mere channels; everyone has the power to heal himself."

Many practitioners of *"medical" massage* claim that their procedures "flush toxins out of the body." Some practitioners claim: "Disorders in the internal organs, acting through the intervention of related nerves, cause pain, numbness, chilling, and stiffness of the skin and muscles. By relieving these symptoms the internal organs can return to sound condition." Neither of these assertions has a scientific basis.

## Negative Ion Therapy

Ions are atoms or groups of atoms bearing electrical charges. Positive ions lack one or more electrons; negative ones possess a surplus of electrons. Polluted air may be lower in negative ions and higher in positive ions. Weather conditions can also affect ion concentrations. According to folklore, an excess of positive ions can cause a variety of physical and emotional problems.

Proponents of negative ion therapy (aeroionotherapy) claim that illness can be prevented by neutralizing positive ions with negative ones produced by small generators. But negative ion generators cannot actually produce enough ions to change the air in a room effectively. Ions have short half-lives; their energy dissipates rapidly as they leave the generators. Scientific studies carried out during the past twenty years have failed to support the claims of negative ion proponents. Moreover, the generators may produce toxic amounts of ozone.

## Nutritional Quackery

Holistic proponents espouse a wide variety of nutritional approaches. Many believe that deficiency states are common and that faulty diet is the major cause of degenerative disease states. A common goal of holistic promoters is to find "the amounts of nutrients that will provide the utmost in health." Many use hair analysis, live-cell analysis, and other questionable diagnostic tests. Most recommend high dosages of vitamins and minerals for the prevention and treatment of disease.

There is no doubt that diet plays a role in the production of some diseases. Obesity is certainly a widespread problem, and dietary composition is related to the development of atherosclerosis, osteoporosis, and several other common health problems. But holistic promoters go far beyond what is proven scientifically.

### Therapeutic Touch

Therapeutic touch was developed during the 1970s by Dolores Krieger, Ph.D., R.N., who for many years was professor of nursing at New York University. Its proponents claim that it is possible to use one's hands to detect when someone is ill, pinpoint areas of pain, reduce anxiety, and stimulate the sick person's recuperative powers. They also claim that their maneuvers produce changes in the body's energy field that can be demonstrated with Kirlian photography, a technique claimed to photograph a person's "energy field" or "aura." As taught by Dr. Krieger, therapeutic touch is said to transfer energy from practitioner to patient. However, there is no scientific evidence that this actually happens. Although anecdotes and poorly designed studies have been reported in various publications, no study of therapeutic touch has been reported in a reputable scientific journal. It is safe to assume that any reactions to the procedure are psychological responses to the laying on of hands. Most practitioners of therapeutic touch are nurses, many of whom consider themselves "holistic."

### Holistic Organizations

Some professionals who call themselves "holistic" have formed interdisciplinary clinics that offer services, and some have joined professional organizations which they hope will enhance their status. The most significant such group is the American Holistic Medical Association (AHMA), which was formed in 1978. Holistic associations have also been formed by dentists, nurses, and veterinarians.

According to its 1989–1990 directory, AHMA is "an organization of physicians dedicated to medicine for the whole person." The directory lists about 350 members, most of whom are medical or osteopathic physicians. AHMA sponsors educational conferences and publishes a bimonthly magazine called *Holistic Medicine*. AHMA is closely affiliated with the American Holistic Medical Foundation, whose primary purpose is to raise funds to support AHMA research and educational projects. However, it appears to have raised little money and sponsored no significant research.

The topics covered at AHMA conferences have included "nutritional therapy," homeopathy, psychoneuroimmunology, neurolinguistic programming, "healing plants as spiritual allies," Ayurvedic medicine, "transformational healing energies," and many other approaches not recognized as valid by the scientific community.

To qualify for the "AMA Physician's Recognition Award," a physician must complete 150 hours of continuing education every three years. Sixty hours must be programs rated "Category I" by an accrediting agency approved by a recognized agency such as the Accreditation Council for Continuing Medical Education. In some states, continuing education is required for license renewal and/or medical society membership.

The purpose of the accreditation system is to ensure high-quality educational programs upon which physicians can rely. For the most part, the system is working well—most accredited programs are sponsored by medical schools and teaching hospitals. However, despite the questionable nature of many of its topics, AHMA conferences are fully accredited for Category I credit. Critics have suggested that "accreditation of nonsense" be stopped by developing lists of treatment approaches and individuals whose lectures should not be certified for continuing education credit. But sponsoring organizations fear that this would trigger expensive lawsuits.

AHMA would like to protect its members from legal difficulty when they use unproven methods. Years ago, an attorney suggested that if AHMA "were to establish a sound membership base and establish official positions on various types of treatment modalities, this provision might come into play and be used to the benefit of physicians who were employing alternative therapy sanctioned by the Association." In 1988, its president wrote to the state attorneys general urging that AHMA be permitted to provide peer review of holistic physicians under investigation by their licensing boards. So far, however, the group's activities do not appear to have had any effect in protecting its members from disciplinary action.

## Conclusion

At one time in the past, the holistic label had a valuable and specific meaning. Today, however, it is a banner around which all manner of questionable practitioners are rallying. It appears to me that the concept of holism has been irretrievably corrupted by confused practitioners and promoters of quackery. The word "holistic" and its associated slogans should therefore be abandoned by scientific practitioners.

# 27

# Prominent Promoters

### Stephen Barrett, M.D.

Adelle Davis. Kurt Donsbach. Carlton Fredericks. Robert Atkins. Gary Null. Jonathan Wright. J.I. Rodale. Linus Pauling. Jeffrey Bland. Earl Mindell. Lendon Smith. Each of them has been a prolific communicator, either in print, or through talk shows, or both. All of them have promoted health methods that the vast majority of medical and nutrition scientists would consider dubious.

## The High Priestess

Adelle Davis was the first "health authority" among modern food faddists who had a professional background. She was trained in dietetics and nutrition at the University of California at Berkeley, and earned an M.S. degree in biochemistry from the University of Southern California in 1938. Despite this training, she promoted hundreds of nutritional ideas that were unfounded. At the 1969 White House Conference on Food and Nutrition, the panel on deception and misinformation agreed that Davis was probably the most damaging source of false nutrition information in the nation. While most of her ideas were harmless unless carried to extremes, some were very dangerous. For example, she suggested magnesium as a treatment for epilepsy, potassium chloride for certain patients with kidney disease, and dangerously high doses of vitamins A and D for various other conditions.

Davis's most popular book was *Let's Eat Right to Keep Fit*. George Mann, M.D., Sc.D., of Vanderbilt University School of Medicine, undertook the fatiguing task of documenting the book's errors and found an average of one mistake per page. In *Let's Get Well*, Davis listed 2,402 references to "document" its thirty-four chapters. However, experts who checked the references have reported that many contained no data to support what she said in the chapter. In Chapter 12, for example, a reference given in her discussion of "lip problems" and vitamins was an article about influenza, apoplexy, and aviation, with no mention of either lips or vitamins. During the early 1970s, Edward Rynearson, M.D., emeritus professor of medicine at the Mayo Clinic, corresponded with eighteen experts whose work had been cited in the book. None liked the book, and many said their views had been misquoted or taken out of context.

In 1971, a four-year-old victim of Davis's advice was hospitalized at the University of California Medical Center in San Francisco. The child appeared pale and chronically ill and was suffering from diarrhea, vomiting, fever, and loss of hair. Her liver and spleen were enlarged, and other signs suggested she had a brain tumor. Her mother, "a food faddist who read Adelle Davis religiously," had been giving her large doses of vitamins A and D plus calcium lactate. Fortunately, when these supplements were stopped, the little girl's condition improved.

Eliza Young was not so fortunate. During her first year of life she was given "generous amounts" of vitamin A as recommended in *Let's Have Healthy Children*. As a result, according to the suit filed in 1971 against Davis and her publisher, Eliza's growth was permanently stunted. The estate of Adelle Davis settled the suit in 1976 for $150,000.

Two-month-old Ryan Pitzer was even less fortunate. According to the suit filed by his parents, Ryan was killed in 1978 by the administration of potassium chloride for colic as suggested in the same book. The suit was settled out of court for a total of $160,000—$25,000 from the publisher, $75,000 from Davis's estate, and $60,000 from the potassium product's manufacturer. After the suit was filed, the book was recalled from bookstores, but it was reissued with changes made by a physician allied with the health food industry. (Of course, thousands of copies of the original book remained in the hands of unsuspecting consumers.).

In 1972, a group of distinguished nutritionists had an opportunity to ask Davis to indicate what scientific evidence she had to back up many of her speculations. Like most food faddists, she did not base her ideas on such evidence. To question after question, she answered, "I will accept your criticism," "I could be wrong," or "I'm not saying it does." But she never told her followers that many of her claims had no factual basis or could be harmful.

Adelle Davis used to say that she never saw anyone get cancer who drank a quart of milk daily, as she did. She stopped saying that when she herself died of cancer in 1974, leaving behind her a trail of ten million books sold and a large and devoted following.

## The "Vitamin King"

In 1982, the *Los Angeles Times* dubbed him the "Vitamin King." In 1985, *Consumer Reports* described his network of organizations as an "empire." The activities and enterprises of Kurt W. Donsbach, D.C., have been so numerous and complex that no one—including Donsbach himself—appears able to document all of them with certainty.

Donsbach (pronounced Dons´-bah) graduated in 1957 from Western States Chiropractic College, in Portland, Oregon, and practiced as a chiropractor in Montana, "specializing in treatment of arthritic and rheumatoid disorders." Later he acquired a license to practice naturopathy in Oregon, based on a degree from the Hollywood College of Naturopathic Medicine. From 1961 to 1965, he worked in "research development and marketing" for Standard Process Laboratories (a division of Royal Lee's Vitamin Products Company) and the Lee Foundation for Nutritional Research, headquartered in Milwaukee, Wisconsin (see Chapter 28). While Donsbach worked for Lee, he lived in California, did literature research, and gave nutrition seminars (primarily to chiropractors) on how to determine nutritional deficiencies. After Lee became ill, Donsbach left his employ and opened Nature's Way Health Food Store, in Westminster, California, and Westpro Laboratories, in Garden Grove, California, which repackaged dietary supplements and a few drugs.

In 1970, undercover agents of the Fraud Division of the California Bureau of Food and Drug observed Donsbach represent to customers in his store that vitamins, minerals, and/or herbal tea were effective against cancer, heart disease, emphysema (a chronic lung disease), and many other ailments. Most of the products Donsbach "prescribed" were packaged by Westpro Labs. Charged with nine counts of illegal activity, Donsbach pleaded guilty in 1971 to one count of practicing medicine without a license and agreed to cease "nutritional consultation." He was assessed $2,750 and served two years' summary probation. In 1973, Donsbach was charged with nine more counts of illegal activity, including misbranding of drugs; selling, holding for sale, or offering for sale, new drugs without having the proper applications on file; and manufacturing drugs without a license. After pleading "no contest" to one of the "new drug" charges, he was ordered to pay a small fine and was placed on two years' summary probation with the provision that he rid himself of all proprietary interest in Westpro Labs. In 1974, Donsbach was found guilty of violating his probation and was fined again.

Donsbach sold the company to RichLife, Inc., of Anaheim, California, for $250,000 plus a promise of $20,000 a year for occasionally conducting seminars and operating the company's booth at trade shows. The agreement also gave RichLife sole right to market Dr. Donsbach Pak Vitamins, which RichLife later described as "specialized formulas" to "help make your life less complicated, more healthy." Among the products were *Arth Pak, Athletic Pak, Dynamite Pak, Health and Beauty Pak,* and *Stress Formula Pak.*

In 1975, after briefly operating another vitamin company, Donsbach began producing a large series of "*DR. DONSBACH tells you everything you always wanted to know about . . .*" booklets on such topics as acne, arthritis, cataracts, ginseng, glandular extracts, heart disease, and metabolic cancer therapies. (According to a current distributor, more than nine million have been sold.) The booklets were published by the International Institute of Natural Health Sciences—operated by Donsbach—which sold distribution rights to RichLife. In 1975, he also began his fourteen years of service as board chairman of the National Health Federation, a group that promotes the full gamut of quackery (see Chapter 28).

In 1980, the District Attorney of Orange County charged RichLife with making false and illegal claims for various products, including some originally formulated by Donsbach. In a court-approved settlement, RichLife paid $50,000 and agreed to stop making the claims. In 1986, RichLife was charged with violating this agreement and was assessed $48,000 more in another court-approved settlement.

In 1984, Donsbach was sued by Jacob Stake, of Urbana, Illinois, who claimed that he became ill and was hospitalized as a result of ingesting large amounts of vitamin A over a two-and-a-half-year period. The suit papers stated that Stake began taking the vitamin at age sixteen because it was recommended in Donsbach's booklet on acne. The case was settled out of court for about $35,000.

During the mid-1970s, Donsbach affiliated with Union University, a nonaccredited school in Los Angeles, where he says he acquired a master's degree in molecular biology and a Ph.D. in nutrition. In a deposition in the Stake case, he said that he also received an honorary doctor of science degree from Christian University (another nonaccredited school that had operated in Los Angeles). However, two reporters have stated that Donsbach told them that his "D.Sc." was obtained from a Midwest bible college. In 1977, Union University formed a Department of Nutrition—"with Kurt Donsbach, Ph.D., Sc.D., as Dean of the Department." Later he launched and became president of his own school, Donsbach University, which in 1979 was "authorized" by California to grant degrees. This status had nothing to do with accreditation or other academic recognition, but merely required the filing of an affidavit that described the school's program and asserted that it had at least $50,000 in assets.

Donsbach University, which operated mainly by mail, initially offered courses leading to B.S., M.S., and Ph.D. "degrees" in nutrition at fees ranging from $1,495 to $3,795, with a 20 percent discount for advance payment. Most of the "textbooks" required for the "basic curriculum" were books written for the general public by promoters of questionable nutrition practices, including Donsbach, Carlton Fredericks, Lendon Smith, and Robert Atkins. The original "faculty" had seven members, including Donsbach and Alan Nittler, M.D., whose California medical license had been revoked for using "nutritional therapies." Nonetheless, ads for the school promised "the finest quality nutrition education available anywhere." Donsbach University also offered courses in iridology, homeopathy, herbal therapy, and chiropractic business administration, as well as a $495 "mini-course" in nutrition for retailers who wanted a "Dietary Consultant" certificate.

In 1980, one of the school's advisors, Benjamin Colimore, was prosecuted by the Los Angeles City Attorney for conduct during the operation of a health-food store owned by him and his wife. Prosecution was initiated after a customer complained that the Colimores had diagnosed a bad heart valve, pancreatic abscesses, and benign growths of her liver, intestine, and stomach—all based on an analysis of her hair—and prescribed two products from the store. After pleading "no contest" to one count of practicing medicine without a license, the Colimores were fined $2,000, given a sixty-day suspended jail sentence, and placed on probation for two years.

In 1979, Donsbach launched the International Academy of Nutritional Consultants, which offered general memberships (to anyone) for $10 per year and "professional memberships" for $50 per year. The $50 fee included a directory listing plus a "beautiful certificate for your office." During 1983, the academy merged with a similar group to become the American Association of Nutritional Consultants. The only requirement for "professional membership" in either of these groups was submission of a name, an address, and a check for $50. Several investigators, including one of my secretaries, had no difficulty in obtaining such membership in the name of a household pet.

In 1985, New York Attorney General Robert Abrams brought actions against Donsbach, his university, and the International Institute of Natural Health Sciences, charging that they lacked legal authorization to conduct business within New York State and that it was illegal to advertise nonaccredited degrees to state residents. Abrams also charged that the institute's Nutrient Deficiency Test was "a scheme to defraud consumers."

This test was composed of 245 yes/no questions about symptoms. When the answers were fed into a computer, a report of supposed nutrient deficiencies and medical conditions was printed out. The questions did not provide a basis for evaluating nutritional status. Moreover, a scientist with the FDA's Buffalo district office who analyzed the computer program found that no matter how the questions were answered, the test reported several "nutrient deficiencies" and almost always recommended an identical list of vitamins, minerals, and digestive enzymes. The questionnaire also contained questions about the subject's food intake during the past week. However, the answers given did not affect the printout of supposed deficiencies.

In 1986, Donsbach and the Institute agreed to: (1) stop marketing in New York State all current versions of its nutrient deficiency questionnaire and associated computer analysis services, (2) place conspicuous disclaimers on future versions of the questionnaire to indicate that the test should not be used for the diagnosis or treatment of any disease by either consumers or professionals, and (3) pay $1,000 in costs. Donsbach and the university agreed to disclose in any direct mailings to New York residents or in any nationally distributed publication that the school's degree programs were not registered with the New York Department of Education and were not accredited by a recognized agency. The university also agreed to pay $500 to New York State.

In 1987, Donsbach abandoned his school, which was renamed and soon ceased operation. He also began operating the newly built Hospital Santa Monica, in Baja, Mexico, "a full care facility specializing in the treatment of chronic degenerative diseases including cancer and multiple sclerosis."

Donsbach has claimed that thousands of people enrolled in his university and that more than 1,000 graduated. As his graduates began representing themselves to the public as nutrition professionals, the American Dietetic Association began striving for passage of state laws to restrict use of the word "nutritionist" to qualified professionals with accredited training. The health-food industry, which does not want the government to help consumers tell the difference between qualified professionals and supplement pushers, has worked hard to thwart passage of such laws. State attorneys general have stopped a few Donsbach graduates from representing themselves as nutritionists and prescribing supplements for the treatment of disease. In 1989, a New Jersey judge who issued such an order referred to a Ph.D. from Donsbach University as "a Mickey Mouse degree."

Donsbach himself was involved in a scandal involving credentials. In June 1988, the Arizona Naturopathic Physicians Board of Examiners revoked the naturopathic license of Jess Franklin Lee after determining that he had used a counterfeit credential to obtain it— a diploma dated "17st June 1961" from the "Hollywood College School of Naturopathy" in Los Angeles. The authorities concluded that no such school had existed and that the "diploma" had been created by making altered photocopies of a 1961 diploma from the Hollywood College School of Chiropractic. Authorities in Oregon then determined that Donsbach and four others had done the same thing to become licensed as naturopaths in Oregon.

Donsbach continues to operate his hospital, market products, issue publications, and serve as a consultant to others in the supplement business. The number of such activities has exceeded my ability to keep up with them.

## The Consultant

Carlton Fredericks (1910–1987) was described on the covers of some of his books as "America's Foremost Nutritionist." He considered himself an expert and gave copious advice in books and in articles for health-food publications. According to the FDA, however, Fredericks had virtually no nutrition or health science training. He graduated from the University of Alabama in 1931 (under his original name: Harold Frederick Caplan) with a major in English and a minor in political science. His only science courses were two hours of physiology and eight hours of elementary chemistry. He had various jobs until 1937 when he began to write advertising copy for the U.S. Vitamin Corporation and to give sales talks, adopting the title of "nutrition educator."

Records of the Magistrates' Court of New York City show that Fredericks began diagnosing patients and prescribing vitamins for their illnesses. After investigation by agents of the New York State Department of Education, Fredericks was charged with unlawful practice of medicine. In 1945, after pleading guilty, he paid a fine of $500 (rather than spend three months in jail). He then enrolled in New York University's School of Education and received a master's degree in 1949, and a night-school Ph.D. (in communications) in 1955, without having taken a single course in nutrition. The title of his doctoral thesis was "A Study of the Responses of a Group of Adult Female Listeners to a Series of Educational Radio Programs." These were his own radio programs—broadcast on New York City's WOR and distributed at times to other stations. The WOR broadcasts alone—which spanned thirty years—were reported to generate thousands of letters a week. Fredericks's thesis analyzed how much of certain things he said on his program was retained by its listeners and how it affected their food-buying habits.

According to an article in *The Reporter* magazine, Fredericks was listed as "Chief Consultant" to Foods Plus, Inc., a vitamin company that ran into trouble with the FDA. In 1960, more than 200,000 bottles of the firm's food supplement preparations were seized as misbranded because literature accompanying them contained false claims that the preparations were useful in treating dozens of diseases. In 1961, the Federal Communications Commission concluded that Fredericks had a contract with Foods Plus to turn over all mail received as a result of public appearances so that the company could use the names for marketing purposes. Fredericks terminated his relationship with Foods Plus in 1962, shortly after the FDA again charged the company with misbranding products. The judge who decided this case in 1965 concluded that Fredericks had been telling a vast radio audience that vitamins and minerals could be used to treat more than fifty problems, including arthritis, epilepsy, multiple sclerosis, and even "lack of mental resistance to house-to-house salesmen." Fredericks' former contract with Foods Plus, the court ruled, made his questionable claims part of the company's product labeling. As an expert witness in the court case, Dr. Victor Herbert described Fredericks as a "charlatan." The defense attorney's objection was overruled after Dr. Herbert read aloud the *Random House Dictionary* definition of charlatan: "one who pretends to more knowledge than he possesses; quack."

Fredericks was one of the originators of the crusade to discredit sugar. He deftly channeled this single theme into a number of variations that reflected and exploited public concerns about alcoholism, emotional disorders, and hypoglycemia (low blood sugar). Once, after being introduced on the Merv Griffin Show as a "leading nutritional consultant," Fredericks was asked to estimate the number of Americans suffering from hypoglycemia. His reply, "twenty million," had no basis in fact. Hypoglycemia is rare. Several years ago, each of the past presidents of the American Diabetes Association was asked to estimate how many patients he had seen with blood sugar disorders. All replies were similar: thousands of patients with diabetes (high blood sugar), but almost none with functional hypoglycemia.

For many years, Fredericks wrote a column for *Prevention* magazine. In 1976, *Prevention* invested $100,000 to sponsor a series of radio programs distributed to stations throughout the United States. Robert Franklin, the show's producer, told me that the programs generated large numbers of letters from desperately ill people, many of whom seemed to think that Fredericks was a medical doctor. (This did not surprise me because generally he was introduced simply as "Dr. Fredericks.") Franklin was so disgusted by the mail that he decided to syndicate a program that gave reputable advice, and the Harvard University School of Public Health agreed to sponsor it for three years. Toward the end of his career, Fredericks did "nutrition consultations" for $200 each at the offices of Dr. Robert Atkins.

In his books and broadcasts, Fredericks attacked the medical profession and the FDA, cited questionable advice, and attributed a myriad of therapeutic qualities to foods and food supplements. He often used humor to illustrate his points and to ridicule those with whom he disagreed. Overall, he encouraged unsafe degrees of self-diagnosis and self-treatment. A heavy smoker, Fredericks died of a heart attack at the age of seventy-six.


## The "Nutrition Doctor"

Robert Atkins, M.D., refers to himself and like-minded colleagues as "the pioneers of Nutrition Medicine who risked their professional standing to develop the methodology that led the Nutrition Breakthrough." Like Carlton Fredericks, whom he regards as his "mentor," Atkins condemns the medical profession as "pill poppers," and drug pushers, but he does not hesitate to recommend large doses of nutritional supplements for a wide variety of diseases and conditions. His books include *Dr. Atkins' Diet Revolution* (1971), *Dr. Atkins' Superenergy Diet* (1977), *Dr. Atkins' Nutrition Breakthrough* (1981), *Dr. Atkins' Health Revolution* (1988), and *Dr. Atkins' New Diet Revolution* (1992).

Atkins founded and directs The Atkins Centers for Complementary Medicine in New York City, which recently moved into a modern six-story building that he owns. He also publishes a newsletter and hosts "Design for Living," the nightly radio talk show on station WOR that Carlton Fredericks had hosted before his death.

In 1991, Atkins testified on behalf of Warren M. Levin, M.D., at a disciplinary hearing held by the New York State Department of Health Board of Professional Conduct. Prior to the hearing, Atkins stated in his newsletter that he used the "same or equivalent practices" as Dr. Levin. During his testimony, Atkins said that about 40 percent of the patients who consulted him had "functional hypoglycemia" and that about one third required treatment for a problem related to *Candida*. (Chapter 9 notes that "hypoglycemia" and "candidiasis hypersensitivity" are fad diagnoses.) The board recommended that Levin's license be revoked (see Chapter 10). In a recent booklet, "6 Alternative Treatments Your Doctor Won't Tell You About," Atkins states that "everyone in America over the age of forty would be very wise to invest in a series of chelation treatments." (See Chapter 9 for information on chelation therapy.)

Patients who consult Atkins typically undergo hair analysis and other tests that are not recognized as valid by the scientific community. Early in 1993, Atkins was consulted by a forty-year-old investigator for the "Geraldo" show who told Atkins she was concerned about her weight and was worried because her thirty-five-year-old brother had recently had a heart attack. Atkins told her she was hypoglycemic and had multiple food allergies. The diagnosis of "hypoglycemia" was based on a glucose tolerance test, which is not a valid test for hypoglycemia. Even if it were, her lowest recorded value was 69 mg per 100 ml, which is not an abnormal level. The "allergies" were diagnosed with cytotoxic testing, which is not a valid test for allergies. The investigator was also told incorrectly that she had a yeast infection that required treatment with a carbohydrate-restrictive diet. The total bill came to about $1,100 for two visits and laboratory tests, plus $129 for supplement products.

The supplements Atkins prescribes are sold at a counter in the lobby of his office building and also by mail. A brochure for "Dr. Atkins' Targeted Nutrition Program" describes it as a regimen in which "building blocks" are added to a "basic formula" to "help the body create its own cures." The seventeen "building blocks" include *Anti-Arthritic Formula, Cardiovascular Formula, Diabetes Mellitus Formula, Heart Rhythm Formula, Hypoglycemia Formula,* and *Urinary Frequency Formula.* (The labels of some of these products do not contain the full name of the product but merely a code—such as *CV* for *Cardiovascular Formula* and *DM* for *Diabetes Mellitus Formula.*) The brochure states that the formulas evolved over twenty-five years of Atkins's experience in using nutrition to treat more than forty thousand patients. It is a federal crime to market a product intended for the treatment of disease unless it is generally recognized by experts as safe and effective for its intended purpose. In his testimony in the Levin case, Atkins denied that the products were intended to treat medical conditions and said they were merely convenient formulations for "managing nutritional deficiencies."

According to an article in *Newsday,* Atkins heads five corporations, including the Robert Atkins Professional Corp., which grossed $3.8 million in 1991; the Atkins Centers, which grossed $5.3 million in 1991; and his private practice, which grossed $320,000 in 1991. However, on the "Geraldo" show, Atkins stated: "We don't have a profit margin. What we charge our patients enables us to break even."

### The "Health Crusader"

Gary Null, whose books bill him as "one of America's leading health and fitness advocates," is one of the nation's leading promoters of dubious treatment for serious disease. He hosts radio and television talk shows, writes books, delivers lectures, and markets supplement products.

According to an article in *East West* magazine, Null became interested in nutrition in his twenties while working as a short order cook in New York City. He researched the subject and wrote *The Complete Guide to Health and Nutrition,* which was published in 1972 and sold briskly after Null appeared on a succession of prominent talk shows. He began hosting radio programs around that time and eventually got his own show on WABC, the flagship radio station of the ABC network. Later he moved to WMCA, which broadcast Null's show on Sunday nights to about two hundred stations across the United States. Currently, he hosts a weekday show on WBAI and a Sunday evening program on WEVD in New York City.

Null is prone to see conspiracies behind many of the things he is concerned about. His favorite target is the pharmaceutical industry, which he says "cannot afford to have an alternative therapy accepted." He promotes hundreds of ideas that are inaccurate, unscientific, and/or unproven. Null has spoken out against fluoridation, immunization, food irradiation, mercury-amalgam fillings, and many forms of proven medical treatment. His series on "The Politics of Cancer," which was published in *Penthouse* magazine in 1979 and 1980, promoted unproven methods that he said were being "suppressed" by the medical establishment. His lengthy series, "Medical Genocide," began appearing in *Penthouse* in 1985 with an article calling our medical care system a "prescription for disaster." Other articles in the series have promoted chiropractic and homeopathy, claimed that effective nutritional methods for treating AIDS were being suppressed, recommended nutritional approaches for arthritis, claimed that chelation therapy was safe and effective for treating heart disease, and endorsed several treatments for cancer that the American Cancer Society recommends against.

Null says that he holds an associate degree in business administration from Mountain State College in West Virginia, a bachelor's degree from Thomas A. Edison State College in New Jersey, and a Ph.D. in human nutrition and public health sciences from The Union Institute in Cincinnati, Ohio. Edison State, a nontraditional school with neither campus nor courses, awards accredited bachelor's degrees based on career experience, equivalency exams, and courses taken at other schools. Union is also accredited, but its degree requirements and standards are vastly inferior to those of traditional universities. Students design their own program, form and chair their own doctoral committee, and are required to attend only an introductory colloquium and a few interdisciplinary seminars. One of the three "adjunct professors" who passed judgment on Null's Ph.D. thesis was Martin Feldman, M.D., a "complementary" physician (and "clinical ecologist") who has pinch-hit for Null as a radio host and helped develop some of Null's books and supplement formulations. When I asked a Union Institute official about the background or location of the other two "adjunct professors," he replied that the information was in storage and was too difficult to obtain.

Traditional universities require that research for a doctoral degree in a scientific discipline make a genuine contribution to the scientific literature. Null's thesis, "A Study of Psychological and Physiological Effects of Caffeine on Human Health," does not appear to do this. His research project compared the effect of a week of caffeine use versus a week without caffeine use among small numbers of volunteers, more than half of whom dropped out or were disqualified for noncompliance.

Null's thesis purports to compare the "adrenal function" of seventeen people who remained in the study for the full two weeks, but his determination was based on invalid tests. The most notable of these involved measurement of the specific gravity, pH (acidity), and surface tension of single samples of the urine—a test used by Emanuel Revici, M.D. Null states that the theory behind the test "is still the subject of debate and has not yet gained wide scientific support." Actually, as noted in Chapter 6 of this book, the test has no medical usefulness whatsoever.

Following forty-one pages of findings, calculations, tables, and graphs, Null concludes that "chronic caffeine users tend to have diminished adrenal function," which he blames on "exhaustion" of the glands. "Fortunately," he observes, "there are non-drug nutritional programs which have the ability to repair or rebalance weakening adrenal glands toward normal." His recommended program includes lifestyle changes plus supplementation with five vitamins and three other products.

The supplements marketed by Null have included *Guard-Ion* (an antioxidant formula claimed to help protect athletes from free radicals the body can't control); *Gary Null's AM-PM Vitamin-Mineral Formula* (a "revolutionary breakthrough in vitamin preparation" that provides the nutrients needed at the best times for the body's anabolic and catabolic activities); *Candida Complex* (to bolster the body's defenses against yeast infection); *Endurance Factor* (containing "all the nutrients and enzymes that have made Bee Pollen famous"); *Energy Plus* (a royal jelly tablet); *Rebalancer* (a "cleansing formulation" for adults exposed to air pollutants, pesticides, or preservatives, or who have "internal metabolic imbalances"); *CoEnzyme $Q_{10}$* ("may reverse deficiencies and improve organ function, especially in the heart); *Sport DMG* (an N,N-dimethylglycine product to "improve cardiovascular function and to enhance the body's natural immune response system); and *Gary Null's Immune*

*Nutrients* ("to nourish and stimulate immune function, not merely at a marginal level of preventing disease and degeneration, but a positive level of striving for wellness and excellence, for optimal health"). Claims made for some of these products are illegal.

A 1991 flyer distributed at Null's booth at a health expo invited people to become distributors for Gary Null Nutritional Products. Participants in Null's "home-based business program" could obtain the products at approximately half price, with a minimum order of $200. The flyer also described Null's annual "Spring Cleansing, Rebuilding, Stress Reduction Program" at a ranch near Dallas, Texas. The week-long program includes aerobic exercise, various sports activities, a fitness assessment, beauty and skin-care treatments, cooking classes, acupressure, applied kinesiology, herbal body wraps, massage, brain-wave stimulation, facials, aromatherapy, reflexology, and loofah apricot scrubs.

In 1992, an Arizona company and its owners agreed to pay $200,000 to settle Federal Trade Commission charges of falsely claiming that bee pollen products could produce weight loss; permanently alleviate allergies; reverse the aging process; and cure, prevent, or alleviate impotence or sexual dysfunction. They were also charged with falsely stating that bee-pollen products cannot result in an allergic reaction. Some of the false claims were made in "infomercials" that were misrepresented as news or documentary programs, even though they were paid ads. One such program ("TV Insiders") featured an interview "by satellite" with "Dr. Gary Null . . . *the* authority on health and nutrition." Null stated that the human body ages because it doesn't produce enough enzymes, and that "you can't get any better food than bee pollen" because it is "loaded" with enzymes and contains a nutrient that "can help the inside of your body prevent the capillaries from aging." Records from the Union Institute indicate that Null "graduated" on August 31, 1989, which, according to an FTC document, was at least three months after broadcasting of the infomercial began. However, Null was not charged with wrongdoing.

## The "Persecuted" Doctor

Jonathan V. Wright, M.D., a Harvard graduate who obtained his medical degree at the University of Michigan, began practicing in 1973 in Kent, Washington, a few miles southeast of Seattle. In *Dr. Wright's Book of Nutritional Therapy* (Rodale Press, 197)], he labels his approach "nutritional biochemistry" and describes how he treats a wide range of health problems with vitamins, minerals, other "natural" substances, and/or dietary measures. He and Alan Gaby, M.D., of Baltimore, give seminars on "Nutrition as Therapy," which present their theories in detail. In 1992, Wright became board chairman of the National Health Federation (see Chapter 28).

Wright has achieved considerable notoriety battling the FDA. The dispute surfaced in July 1991 when law enforcement officers seized 103 bottles of L-tryptophan from the For Your Health Pharmacy adjacent to Wright's clinic. The FDA had banned the marketing of L-tryptophan after it was implicated in an outbreak of eosinophilia-myalgia syndrome (see Chapter 2), but Wright continued to prescribe it. In August 1991, he filed suit, asserting that the outbreak was due to a contaminant and that his tryptophan was safe and therefore legal to dispense. The suit also asked the court to return the product and bar the FDA from "unreasonably interfering" with Wright's ability to exercise clinical judgment in treating patients.

During the same month, according to an FDA affidavit, FDA investigators observed mold in some glass vials at the pharmacy and were informed that the products had been made at a laboratory adjacent to Wright's clinic. Further investigation indicated that Dr. Wright and the pharmacist were co-owners of the laboratory and clinic and that a clandestine manufacturing facility was being constructed in a vacant business next to the pharmacy. When the investigators went to the laboratory, Wright would not permit them to conduct a full inspection. During the next few months, however, illegally marketed products were identified by inspecting trash from the clinic and pharmacy.

In December 1991, an FDA inspector posing as a patient was diagnosed with an Interro device. He reported that the woman who operated the device probed points on one of his fingers while selecting items on the screen that were said to represent substances to which he might be allergic. The woman explained that the height of a vertical bar that appeared when she probed his finger would indicate whether or not he was sensitive to the item being tested. After the test was completed, a printer next to the monitor printed a list of foods, chemicals, and other substances, with numerical values corresponding to readings on the Interro screen. Then the inspector was given several homeopathic medicines, instructions for using them, and an article stating that they would result in dramatic relief of his allergic symptoms. The Interro is a computerized galvanometer that measures changes in the skin's electrical resistance and depicts them on the screen of a monitor. The reading on the screen is determined by how hard the probe is pressed against the patient's finger; the harder the pressure, the less skin resistance and the higher the reading (see Chapter 13). The FDA Center for Devices and Radiologic Health has said that the device is "adulterated and misbranded" and can have no legal medical use.

In February 1992, Wright's clinic posted a notice claiming that state-licensed physicians are "exempt from the restrictions and regulations of the federal Food and Drug Administration as a matter of federal law." The notice also stated that "no employee, agent or inspector of the FDA shall be permitted on these premises."

In May 1992, a U.S. Magistrate issued warrants authorizing the FDA to conduct criminal searches at Wright's Clinic and the adjacent pharmacy. Two days later, FDA agents accompanied local police officers who broke down the front door of Tahoma clinic. Wright and his supporters claim that the search party entered with guns drawn and terrorized the clinic staff. However, federal officials state that the police broke down the door because the clinic staff had refused to open it when they knocked. The officials also state that a single gun was drawn because the officers suspected that those inside might be hostile, but the gun was never pointed at anyone and was reholstered as soon as the area was deemed safe. The authorities seized products, patient files, computer records, and Interro devices from the clinic and additional materials from the pharmacy. Two weeks later, the state pharmacy board summarily suspended the pharmacy's license, an action taken only when the board feels that public health may be endangered.

Wright and his allies have characterized the search procedure as "the Vitamin-B Bust" and sold videotapes showing part of the raid, the reaction of several clinic employees, and demonstrations staged by Wright supporters. However, Sherman L. Cox, Assistant Secretary for Licensing and Certification for the State of Washington, has stated that the items seized "were not just injectable vitamins but included a number of unapproved drugs." He did concede that the police officers' fear of danger was the result of assuming that the FDA definition of "illegal drugs" was the same as the county's definition (which covered heroin, cocaine, etc.).

On the "Larry King Live" television show, an FDA official said that the agency became interested in Wright's activities after someone complained that he was prescribing L-tryptophan and sending people to the pharmacy to have the prescriptions filled. Wright maintained that he had a right to do this because his supply was not contaminated. When Larry King asked why he thought the FDA ban did not apply to him, Wright replied, "My lawyer said I could use it."

The health-food industry is attempting to arouse public sympathy and fire up its own supporters by claiming that the authorities used excessive force— that Wright "had committed no crime but was only providing his patients with nutritional supplements and non-toxic, natural therapeutics." Wright and his supporters have generated extensive press coverage of their version of the controversy and have also established a legal defense fund. The Nutritional

Health Alliance, a group campaigning to weaken FDA jurisdiction over vitamins, has donated $50,000 to the fund.

In August 1992, Dr. Wright signed an agreement consenting to the destruction of the 103 bottles of L-tryptophan that had been seized and agreeing to pay at least $850 to cover court costs and fees associated with the action. But he has also filed a suit seeking to stop the FDA from regulating what he does. In a recent interview he stated that the pharmacy had given up its license and gone out of business, but that he has continued to operate his clinic. For Your Health is now operating as a health food store. A grand jury convened to determine whether Wright should be criminally prosecuted for violating FDA drug laws has not yet reported its findings.

## The Magazine Salesmen

> Man has been a creature of fallacy ever since time began. It seems to be inherent in his nature to believe in false things. . . . In the field of medicine, especially, man seems to delight in being completely taken in.

J.I. Rodale, who wrote this in 1954, seemed to understand how gullible people can be. Like Carlton Fredericks, Rodale had changed his original name (Jerome Irving Cohen) to one that was more promotable. Rodale was a shrewd businessman. His financial success attracted considerable attention in the early 1970s, and the publicity he received boosted his profits even more. He died in 1971, leaving a publishing empire to his son Robert. In 1991, Rodale Press's reported gross income was $289 million and the circulation of its leading magazine, *Prevention,* was over three million. Robert remained head of the company until 1990, when he was killed in a traffic accident while visiting the Soviet Union.

For many years, *Prevention* was the leading magazine promoting the health-food industry's viewpoints. It attacked ordinary foods and recommended supplements and health foods with claims that often were ludicrous. J.I. Rodale imagined many dangers lurking in our food supply. He accused sugar of "causing criminals," and blamed bread for colds, stomach irritation, bronchitis, pneumonia, conjunctivitis, rickets in children, and steatorrhea (passage of large amounts of fat in the feces) in adults. He warned that cola drinkers would become sterile. Even roast beef, pickles, ice cream, and bagels aroused his concern. An article in the *New York Times Magazine* reported that each day, J.I. took seventy food supplement tablets and would spend ten to twenty minutes under a short-wave machine "to restore his body electricity." He would live to one hundred, he told the reporter, unless he was run down by "a sugar-crazed taxi driver." But a few weeks later, at age seventy-two, he died of a heart attack while taping a TV interview for the Dick Cavett show.

Before J.I. Rodale's death, *Prevention* was filled with nonsense promoting dietary supplements—and ads from mail-order companies offering them for sale. Readers were told that our food supply was depleted of nourishment. News of nutritional "discoveries" was slanted to suggest that people who took food supplements were likely to benefit from discoveries that were just around the corner. Many articles contained therapeutic claims that would be illegal on product labels. Each issue also contained two dozen or so letters from readers telling how nutritional remedies had supposedly helped them. A 1973 survey reported that families that subscribed to *Prevention* spent an average of $190 per year for vitamin supplements and health foods—which I estimated was five to ten times as much as it would cost to supply an average family with a well-balanced multivitamin/mineral product (which they probably didn't need anyway).

Although water fluoridation is an extremely valuable way to supplement the diet to prevent disease (tooth decay), J.I. Rodale adamantly opposed it. Before his death, most issues of *Prevention* contained vicious attacks on fluoridation in articles, editorials, and letters to the editor. Communities around Rodale's headquarters in Emmaus, Pennsylvania, were subjected to an even greater amount of antifluoridation propaganda; in 1961, for example, Rodale Press spent more than $10,000 on a scare campaign which defeated a fluoridation referendum in nearby Allentown. The fears that were aroused still prevent Allentown from being fluoridated today. Following J.I.'s death, *Prevention* stopped attacking fluoridation and making ridiculous claims for dietary supplements. However, it continued to recommend supplements for everyone.

During the 1980s, *Prevention* shifted toward the scientific mainstream. In 1985, it dropped Carlton Fredericks and Jonathan Wright as columnists. During the next two years it acquired a prominent editorial advisory board and began sending many of its articles to experts (including me) for prepublication review. Partly in response to these changes, ads for vitamins and other supplements dropped from forty or fifty pages per issue to perhaps four or five, and some health-food industry writers even complained that *Prevention* had "sold out to the establishment." Today *Prevention* emphasizes healthy food choice, appropriate exercise programs, and other health-promoting activities. However, although its advice on most topics is accurate, it still tends to encourage unnecessary use and undue experimentation with dietary supplements. And ads for dubious products and/or services still appear in most issues despite considerable effort on my part to persuade them to screen them out. (See Chapter 31 for my comparison of *Prevention* with other health magazines.)

In recent years, Rodale's book division and the Prevention Book Club have marketed some books that are authoritative and others that espouse quack ideas. Ads for some books are even more blatant than the books themselves. For example, a mailer for *The Doctor's Vitamin and Mineral Encyclopedia*, by Sheldon Saul Hendler, M.D., was headlined "The World's Most Powerful Healing Vitamins and Minerals" and promised information on "a substance that reverses the aging process," a "heavy duty smart pill" that "stops the aging process and dramatically improves your memory," and a daily supplement that "could dramatically reduce your chances of breast cancer." The pertinent passages in the book reported speculations based on preliminary or anecdotal evidence.

In 1989, Rodale Press sent *Prevention*'s readers an ad for *Nutrition Prescription,* by Brian Morgan, Ph.D. The ad promised that the book would provide "a 'crystal ball' that gives us advance warning of the diseases we are most vulnerable to" plus a nutritional program "specifically designed to defeat the disease, reverse the symptoms and change your medical future for the better." The ad also described Morgan as "America's leading authority on nutrition." Calling the book "an inseparable mixture of good and poor advice," I urged the National Advertising Division (NAD) of the Council of Better Business Bureaus to ask Morgan whether he considered himself "America's leading authority." I did not see Morgan's reply; but, after reviewing his resumé, NAD concluded he was not.

## The Theoretician

The widespread public belief that high doses of vitamins are effective against colds and other illnesses is largely attributable to Linus Pauling, Ph.D., winner of the Nobel Prize for chemistry in 1954 and for peace in 1962. In 1968, Pauling postulated that people's nutrient and vitamin needs vary markedly and that to maintain good health, many people need amounts much greater than the Recommended Dietary Allowances (RDAs). And he suggested that mega-doses of certain vitamins and minerals might well be the treatment of choice for some forms of mental illness. Pauling termed this approach "orthomolecular," meaning "right molecules." Since that time, he has steadily expanded the number of illnesses he thinks can be influenced by "orthomolecular" therapy and the number of nutrients that are suitable for such use. The vast majority of medical and nutrition scientists do not share these views.

In 1970, Pauling proclaimed in *Vitamin C and the Common Cold* that taking 1,000 mg of vitamin C daily will reduce the incidence of colds by 45 percent for most people but that some people need much larger amounts. (The RDA for vitamin C is 60 mg.) The 1976 revision of the book, retitled *Vitamin C, the Common Cold and the Flu*, suggested even higher dosages. Another book, *Vitamin C and Cancer* (1979) claims that high doses of vitamin C may be effective against cancer. Pauling himself reportedly takes 12,000 mg daily and raises the amount to 40,000 mg if symptoms of a cold appear.

Scientific fact is established when the same experiment is carried out repeatedly with the same results. To test the effect of vitamin C on colds, it is necessary to compare groups that get the vitamin to similar groups that get a placebo (a dummy pill that looks and tastes like the real thing). This is the only way to determine whether taking vitamin C is more effective than doing nothing. Since the common cold is a very variable illness, proper tests must involve hundreds of people for significantly long periods of time. At least sixteen well-designed, double-blind studies have shown that supplementation with vitamin C does not prevent colds. Slight symptom reduction may occur as the result of an antihistamine-like effect, but whether this has practical value is a matter of dispute. Pauling's views are based on analysis of the same studies as other scientists, but his conclusions are different.

The largest clinical trials, involving thousands of volunteers, were directed by Dr. Terence Anderson, professor of epidemiology at the University of Toronto. Taken together, his studies suggest that extra vitamin C may slightly reduce the severity of colds, but it is not necessary to take the high doses suggested by Pauling to achieve this result. Nor is there anything to be gained by taking vitamin C supplements year-round with the hope of preventing colds.

Another important study was reported in 1975 by scientists at the National Institutes of Health, who compared vitamin C pills with a placebo before and during colds. The experiment was supposed to be double-blind, with neither experimenters nor subjects able to tell who got the vitamin and who got the placebo; however, half the subjects did correctly guess which one they had received. When the results were tabulated with all subjects lumped together, the vitamin group reported fewer colds per person over a nine-month period. But among the half who guessed incorrectly, no difference in the incidence or severity was found. This illustrates how people who think they are doing something effective (such as taking a vitamin) can report a favorable result even when none exists.

In 1976, Pauling and Dr. Ewan Cameron, a Scottish physician, reported that a majority of one hundred terminal cancer patients treated with 10,000 mg of vitamin C daily survived three to four times longer than similar patients who did not receive vitamin C supplements. However, Dr. William DeWys, chief of clinical investigations at the National Cancer Institute, found that the study was poorly designed because the patient groups were not comparable. The vitamin C patients were Cameron's, while the other patients were under the care of other physicians. Cameron's patients were started on vitamin C when he labeled them "untreatable" by other methods, and their subsequent survival was compared to the survival of the "control" patients after they had been labeled untreatable by *their* doctors. DeWys reasoned that if the two groups were comparable, the lengths of time from entry into the hospital to being labeled untreatable should be equivalent in both groups. However, he found that Cameron's patients were labeled untreatable much earlier in the course of their disease—which means that they entered the hospital less sick than the other doctors' patients and would naturally be expected to live longer.

Nevertheless, to test whether Pauling might be correct, the Mayo Clinic conducted three double-blind studies involving a total of 367 patients with advanced cancer. The studies, reported in 1979, 1983, and 1985, found that patients given 10,000 mg of vitamin C daily did no better than those given a placebo.

Science aside, it is clear that Dr. Pauling is politically aligned with the promoters of unscientific nutrition practices. He says his initial interest in vitamin C was aroused by a letter from biochemist Irwin Stone, with whom he subsequently maintained a close working relationship. Although Stone was often referred to as "Dr. Stone," his only credentials were a certificate showing completion of a two-year chemistry program, an honorary chiropractic degree from the Los Angeles College of Chiropractic, and a "Ph.D." from Donsbach University.

In *Vitamin C and the Common Cold,* Pauling attacked the health-food industry for misleading its customers. Pointing out that "synthetic" vitamin C is identical with "natural" vitamin C, he warned that higher-priced "natural" products are a "waste of money." And he added that "the words 'organically grown' are essentially meaningless—just part of the jargon used by health-food promoters in making their excess profits, often from elderly people with low incomes." But *Vitamin C, the Common Cold and the Flu,* issued six years later, contained none of these criticisms. This omission was not accidental. Pauling informed me that, after his first book came out, he was "strongly attacked by people who were also attacking the health-food people." His critics were so "biased," he decided, that he would no longer help them attack the health-food industry while another part of their attack was directed at him.

The Linus Pauling Institute of Medicine, founded in 1973, is dedicated to "orthomolecular medicine." Its largest corporate donor has been Hoffmann-La Roche, the pharmaceutical giant that is the dominant factor in worldwide production of vitamin C.

During the mid-1970s, Pauling helped lead the health-food industry's campaign for passage of the Proxmire Bill, which weakened FDA protection of consumers against misleading nutrition claims (see Chapter 28). In 1977 and 1979, Pauling received awards and presented his views on vitamin C at the annual conventions of the National Nutritional Foods Association (NNFA), the major trade association of health food retailers, distributors, and producers. In 1981, he accepted an award from the National Health Federation (NHF) for "services rendered in behalf of health freedom" and gave his daughter a life membership in this organization. Pauling has also appeared as a speaker at a Parker School for Professional Success Seminar, a meeting where chiropractors were taught highly questionable methods of building their practices (see Chapter 12). An ad for the meeting invited chiropractors to pose with Dr. Pauling for a photograph (which presumably could be used for publicity when the chiropractors returned home). In 1993, NNFA set up an annual Linus Pauling Award and announced that Pauling would be its first recipient.

Pauling has also helped to defend individuals accused of improper practices. In 1983, he and Irwin Stone testified at a hearing on behalf of Oscar Falconi, a vitamin promoter charged by the Postal Service with making false claims for several products. Pauling supported Falconi's contentions that vitamin C was useful not only in preventing cancer, but also in curing drug addicts and destroying both viruses and bacteria. In 1984, Pauling testified before the California Board of Medical Quality Assurance in defense of Michael Gerber, M.D., who was accused of improperly administering to patients. One was a fifty-six-year-old woman with treatable cancer who—the Board concluded—had died as a result of Gerber's neglect while he treated her with herbs, enzymes, coffee enemas, and chelation therapy. The other patients were three-year-old twin boys with ear infections for which Gerber had prescribed 70,000 or more units of vitamin A daily and coffee enemas twice daily for several weeks. Gerber lost his license to practice medicine as a result of the hearings. In 1992, Pauling testified in behalf of "clinical ecologist" Warren Levin, M.D., during hearings that culminated in a recommendation by New York State authorities that Levin's license be revoked for "gross negligence," "fraudulent practice," and "moral unfitness" (see Chapter 10).

A flyer distributed in 1991 by the Linus Pauling Institute recommends daily doses of 6,000 to 18,000 mg of vitamin C, 400 to 1,600 IU of vitamin E, and 25,000 IU of vitamin A, plus various other vitamins and minerals. These dosages have no proven benefit and can cause troublesome side effects.

## The Interpreter

Jeffrey S. Bland, Ph.D., is undoubtedly the health-food industry's most prolific publicist and interpreter of nutrition-related scientific developments. His interpretations consistently favor the use of supplements. A former biochemistry professor, Bland appears frequently at trade shows, writes books and articles, produces audio and video tapes, markets nutritional products and home study courses, conducts seminars for health professionals and health-food retailers, and serves as a consultant to organizations that share the supplement industry's views. Bland is president of HealthComm (originally called J.S.B. and Associates), which he formed in 1984 "to educate doctors about nutrition." He has also been a research associate at the Linus Pauling Institute of Medicine and has directed its nutrient analysis laboratory. Bland has a B.S. in biology from the University of California at Irvine and a Ph.D. in chemistry from the University of Oregon.

Bland's advice to health-food retailers was vividly described in *Nutrition Forum* by science writer Odom Fanning, who attended a seminar called "Nutritional Selling: A Powerful Customer Service," at a trade show held in 1985 in Washington, D.C. The seminar, led by Bland, included several skits in which he played storekeeper and three retailers played customers. Members of the audience were also invited to act as customers and ask their "toughest question" to the four panelists acting as clerks. Bland's delivery was rapid-fire, with frequent use of biochemical concepts and "emerging" research findings that he considered relevant and encouraging.

Much of the seminar concerned how product information might be communicated without "prescribing," which would be practicing medicine without a license. Bland said he would try to make it clear to customers that he was merely "trying to support them with nutritional information adjunct to traditional medical care." He also warned that requests for specific product information should be handled cautiously to avoid being "nailed for prescribing." When a retailer asked about the limits of advice, Bland replied:

> If a client asks a question that specific, you need to decide whether he is a client or a friend, and how well you know him. If he is a friend, then I would take him out to lunch, away from your store, and talk to him

as a friend. Don't talk as the store proprietor because that would be diagnosis and treatment. No matter what you think you are offering as a service, you are really, by the letter of the law, doing things that could be interpreted as diagnosis and treatment. However, if, as a friend, you anecdotally talk about your experience as a human being, there's no law that prevents freedom of speech.

When asked what retailers should become knowledgeable about, Bland rattled off a long list of biochemical terms and tidbits related to amino acids— "things you should have in the back of your mind even though you're not going to prescribe for treatment." At another point, he described how to question a customer who asks about a breast lump in order to assess whether it might be amenable to nutritional intervention.

One of Bland's educational products is "Why Nutrient Supplementa- tion?," a twenty-minute videotape or slide/audiocassette program intended for in-store customer viewing. In it Bland claims that: (1) "marginal deficiencies" are common in the United States; (2) many people who presume they are healthy because they are not diseased would actually benefit from higher levels of health by taking a regular nutritional supplement; (3) if you eat a balanced diet, the need for supplementation may be reduced; and (4) "prudent nutritional supplementation" can "optimize nutrient quality" to help augment health and prevent disease. Bland also lists ten situations where supplements are suppos- edly needed, but says nothing about how individuals can determine whether they fit these supposed categories. (Presumably, those listening to the tape will either "play it safe" by buying a supplement or ask the retailer for advice on "optimization.")

Bland's other informational products are so voluminous and complex that I have neither the time nor the expertise to evaluate them. Regardless of their accuracy, however, I doubt that most retailers, unconventional physicians, chiropractors, and naturopaths can utilize the information in a rational and responsible way.

Bland is also president of Nu-Day Enterprises, which markets a diet program. In 1991, the Federal Trade Commission (FTC) charged Bland and Nu-Day with falsely claiming that their program could cause weight loss by "tuning up the body's heat-producing machinery." The program, which cost $59.95 for a two-week supply, contained a meal-replacement formula; *Nu-Day Herbulk* (said to be a "natural appetite suppressant" that provides fiber and "cleanses the digestive system"); an instructional booklet; and an audiocassette. It had been promoted with a thirty-minute television infomercial titled "The Perfect Diet," which offered "amazing true stories of people like yourself losing twenty, thirty, fifty pounds or more, safely, quickly, and naturally." Without admitting wrongdoing, Dr. Bland signed a consent agreement to pay $30,000 for redress and to refrain from making unsubstantiated claims that the Nu-Day Diet Program, or any similar program, would cause weight loss by altering the body's metabolism.

**The Bible Maker**

Earl Mindell, R.Ph., helped found the Great Earth chain of health food stores, which, numbering about two hundred, is now the nation's second largest. He has also written *Earl Mindell's Vitamin Bible for Your Kids, Earl Mindell's Pill Bible, Earl Mindell's Quick & Easy Guide to Better Health, Earl Mindell's Shaping Up with Vitamins, Unsafe at Any Meal,* and *Earl Mindell's Herb Bible*—books whose total sales are in the millions.

Mindell's *Vitamin Bible* was written while he was working toward a "Ph.D." at the University of Beverly Hills, a nonaccredited school that lacked a campus or laboratory facilities. Mindell also obtained a "Ph.D." in nutrition from nonaccredited Union University. Both schools ceased operations in 1986.

The advisor for Mindell's Beverly Hills project was James Kenney, Ph.D., R.D., a genuine expert who is now a nutritionist at the Pritikin Longevity Center in Santa Monica, California. Kenney reviewed Mindell's manuscript and told him that it contained over four hundred errors, more than one hundred of which were important. Kenney says that most of the errors remain in the published version. The acknowledgments section of the book recognizes Kenney for his help and thanks the American Medical Association, the National Academy of Sciences, the National Dairy Council, the American Academy of Pediatrics, and the Nutrition Foundation, "without whom a project of this scope could never have been completed." However, the fact that all these prestigious organizations would strenuously disagree with information in the book is not mentioned. *Shaping Up with Vitamins* thanks these groups plus the American Dietetic Association, which Mindell surely must know disagrees with his views on supplementation.

In a section of *Vitamin Bible* titled "The Whole Truth," Mindell tells what each vitamin and mineral can supposedly do for you and gives advice for self-treatment with supplements of many of them. For example, he suggests pantothenic acid for tingling hands and feet, vitamin D for conjunctivitis, and calcium for menstrual cramps. This section also promotes substances that Mindell calls "vitamins" $B_{10}$, $B_{11}$, $B_{13}$, $B_{15}$, $B_{17}$, P, T, and U. There is no evidence that any of these substances are essential to humans or that supplements of any of them are beneficial; furthermore, $B_{15}$ (pangamic acid) and $B_{17}$ (laetrile) pose health risks. Another section of the book recommends self-treatment with supplements for more than fifty ailments and conditions, including acne, bad breath, baldness, headaches, measles, mumps, prostatitis, syphilis, gonorrhea, and warts. Despite all this, the book's jacket refers to Mindell as "America's #1 Vitamin Expert."

In *Vitamin Bible for Kids,* Mindell advises parents who suspect that their child is deficient in any nutrient to consult a "nutritionally oriented doctor" or (if mineral deficiency is suspected) obtain a hair analysis. Among other things, the book recommends vitamin supplements for acne, bronchitis, athlete's foot, canker sores, chicken pox, clumsiness, colitis, dandruff, diabetes, forgetfulness, impetigo, insect bites, prickly heat, poison ivy, stomach aches, tonsillitis, and warts. For multiple sclerosis, it recommends orotic acid, which Mindell refers to as vitamin $B_{13}$. And for children whose "little white lies are growing darker," he recommends eliminating sugars, refined starches, and junk food from the diet and supplementing with B-complex vitamins.

*Earl Mindell's Herb Bible* is full of misinformation. Herb expert Varro Tyler, Ph.D., has noted that the book misidentifies many plants and makes many unproven and inaccurate assertions about their usefulness. In the September/ October 1992 issue of *Nutrition Forum,* Tyler concluded: "As a sales tool for health food stores it undoubtedly will do well. As a bible, it fails miserably."

Mindell co-edited Keats Publishing Company's "Good Health Guides," a large series of booklets promoting dozens of questionable supplements. His fellow editor was Richard A. Passwater, whose "Ph.D." is from Bernadean University, a correspondence school that was never accredited or legally authorized to grant any degrees.

Mindell has also written information sheets that for many years were distributed as educational material in health-food stores. Although all of them warned that the information they contained was "not intended as medical advice but only as a guide in working with your doctor," it is clear that they were used to boost product sales by making claims that would be illegal on product labels. Some described how various vitamins, minerals, and amino acids function in the body and provided tidbits on research involving these substances. Others promoted such products as ginseng, bee pollen, chelated minerals, L-tryptophan, kelp (to help the thyroid gland), yucca extract tablets (for arthritis), papaya (to help digestion), octacosanol ("the amazing energy sustainer"), and goldenseal root (for stomach and liver troubles).

I have reviewed more than sixty of these flyers dated between 1980 and 1984, and found that most were misleading and many contained errors. In #63, for example, Mindell stated that research done at Temple University in Philadelphia found that rats fed dehydroepiandrosterone (DHEA) lost weight. What actually happened, however, was that rats who received dosages fifty times greater than those marketed for humans did not lose weight but merely gained less than expected. Great Earth was one of many companies selling DHEA pills as a "fat fighter" until the FDA ordered all DHEA products off the market in the spring of 1985.

Flyer #44B suggested that supplements of glucomannan (a plant fiber) are an effective appetite suppressant—which they are not. A previous version of this flyer claimed that studies conducted by Judith Stern, D.Sc., of the University of California at Davis, showed that subjects taking glucomannan lost more weight than control subjects. Actually, no significant differences were found between the two groups, and mention of Dr. Stern was deleted after she threatened to take legal action.

Flyer #4B suggested that supplementation with lecithin can prevent heart disease, aid anemia, strengthen weak muscles, reverse psoriasis, improve memory and balance, and even "appears to help multiple sclerosis." Mindell has also called lecithin "the Roto-Rooter of the nutritional world" because "it cleans out blood vessel walls"—an untrue claim.

Flyer #31 claimed that superoxide dismutase (SOD) is an "anti-aging enzyme" that may be effective against arthritis, atherosclerosis, cancer, and senility. Even if this were true, SOD in pill form could not possibly be effective. Tests on animals have shown that oral supplementation does not affect tissue SOD activity—a finding easily predictable from the fact that SOD, like all other proteins, would be digested rather than absorbed intact into the body.

Flyers #9A and #9B endorsed the theory of Benjamin Frank, M.D., that increasing intake of RNA and DNA through dietary measures or supplements will "reverse the aging process." (*Dr. Frank's No-Aging Diet,* popular fifteen years ago, recommended eating sardines, yeast, and other foods rich in these nucleic acids.) Nucleic acids, found in all living matter, are basic to cell reproduction. Like SOD, however, those that are eaten are digested and never reach the cells intact. Moreover, nucleic acids are like specific blueprints. If DNA and RNA from yeasts or sardines could actually work in humans, they would turn them into young yeasts or baby sardines.

Mindell advises that everyone should take supplements. He claims that foods from the grocery store are depleted of vitamins and minerals and, therefore, are nutritionally inadequate. He says that smokers need extra vitamin C, those who drink alcohol need extra B-vitamins, and that women taking birth control pills need extra $B_6$.

During a lecture in Tucson several years ago, Mindell said he personally took "twenty-odd" supplements twice daily. He also stated that "natural" vitamins, such as natural vitamin C with rose hips, are better than synthetic ones. Mindell's lecture included advice that was potentially dangerous. He said, for example, that vitamin A is safe in amounts up to 100,000 IU per day and that any potentially toxic doses carry warnings. Neither of these statements is true. At one point during his talk, Mindell tried to persuade a member of the audience to follow his advice rather than that of his doctor by claiming that medical doctors are ignorant about vitamins.

Now retired from active management of his stores, Mindell spends much of his time writing, lecturing, and appearing on talk shows. Despite the astonishing number of inaccuracies he has promoted—his ideas are rarely questioned by members of the media who encounter him.

**The Children's Doctor**

Pediatrician Lendon H. Smith, M.D., contends that nutrition plays a major role in behavior and that nutritional remedies are helpful for a wide range of diseases and conditions. He claims, for example, that allergies, alcoholism, insomnia, hyperactivity in children, and many other ailments result from enzyme disturbances that can be helped by dietary changes. He recommends a variety of food supplements and avoidance of white sugar, bleached flour, pasteurized milk, and other foods that are not "natural." For many years, Smith's ideas were promoted widely on his own syndicated TV program and through guest appearances on other shows. During Smith's heyday, a Donahue show executive said, "Unlike other M.D.s, Smith presents well on the air and has a special rapport with parents. He's funny, interesting and makes people feel good about themselves and their children."

Smith's books include: *The Children's Doctor, Feed Your Kids Right, Improving Your Child's Behavior Chemistry, Encyclopedia of Baby and Child Care, Feed Yourself Right, Foods for Healthy Kids, Dr. Smith's Low Stress Diet,* and *Dr. Smith's Diet Plan for Teenagers.* Most were published by the trade division of McGraw-Hill, a leading publisher of college textbooks.

In *Improving Your Child's Behavior Chemistry,* Smith writes how "It is amazing how children's behavior can be turned around 180 degrees by a vitamin C and B injection. Overnight, they sleep better, begin to eat, and are cheerful, calm and cooperative the next day." (If true, I suspect that the reason for any such behavior change is not nutritional but fear of having more shots.)

In *Feed Your Kids Right,* Smith suggested that a daily dose of 15,000 to 30,000 units of vitamin A is "about right for most of us." He also recommends a "stress formula" which includes up to 10,000 mg of vitamin C and 50,000 units of vitamin A each day for a month. These dosages, of course, are dangerous—particularly to children.

In 1973, the Oregon State Board of Medical Examiners placed Smith on probation for prescribing medication that was "not necessary or medically indicated" for six (adult) patients, one diagnosed as hyperactive and the other five as heroin addicts. His probation lasted until 1981. Shortly after the board's action, Smith turned to "nutritional therapy" and allied himself with naturopaths, homeopaths, and chiropractors. Later he became the first physician named to the board of the Portland-based National College of Naturopathic Medicine. He has been a frequent speaker at health-food industry seminars and dental meetings.

In 1987, Smith permanently surrendered his medical license rather than face Board action on charges of insurance fraud. According to press reports, the trouble arose because he had signed documents authorizing insurance payments for patients he had not seen. The patients had actually been seen by chiropractors, homeopaths, and other practitioners at "nutrition-oriented" clinics in which Smith had worked.

Since this trouble occurred, Smith has been far less visible in both the general and "alternative" media. He has written columns for health-food and chiropractic publications and has published a newsletter called *The Facts.* In the November 1989 issue of the latter, Smith advised readers to smell the vitamins and minerals they take. (This "really works, he says. "No one over- or underdoses.") According to Smith's theory, if a multivitamin obtained in a health-food store becomes malodorous, "it means the customer has taken enough of the tablets and his body is now saying he had had enough." In a column in *Total Health,* Smith advised parents that if a child who has a good self-image shows symptoms of depression, they should consider inappropriate diet as an explanation: "My rule is, if a person likes something and they must have it everyday, it is probably causing the symptoms. If depression comes and goes, then diet is surely the inciting agent."

In 1988, after I mentioned Smith in *Nutrition Forum,* he sent me a cordial letter, which ended: "I would like to keep in touch with you because you are right, we must get rid of the quacks and charlatans, but I find it very difficult to tell where to draw the line. Please help me." I replied: "I prefer to think of quackery rather than quacks; most people who promote it are not charlatans but sincere individuals who reply on personal experience and not enough on testing their theories. I'm not sure I can help you sort things out."

## Crusading Groups

Promoters of questionable health practices often form organizations to multiply their effectiveness. How can one tell which groups are reliable and which are not? There is no sure way, but six precautionary questions may help:

1. *Are its ideas inside the scientific mainstream?* Some groups admit that they were formed because their founders felt alienated from the scientific community. One group that made no secret of this was actually called the American Quack Association, whose main purposes were to provide emotional support to its members, poke fun at their critics, and stimulate positive public feelings toward unconventional practitioners. The group was founded in 1985 by Jonathan Wright, who became its president, and Roy Kupsinel, M.D., a "holistic" practitioner from Florida, who became its vice-president. It attracted about three hundred members but no longer appears active.

2. *Who are its leaders and advisors?* The International Society for Fluoride Research may sound respectable but it is actually an antifluoridation group. The International Academy of Preventive Medicine (now called the International Academy of Nutrition and Preventive Medicine) numbered among its leaders Carlton Fredericks, Linus Pauling, Lendon Smith, and other promoters of questionable nutrition practices. The Health Resources Council is an advocacy group founded by Gary Null to promote "alternative" health methods.

3. *What are its membership requirements?* Is scientific expertise required—or just a willingness to pay dues? An organization open to almost anyone may be perfectly respectable (like the American Association for the Advancement of Science), but don't let the fact that an individual belongs to it impress you. The International Academy of Nutritional Consultants and the American Association of Nutritional Consultants issued attractive certificates, but their only requirement for "professional membership" was payment of a $50 fee. Some "institutes" are simply names adopted by an individual or a few individuals who wish to make their work sound more respectable.

4. *Does it promote a specific treatment or treatments?* Most such groups should be highly suspect. A century ago, valid new ideas were hard to evaluate and often were rejected by the medical community. But today, effective new treatments are quickly welcomed by scientific practitioners and do not need special groups to promote them. The American College of Advancement in Medicine (formerly called the Association for Chelation Therapy) falls into this category. So do the World Research Association and various other groups that promote questionable cancer therapies; the American Academy of Environmental Medicine (which promotes "clinical ecology"); the American Schizophrenia Association (which promotes megavitamins); and the latter's parent organization, the Huxley Institute for Biosocial Research. And we may add the National Wellness Coalition, whose stated mission is "to promote wellness principles, policies and practices as the key to affordable, effective health care and a healthy prosperous nation." Despite the rhetoric,

however, the coalition pays very little attention to proven health methods and promotes a broad spectrum of unscientific approaches.

5. *Does it espouse a version of "freedom of choice" that would abolish government regulation of the health marketplace?* Such "freedom" is nothing more than a ploy to persuade legislators to permit the marketing of quack methods without legal restraints. Several groups with this philosophy are discussed in Chapter 28.

6. *How is it financed?* The Council for Responsible Nutrition, despite its respectable-sounding name, is a Washington, D.C., group that represents manufacturers and distributors of food supplements and other nutritional products. Don't assume, however, that funding by an industry makes an organization unreliable. Reliability should be determined by judging the validity of a group's ideas rather than its funding. The National Dairy Council and the Institute of Food Technologists are highly respected by the scientific community for their accurate publications on nutrition.

**The Bottom Line**

All of us are exposed daily to many ideas about health, some of which are accurate and some not. Promoters of unproven and unscientific methods are working hard to gain your allegiance. When you are well, unless you are taken in to an extreme degree, what you believe may not matter much. But if you have a health problem—particularly a serious one—misplacing your trust can kill you or others who rely upon your judgment.

# 28

# "Health Freedom" Crusaders

## Stephen Barrett, M.D.

This chapter describes the activities of four groups that want to weaken or destroy government regulation of health practitioners and products. The National Health Federation (NHF) and the Foundation for the Advancement of Innovative Medicine (FAIM) are alliances of promoters and followers who engage in lobbying campaigns and many other activities. The Committee for Freedom of Choice in Medicine (CFCM) is the political arm of several interlocking corporations promoting and/or marketing questionable remedies for cancer and other serious diseases. The People's Medical Society (PMS) is a "consumer group" that publishes reports and engages in letter-writing campaigns. All four groups are antagonistic toward established medical practices and use the words "alternative," and "freedom" to suit their own purposes.

### The National Health Federation (NHF)

NHF is headquartered in Monrovia, California. Its members pay from $36 per year for "regular" membership to a total of $1,000 or more for "perpetual" membership. NHF members receive occasional mailings and a monthly magazine called *Health Freedom News* (formerly called *Public Scrutiny* and the *NHF Bulletin*). In 1991, it had about 6,600 members.

    Since its formation, NHF's stated purpose has been to promote "freedom of choice" by consumers. As expressed for years in its *Bulletin*:

> NHF opposes monopoly and compulsion in things related to health where the safety and welfare of others are not concerned. NHF does not

oppose nor approve any specific healing profession or their methods, but it does oppose the efforts of any one group to restrict the freedom of practice of qualified members of another profession, thus attempting to create a monopoly.

At first glance, this credo may seem "democratic" and somehow related to unfair business competition. What NHF really means, however, is that government should not help scientifically based health care to drive unproven methods out of the marketplace. NHF wants anyone who merely *claims* to have an effective treatment or product to be allowed to market it without scientific proof that it works.

NHF promotes questionable health methods and has little interest in scientifically recognized methods. *Health Freedom News* contains ads for questionable treatments and products that are being marketed illegally. Nutritional fads, myths, and gimmicks are mentioned favorably by NHF publications and convention speakers. Worthless cancer treatments, particularly laetrile, have been promoted in the same ways. Articles in NHF publications have looked with disfavor on such proven public health measures as pasteurization of milk, immunization, water fluoridation, and food irradiation. Use of nutritional supplements is encouraged by claims that modern food processing depletes our food supply of its nutrients. "Natural" and "organic" products have been promoted with suggestions that our food supply is "poisoned." Chiropractic, naturopathy, and homeopathy are regarded favorably. Books that promote questionable health concepts are given favorable reviews. Antiquackery legislation is condemned. Underlying all these messages is the idea that anyone who opposes NHF's ideas is part of a "conspiracy" of government, organized medicine, and big business against the little consumer.

NHF has been very active in the political arena. It presents testimony to regulatory agencies and sponsors legislation aimed at minimizing government interference with the health-food industry. To bolster the influence of its lobbyists, it generates letter-writing campaigns that urge legislators and government officials to support NHF positions. These campaigns typically include charges of persecution, discrimination, and conspiracy. NHF also has filed lawsuits against government agencies and helped to defend people prosecuted for selling questionable "health" products or services.

### NHF's Leaders

Not surprisingly, most of NHF's leaders have been economically involved with the issues it has promoted—and at least twenty have been in legal difficulty for such activities. NHF's officers and board members have included the following people.

• Fred J. Hart, who founded NHF in 1955, was president of the Electronic Medical Foundation, a company that marketed quack devices. In 1954, Hart and his foundation were ordered by a U.S. District Court to stop distributing thirteen devices with false claims that they could diagnose and treat hundreds of diseases and conditions. In 1962, Hart was fined by the court for violating this order. He died in 1976.

• Royal S. Lee, D.D.S., a nonpracticing dentist who died in 1967, helped Hart found NHF and served on its board of governors. Lee owned and operated the Vitamin Products Company, which sold food supplements, and the Lee Foundation for Nutritional Research, which distributed literature on nutrition and health. One of the vitamin company's products was *Catalyn,* a patent medicine composed of milk sugar, wheat starch, wheat bran, and other plant material. During the early 1930s, a shipment of *Catalyn* was seized by the FDA and destroyed by court order because it had been marketed with false claims of effectiveness against serious diseases. In 1945, the FDA ordered Lee and his company to discontinue illegal claims for *Catalyn* and other products. In 1956, the Post Office Department charged Lee's foundation with fraudulent promotion of a book called *Diet Prevents Polio.* The foundation agreed to discontinue the challenged claims. In 1962, Lee and the Vitamin Products Company were convicted of misbranding 115 special dietary products by making false claims for the treatment of more than five hundred diseases and conditions. Lee received a one-year suspended prison term and was fined $7,000. In 1963, a prominent FDA official said Lee was "probably the largest publisher of unreliable and false nutritional information in the world."

• Jonathan V. Wright, M.D., who became NHF's board chairman in 1992, is embroiled in disputes with the FDA involving nutritional products that the FDA seized in a much-publicized raid on Wright's clinic and an adjacent pharmacy (see Chapter 27).

• Kurt W. Donsbach, D.C., a protégé of Lee, replaced Fred Hart as NHF's board chairman in 1975 and held that position until 1989. In 1971, after agents of the California Bureau of Food and Drug observed Donsbach tell customers at his health food store that vitamins, minerals, and/or herbal tea were effective against several serious diseases, he pled guilty to one count of practicing medicine without a license and agreed to cease "nutritional consultation." In the ensuing years, Donsbach has marketed supplement products, issued publications, operated nonaccredited correspondence schools, marketed a bogus "nutrient deficiency" test, and administered dubious treatments at Mexican cancer clinics. (See Chapter 27 for further details.)

• During NHF's early years, Andrew S. Rosenberger served as the group's "nutrition chairman" and spoke at NHF conventions. For many years, he and his brother Henry operated a large chain of health-food stores called Nature Food Centers. In 1938, their firm made an agreement with the FTC to stop making therapeutic claims for more than twenty products. During the 1950s, the Post Office Department filed several complaints against the firm for making false therapeutic claims for various products; in each case, the company agreed to discontinue the claims. In 1962, the Rosenberger brothers were fined $5,000 each and given six-month suspended prison sentences for misbranding dietary products. Nature Food Centers was fined $10,000.

• Clinton Miller was NHF's legislative advocate from 1962 through 1989 and has also served as NHF's executive director. Before coming to NHF, Miller chaired the antifluoridation committee of Utah, which helped make Utah the least fluoridated state in the U.S. In the 1960s and early 1970s, he operated Clinton's Wheat Shop (a health-food store) in Bountiful, Utah, and Miller's Honey Company in Salt Lake City. During this period the FDA took seven enforcement actions (two citations and five seizures) involving products marketed by these companies. One was a seizure from the wheat shop in 1962 of some "dried Swiss whey," which the FDA considered misbranded when claimed as effective in treating intestinal disorders. The whey was returned when Miller agreed to change its labeling. In 1976, he was an unsuccessful candidate for the U.S. Senate.

• Maureen Kennedy Salaman, NHF's president from 1982 to 1992, hosts a radio talk show and has been very active in promoting questionable cancer remedies. Her 1983 book, *Nutrition: The Cancer Answer,* claims that "the American Cancer Society advocates treating cancer rather than preventing it." In 1984, she ran for vice-president on the Populist party ticket.

• David Ajay was president of the National Nutritional Foods Association (NNFA), a trade association that represents health food retailers, distributors, and producers.

• Norman J. Bassett was publisher of *Let's Live,* a magazine that promotes questionable health methods.

• Walter Douglas Brodie, M.D., was convicted twice of failing to file income tax returns. In 1977, he was sentenced to six months in prison, and in 1987 he was fined $10,000 and sentenced to one year in prison and five years' probation. In a 1983 letter describing how he has prescribed laetrile and other "alternative" cancer treatments, Brodie stated that he had moved his practice to Nevada after "political persecution" by the California State Board of Medical Quality Assurance, which had unsuccessfully attempted to discipline him several times.

• Kirkpatrick Dilling, who was NHF's general counsel for many years, is an attorney who specializes in the issues in which NHF has been involved. He has also been the attorney for the Cancer Control Society, a group that promotes questionable methods of cancer treatment.

• H. Ray Evers, M.D., who died in 1990, was a leading practitioner of "chelation therapy" (see Chapter 9). During his career he claimed to have treated more than twenty thousand patients and supervised more than 500,000 chelation treatments. In 1976, at the FDA's request, a Louisiana federal judge prohibited Evers from using chelation therapy in Louisiana. Testimony in the case suggested that at least fourteen patients had died from this therapy at Evers' hospital. Later that year, Evers was given a suspended prison sentence and two years' probation after pleading guilty to "intimidating and impeding officers of the Internal Revenue Service." According to the IRS agents' report, Evers had cursed at them, threatened their lives, and attempted to run one of them down with his car when they visited his property in connection with a tax matter.

Evers then moved to Montgomery, Alabama, where, despite FDA efforts, a judge allowed him to continue doing chelation therapy. In 1980, he opened the ninety-bed Evers Health Center in Cottonwood, Alabama. His letter to prospective patients stated that his practice was "limited to the diagnosis and treatment of chronic degenerative diseases by the nutritional, non-toxic, metabolic method including chelation therapy" and offered "special regimes of treatment" for arthritis, amyotrophic lateral sclerosis, multiple sclerosis, diabetes, cancer, Parkinson's disease, and other diseases. According to the clinic brochure, a patient's typical day would include a visit with Dr. Evers, spinal manipulation by his chiropractic associate, chelation therapy (three hours), and other therapies such as hyperbaric oxygen and colonic irrigation.

In December 1986, the Alabama Medical Licensure Commission revoked Evers's medical license. According to an article published by his son Michael, the proceedings were based on Evers's use of an herbal salve to treat a thirty-year-old woman who had cancer and died several months later, presumably of her disease. The revocation was for "engaging in the practice of medicine in such a manner as to endanger the health of [the patient]," "using untruthful or deceptive or improbable statements concerning the effects or results of his proposed treatment," and "demonstrating unprofessional conduct in the treatment of [the patient]." The commission also concluded that Evers's actions constituted "gross malpractice." After the appeals process ended, Evers moved his practice to Mexico.

• Michael Gerber, M.D., had his California medical license revoked after hearings before the California Board of Medical Quality Assurance in which he was accused in 1984 of improperly administering to patients. One patient was a fifty-six-year-old woman with treatable cancer who had allegedly died as a result of Gerber's neglect while he treated her with herbs, enzymes, coffee enemas, and chelation therapy. The other patients were three-year-old twin boys with ear infections for which Gerber had prescribed 70,000 or more International Units of vitamin A daily and coffee enemas twice daily for several weeks. After his medical license was revoked, Gerber acquired a homeopathic licence and began operating a chain of clinics in Nevada.

• Garry Gordon, M.D., has been president of the American Academy of Medical Preventics (currently called the American College of Advancement in Medicine), a group of doctors who do chelation therapy. He has also been medical director and board chairman of Mineralab (a large commercial hair analysis laboratory) and director of a subsidiary that sold questionable nutritional products.

• Bruce Halstead, M.D., was convicted in 1985 of twenty-four counts of cancer fraud and grand theft for selling an herbal tea called ADS to ten patients with cancer and other serious diseases for $125 to $150 per quart. Although he maintained that ADS was a "nutritional supplement," analysis showed it to be 99.4 percent water and a brownish sludge composed mainly of coliform bacteria (the same bacteria found in human feces). Halstead, who operated the Halstead Preventive Medicine Clinic in Colton, California, has been a leading promoter of laetrile, chelation therapy, and many other questionable practices. Following the trial, which lasted for five months, Los Angeles County Deputy District Attorney Hyatt Seligman called Halstead "a crook selling swamp water." He was fined $10,000 and sentenced to four years in prison, but remains free during the appeals process. According to an article published by Michael Evers, Halstead maintained during his trial that he was the target of a "Medical Gestapo" out to destroy health practitioners who deviate from orthodox cancer therapies such as surgery, radiation and chemotherapy. In 1992, his license to practice medicine in California was revoked. He is still vice-president of the Committee for Freedom of Choice in Medicine.

• Bruce Helvie had vitamin and mineral products seized by the FDA because they were marketed with false and misleading claims for the treatment of more than twenty-five diseases and conditions. The seized products were destroyed by consent decree in 1960.

• Bob Hoffman, who died in 1985, published bodybuilding magazines and sold bodybuilding equipment and food supplement products through his company, York Barbell Co., of York, Pennsylvania. In 1960, the company was charged with misbranding its *Energol Germ Oil Concentrate* because literature accompanying the oil claimed falsely that it could prevent or treat more than 120 diseases and conditions, including epilepsy, gallstones, and arthritis. The material was destroyed by consent decree. In 1961, fifteen other York Barbell products were seized as misbranded. In 1968, a larger number of products came under attack by the government for similar reasons. In the consent decree that settled the 1968 case, Hoffman and York Barbell agreed to stop a long list of questionable health claims for their products. In 1972, the FDA seized three types of York Barbell protein supplements, charging that they were misbranded with false and misleading bodybuilding claims. A few months later, the seized products were destroyed under a default decree. In 1974, the company was again charged with misbranding *Energol Germ Oil Concentrate* and protein supplements. The wheat germ oil had been claimed to be of special dietary value as a source of vigor and energy. A variety of false bodybuilding claims had been made for the protein supplements. The seized products were destroyed under a consent decree.

Despite his many brushes with the law, Hoffman achieved considerable professional prominence. During his athletic career, first as an oarsman and then as a weightlifter, he received over six hundred trophies, certificates, and awards. He was the Olympic weightlifting coach from 1936 to 1968 and was a founding member of the President's Council on Physical Fitness and Sports. These activities helped make Hoffman a major factor in the growth of nutritional fads for athletes.

• Max Huberman was president of the National Nutritional Foods Association and a board member of the American Natural Hygiene Society.

• Victor Earl Irons, who was vice chairman of NHF's board of governors for more than twenty years, received a one-year prison sentence in 1957 for misbranding *Vit-Ra-Tox*, a vitamin mixture sold door to door. In 1959, shipments of eight products and accompanying literature shipped by V.E. Irons, Inc., were destroyed under a consent decree because the products were promoted with false or misleading claims. Other seized products were ordered destroyed in 1959 and 1960. Irons has claimed that virtually everyone has a "clogged colon," that deposits of fecal material cause "toxins and poisonous gases" to "seep into your blood and poison all your organs and tissues," and that "if every person in this country took 2–3 home colonics a week, 95% of the doctors would have to retire for lack of business." Literature from V.E. Irons, Inc., has stated that "the most important procedure toward regaining your Health is the COMPLETE and THOROUGH cleansing of the colon, no matter what or how long it takes." This is the goal of the "Vit-Ra-Tox Seven Day Cleansing Program," which involves eating no food, drinking a quart or more of water daily, using herbal laxatives and various supplement products, and taking at least one strong black coffee enema each day. Ten years ago, products for this program cost $60, while those for maintenance after the seventh day cost about $100 per month.

• Bernard Jensen, D.C., is a leading proponent of iridology, a pseudo-scientific system of diagnosis based upon examination of the eye (see Chapter 26). He formulated the products and was chairman of the health advisory board of Nova Nutritional Products, Inglewood, California, a multilevel company that called itself "the ultimate in nutritional science." Nova's products included *Stress-Buster, Immune Forte,* and *Endurance Plus.* Jensen also helped found and was board chairman of Vitality International, a Seattle-based multilevel marketing company whose products included a "life extension formula" called *New Youth.*

• Terence Lemerond is president of Enzymatic Therapy, Inc., of Green Bay, Wisconsin, which has marketed hundreds of formulas containing vitamins, minerals, herbs, amino acids, and/or glandular tissue. The company has made illegal claims for these products in advertisements, newsletters, "confidential reports," testimonial messages, "research bulletins," "health guides," and other materials given to health food retailers for distribution to their customers. Company publications state that Lemerond studied nutrition for twenty years and was a nutritional consultant for nine years.

During the late 1980s, the company held seminars whose attendees received a loose-leaf manual describing how Enzymatic Therapy products could be used to treat more than eighty diseases and conditions. The manual also contained "protocols" for using various products to combat AIDS, multiple sclerosis, cancer, arthritis, and other serious health problems. In 1991, after five years of investigation and several warnings, the FDA took Lemerond and Enzymatic Therapy to court. In 1992, the case was settled with a consent degree barring the company from marketing products with unproven therapeutic claims. The court order also lists fifty-six items that cannot be marketed or manufactured unless new promotional material for them is approved by the FDA.

• Andrew R.L. McNaughton was a central figure in the worldwide promotion of laetrile. In 1977, he was placed on two years' probation after pleading guilty to a criminal charge of conspiracy to facilitate the transportation of smuggled laetrile. He had a prior conviction in Canada for a stock fraud.

• Robert S. Mendelsohn, M.D., who died in 1988, was NHF's president from 1981 to 1982. He spoke frequently at NHF conventions and produced a newsletter and a syndicated newspaper column, both called *The People's Doctor.* Although he had taught at several medical schools and been chairman of the Illinois state licensing board, Mendelsohn considered himself a "medical heretic." He opposed water fluoridation, immunization, licensing of nutrition-ists, and screening examinations to detect breast cancer. One of his books charged: "Modern Medicine's treatments for disease are seldom effective, and they're often more dangerous than the diseases they're designed to treat"; that "around ninety percent of surgery is a waste of time, energy, money and life"; and that most hospitals are so loosely run that "murder is even a clear and present danger."

Mendelsohn was also president of the New Medical Foundation, a tax-exempt organization formed in the late 1970s to support "innovative forms of medical education of the public and the medical profession." At a meeting sponsored by this group in 1984, he said:

> Doctors complain that quacks keep patients away from orthodox medicine. I cheer! Since all the treatments, both orthodox and alterna-tive, for cancer, coronary heart disease, hypertension, stroke, and arthritis, are equally unproven, why would a sane person choose treatment that can kill the patient?

In 1986, the National Nutritional Foods Association gave Mendelsohn its annual Rachel Carson Memorial Award for his "concerns for the protection of the American consumer and health freedoms."

• Betty Lee Morales, who died in 1987, was president of the Cancer Control Society. She published two newsletters, owned a health food store, and was co-owner of Eden Ranch, the company that marketed Betty Lee Morales Signature Brand food supplements. Promotional material from Eden Ranch suggested that Americans who did not use food supplements ran a significant risk of developing deficiency diseases. Among its many supplement products were *Lipotropic Plus,* to relieve "liver stress," and *Nia-Flex,* for stiff joints.

During her career, Mrs. Morales also provided "nutritional consultations" by telephone and by mail. In 1976, the Lehigh Valley (Pa.) Committee Against Health Fraud (LVCAHF) tested the quality of her advice after answering an ad in *Let's Live* magazine for Eden Ranch products. The reply contained a two-page health questionnaire which LVCAHF returned, indicating that the writer, "age 61," was in good health except that:

> For several years I have had (on and off) pain and swelling in the joints of my fingers and toes. During the past few months, I have had attacks of blurred vision. Sometimes my eyes ache and I see halos around lights at night. Your suggestions would be most welcome.

The arthritis symptoms, while not specific, were compatible with a diagnosis of gout, a type of arthritis that can sometimes benefit from a special diet. The eye symptoms were taken from a textbook description of glaucoma, a condition that could soon lead to blindness if not medically treated. Mrs. Morales' reply contained a disclaimer that her advice was for:

> public education . . . and to assist individuals to cooperate with the doctors of their choice in building better health. . . . In the event that the information is used without the supervision or approval of a doctor, that is prescribing for yourself, which is your constitutional right, but we assume no responsibility.

Her "highly personalized nutrition program" consisted of "detoxification" with a special diet and enemas, plus fifteen different food supplements that could be purchased from Eden Ranch or a health-food store. Based on an enclosed price list, the supplements would cost more than $40 per month; however, they had no medically recognized benefit for either arthritis or visual difficulty. Mrs. Morales did not appear to recognize that the writer's symptoms might be serious or require urgent medical attention.

• Roy F. Paxton headed a firm that marketed *Millrue* through agents, health food stores, and ads in an NHF publication. In addition, Paxton consulted personally with prospective customers, diagnosing them and recommending *Millrue* for such diseases as cancer, arthritis, and diabetes. In 1958, he and his company were fined a total of $1,200 for false and misleading labeling claims for *Millrue*. When they persisted in selling the product and promoting it through an NHF publication, the FDA again brought prosecution for misbranding. In 1963—the year that Paxton's term as NHF governor expired—he and the company were fined a total of $4,000 and he was sentenced to three years in prison.

• Donald F. Pickett founded and was board chairman of the Neo-Life Corporation, a multilevel company that sells dietary supplements and various other products. The company magazine has advised Neo-Life distributors that people who complain about being tired, sluggish, or listless might be lacking in essential nutrients. To induce sales, the magazine suggested telling prospects that "food low in nutrients will have the same long-term effects on the body as used oil does to the automobile—lower performance and greater wear and tear."

• James R. Privitera, Jr., M.D., was convicted in 1975 and sentenced to six months in prison for conspiring to prescribe and distribute laetrile. In 1980, after the appeals process ended, he served fifty-five days in jail. Then, because he had been prescribing unapproved substances (including laetrile, calcium pangamate, and DMSO) for the treatment of cancer, the California Board of Medical Quality Assurance suspended Privitera's medical license for four months and placed him on ten years' probation under board supervision. During the probationary period, Privitera was "prohibited from making any representation that he is able to cure cancer through nutrition." He was also forbidden to tell a patient he had cancer unless the diagnosis had been confirmed in writing by an appropriate board-certified specialist.

Privitera founded two companies that have marketed devices for doing "live cell analysis," a procedure in which blood obtained from a patient's finger is placed under a dark-field microscope to which a television monitor has been attached, so that both the practitioner and the patient can examine cells and particles in the blood. Proponents claim that this method can be used to detect "multiple vitamin and mineral deficiencies, toxicity, tendencies toward allergic reaction, excess fat circulation, liver weakness, and arteriosclerosis." However, the test has little or no value in diagnosing such conditions.

• John N. Ritchason, N.D., wrote *The Vitamin and Health Encyclopedia* (1986) and *The Little Herb Encyclopedia* (1982), both of which recommend vitamins, minerals and/or herbs for more than 150 health problems. The books state that Ritchason had a Ph.D. from Donsbach University and was a naturopath, iridologist, herbalist, Touch-for-Health Instructor, and Registered Healthologist.

• Frank Salaman, a current board member and former husband of NHF president Maureen Salaman, was convicted in 1977 of conspiring to smuggle laetrile.

• Emory Thurston, who died in 1981, was an active promoter of laetrile and displayed pamphlets he had edited at a booth at NHF conventions. At a 1973 convention, when approached by an agent of the California Bureau of Food and Drug who said she had cancer of the uterus, Thurston offered to supply her with laetrile. He instructed the agent to contact him at his office at the Institute for Nutritional Research in Hollywood. He later sold laetrile to the agent and advised her not to have surgery. After additional evidence was gathered, Thurston was convicted, fined, and placed on probation for two years.

• Paul J. Virgin, who has served as NHF treasurer, was public relations director of the Alta-Dena Dairy, the leading producer of certified raw (unpasteurized) milk. This dairy has been implicated repeatedly as a source of salmonella infection in raw milk consumers in California. In 1989, a California judge ordered the dairy (then operating as Steuve's Natural) to stop making false and misleading claims that its unpasteurized products were safer and nutritionally superior to pasteurized milk products. The judge also ordered the dairy to place a warning label on its raw milk cartons.

• Floyd Weston is a former insurance executive who stated in an interview in NHF's *Public Scrutiny* that he had organized a group of businessmen in 1975 "to conduct a worldwide search for the answer to good health." One of his "discoveries" was an "electrodiagnosis" machine based on the theory that there is "an electric wiring system in the body—each organ having a wire that goes to a standard location in the hands and feet." Weston claimed that such devices can "verify the exact condition of individual organs throughout the body," "differentiate between acute, chronic, or degenerative stages," and "discover these pathological processes when regular clinical diagnoses cannot detect them." Treatment is then administered with homeopathic remedies, vitamins, and/or minerals (see Chapter 13). At various times, Weston has shared ownership of a homeopathic clinic and marketed electrodiagnostic devices and homeopathic remedies. California authorities are currently trying to stop him from marketing such devices.

Other NHF board members have included Sid Williams, D.C. (see Chapter 12), and Robert Atkins, M.D. (see below and Chapter 27).

### NHF's "Vitamin Bill"

NHF's most notable campaign occurred during the 1970s with a bill to weaken FDA jurisdiction over vitamins. In 1972, after lengthy study, the agency had proposed that food products be labeled so that ingredients, nutrient content, and other information would be displayed in a standard format. These provisions became regulations with little controversy .

The FDA proposal also said that labeling could neither state nor imply that a balanced diet of ordinary foods cannot supply adequate amounts of nutrients. Because this struck at the heart of health food industry propaganda, NHF filed lawsuits and proposed legislation to remove FDA jurisdiction over vitamins. Crying "Fight for your freedom to take vitamins!" NHF organized its members and allies into unprecedented political activity. Article after article urging support of the anti-FDA bill appeared in the *NHF Bulletin,* in various health-food industry magazines, and in chiropractic journals. Letter-writing kits were distributed by chiropractors, by health-food stores, and in special NHF mailings. At a Congressional hearing on this issue, several Congressmen reported that they had received more mail about vitamins than about Watergate.

In 1976, as a result of this pressure, Congress passed the Proxmire Amendment to the federal Food, Drug, and Cosmetic Act. Though not as restrictive as NHF's proposal, this law prevents the FDA from regulating food supplements unless they are inherently dangerous or are marketed with illegal claims that they can prevent or treat disease.

NHF has also promoted "Medical Freedom of Choice" and "Foods Are Not Drugs" bills. Federal laws now require that all new drugs be proven both safe and effective before they are marketed. NHF's proposed bills, which would remove the efficacy requirement, would open the door to any supposed "remedy" that doesn't kill people on the spot. Such bills are a snake-oil salesman's dream.


## The Promotion of Laetrile

Because laetrile lacks FDA approval, it is illegal to market it in interstate commerce. In 1977, a federal court set up an "affidavit" system under which personal supplies of laetrile could be imported into the United States by cancer patients certified by a physician as "terminal." The plaintiff in the case was Glen Rutherford, a Kansas seed salesman who believed that laetrile was needed to keep him alive. Although the U.S. Supreme Court ruled against Rutherford in 1979, the affidavit system was not dismantled until 1987. During the appeals process, Rutherford became an NHF governor, Kirkpatrick Dilling became one of his lawyers, and NHF took care of his attorney fees.

From 1978 to 1982, NHF published *Public Scrutiny,* a monthly newspaper (later converted to a magazine) whose primary focus was on laetrile and "metabolic therapy." Most of its original staff members were prominent promoters of laetrile, and three of its advisers had been convicted of laetrile-related crimes. Each issue of *Public Scrutiny* contained a full-page ad from the Laetrile Information Center, a company near the Mexican border that would arrange for legal importation. Mexican clinics and other sellers of laetrile also advertised regularly in *Public Scrutiny.*

After NHF governor James Privitera, M.D., was charged with a laetrile-related offense, appeals in *Public Scrutiny* raised more than $5,000 to help defend him; and after he was convicted, NHF generated more than 10,000 form letters asking California governor Jerry Brown to pardon him (which he did). NHF also contributed $5,000 toward the legal expenses of the parents of Chad Green, a three-year-old boy with leukemia; and an NHF governor served as a lawyer for the parents.

Chad attracted nationwide attention when his family moved to Mexico to defy a Massachusetts court order that the boy receive proper therapy and stop getting laetrile. The October 1979 issue of *Public Scrutiny* described how Chad was thriving, how his father was studying for a career as a "nutrition consultant," and how Chad's mother had stopped his chemotherapy without telling the Mexican clinic doctor. A few days after the newspaper was distributed, Chad died. His parents continued to promote laetrile and to claim that Chad died because he had "lost the will to live." However, the autopsy showed recurrent leukemia, and cyanide (a breakdown product of laetrile) in his liver and spleen.

NHF also assisted the parents of Joey Hofbauer, an eight-year-old boy with Hodgkin's disease, a form of cancer usually curable in its early stages. In 1977, New York State authorities sought custody of Joey because his parents chose laetrile over effective treatment for the boy. With NHF attorney Kirkpatrick Dilling representing the parents, the court ruled that they were "concerned and loving" and "not neglectful" in rejecting conventional treatment. After eighteen months of laetrile and megavitamin treatment from Michael Schachter, M.D. (a New York psychiatrist who occasionally lectures at NHF conventions), Joey was moved to the Bahamas for another type of questionable treatment. He died in 1980 with lungs full of tumors.

A bill to exempt laetrile from FDA jurisdiction was introduced by *Public Scrutiny*'s legislative advisor, physician-Congressman Larry McDonald (D-GA). In 1979, a malpractice suit against him by survivors of a patient he had treated with laetrile was settled for $30,000. NHF's efforts to exempt laetrile petered out after McDonald was killed in the crash of the Korean airliner shot down by the Soviets in 1983.

## Opposition to Fluoridation

Adjusting community drinking water to about one part fluoride to one million parts of water is a safe, simple, and inexpensive way to help prevent tooth decay. Although NHF's leaders claim to be interested in preventing disease by "proper nutrition," they are rigidly opposed to fluoridation.

Over the years, NHF has assembled many documents which it claims are "proof" that fluoridation is dangerous (which it is not). Close examination of these documents shows that they contain reports of poorly designed "experiments," twisted accounts of actual events, statements by respected scientists taken out of context to change their meaning, misinterpreted statistics, and other forms of falsification. Given enough publicity, however, these items have convinced many communities that fluoridation is too risky.

In 1972, NHF granted $16,000 for a fluoridation study to the Center for Science in the Public Interest (CSPI), a group led by former associates of Ralph Nader. To help raise this money, a special mailing to NHF members announced that a clinically controlled test was being conducted by "FRIENDS of indisputable, scientific reputation." The mailing claimed that the study would arm NHF with "unassailable, up-to-date, scientific data to help defeat fluoridation." When CSPI learned about this message, it protested, stating that the study would be a scientific review whose outcome was certainly not fixed against fluoridation. NHF apologized, claiming that the fundraiser had been mailed "without being cleared by appropriate officials" and contained "serious errors" about the study's nature. NHF members were never told of these errors, however. Nor were they notified when the study concluded that "the known benefits of fluoridation far outweigh any risks which may be involved."

In 1974, NHF announced that opposing fluoridation would be its number two priority and that a biochemist named John Yiamouyiannis had been hired to "break the back" of fluoridation. Yiamouyiannis soon began issuing reports based on misinterpreted government statistics, claiming that fluoridation causes cancer (see Chapter 21). He was joined in this effort by Dean Burk, a retired National Cancer Institute employee who was also a leading promoter of laetrile. In 1980, Yiamouyiannis left NHF and founded another group whose structure and activities were similar. Although NHF remains opposed to fluoridation, it has had little political involvement since Yiamouyiannis departed.

### Recent Friction

In 1986, a company controlled by Kurt Donsbach published *The Great Medical Monopoly Wars,* a book which claimed that the American Medical Association, the FDA, drug companies, and various individuals were conspiring to "destroy the American free-enterprise system in the health care field." The book contained false and defamatory statements about antiquackery activists John H. Renner, M.D., and Victor Herbert, M.D., J.D. Despite warnings from the pair's attorney, NHF and several allied individuals, organizations, and publications promoted the book and made additional defamatory remarks. Dr. Renner filed suit in Missouri against six defendants and wound up collecting $60,000 in an out-of-court settlement with Donsbach, Clinton Miller, and Maureen Salaman. Dr. Renner's suit against the book's author, P.J. Lisa, is still pending. Dr. Herbert filed suit in Iowa against twenty-six defendants, twenty-two of whom were dismissed by the judge because he felt that they were not doing enough business in Iowa for his court to have jurisdiction. Dr. Herbert has appealed the dismissal. The case involving the four remaining defendants is scheduled for trial in 1993.

These lawsuits appear to have caused considerable strife among NHF's leaders, some of whom had been upset with each other anyway. In 1989, Donsbach left under bitter circumstances and launched a new organization. A special NHF report distributed in July 1990 stated that Clinton Miller had been fired for setting up an unauthorized bank account, and that attorney Dilling was suing NHF for $64,633.17 for allegedly unpaid fees in the Herbert and Renner cases. NHF wound up suing Donsbach, Miller, and various other former NHF members. These difficulties, added to other financial problems and decreased membership, appear to have greatly weakened NHF.

### Foundation for the Advancement of Innovative Medicine (FAIM)

FAIM was formed in 1986 "as a voice for innovative medicine's professionals, physicians, patients, and suppliers." Now headquartered in Suffern, New York, it had about 2,400 members in September 1992. Its professional members, about sixty of whom have been identified in the group's publications, include medical doctors, osteopaths, chiropractors, dentists, and psychologists, almost all of whom practice in New York or New Jersey.

FAIM defines innovative medicine as "a treatment or therapy of empirical benefit that is yet outside the mainstream of conventional medicine." According to several flyers:

> FAIM's mission is to secure free choice in health care. Our first goal is the development of a membership to serve as both a forum for exchange and a constituency for change. The second goal is to educate both those within the field and the general public as to the benefits and issues of innovative medicine. This activity includes the collection of statistical data with which to advocate our position. The third goal is guaranteed reimbursement for the patients, be it through legislation, litigation or negotiation with state and insurance agencies. And lastly, in laying the groundwork for a climate receptive to medical innovation, we encourage research and development of promising new approaches.

FAIM's quarterly magazine, *Innovation,* has carried articles promoting "alternative" cancer therapies, chelation therapy, homeopathy, shark cartilage for arthritis and for protection against tumor growth, and an oral bacterial preparation for chronic fatigue syndrome. One article describes how to sue insurance companies in small claims court when they deny claims for "complementary" treatment. Other articles blast fluoridation, mercury-amalgam fillings, and sugar (for allegedly causing digestive problems).

FAIM's educational fund (FAIM ED) was incorporated in 1991 "to promote the American health care consumer's access to information and education regarding health care alternatives" and "to support promising research projects that may not currently be the focus of government and private efforts." Each year, FAIM (and/or FAIM ED) sponsors several symposia featuring prominent practitioners and promoters of "alternative" medicine. Exhibitors at these meetings have included marketers of supplements, homeopathic remedies, herbs, and other products that are promoted with unproven claims that would not be legal to place on their labels.

FAIM's current board of trustees is composed of eight medical doctors and one dentist. The board's president—and a FAIM co-founder—is Robert C. Atkins, M.D., who operates a large clinic, hosts a radio talk show, publishes a newsletter, markets supplement products, and has written several books on his unconventional methods (see Chapter 27). FAIM has been lobbying actively to persuade the New York State legislature to enact a bill to ensure that "unconventional" practitioners participate in the judging of colleagues who are accused of professional misconduct. This bill is intended to protect FAIM's professional members by placing one on the state board that has the power to revoke licenses. One impetus for this bill was the license revocation proceeding against FAIM board member Warren Levin, M.D. (see Chapter 10).

## Committee for Freedom of Choice in Medicine (CFCM)

CFCM was launched in 1972 as the Committee for Freedom of Choice in Cancer Therapy (CFCCT) and assumed its current name in 1984. The committee is one of several interlocking organizations involved in the promotion of questionable treatments.

Proponent literature states that CFCCT's formation was triggered by the arrest of John A. Richardson, M.D., a physician in Albany, California. Richardson, who frequently prescribed laetrile, was charged with multiple violations of the state's "cancer quackery" statutes. According to proponents, Richardson was a prominent member of the John Birch Society, a right-wing group founded in 1958 to oppose what it considered a Communist plot for world domination. Although the society itself took no official position on laetrile, many of its members "grouped in a complex of ad hoc committees collectively known as the Committee for Freedom of Choice in Cancer Therapy." Although Dr. Richardson was not convicted, the California Board of Medical Quality Assurance revoked his medical license in 1976 for "extreme departure from the standard practice of medicine."

During the 1970s, CFCCT held seminars and "doctors' workshops" and distributed books, pamphlets, and other information on methods of cancer management considered questionable by the scientific community. The group also generated letter-writing campaigns in support of these methods and the practitioners who used them. The primary political goal appeared to be the passage of state and federal laws to legalize the use of laetrile. In recent years, CFCM has opposed both a California bill to permit forfeiture of property in certain cases of health fraud and a federal nutrition labeling bill provision to restrict claims for nutritional supplements. The Committee has also expressed interest in laws that would make it more difficult for state boards to discipline "alternative" practitioners.

CFCCT was organized by Robert W. Bradford, who also founded and heads the Robert Bradford Research Institute; the Robert W. Bradford

Foundation; American Biologics–Mexico (a hospital in Tijuana); and two pharmaceutical firms, American Biologics and Choice Metabolics. All except the hospital are now located in Chula Vista, California. According to a Stanford University official, Bradford graduated from San Jose State University and worked from 1963 to 1976 as an electronics engineer for the Stanford University Linear Accelerator Center. Bradford is also said to have received two honorary degrees: a "cultural doctorate in nutritional science" in 1983 from the World University and a "doctor of biochemistry degree" in 1984 from Medicina Alternativa, an "international holistic medical group" in Sri Lanka. Although these degrees have no academic standing, the publications of both the Committee for Freedom of Choice in Medicine and the Bradford Institute identify him as "Dr. Bradford" or "Robert Bradford, DSc." In 1977, Bradford, Frank Salaman (then CFCCT vice-president), Dr. John Richardson, and Richardson's office manager, Ralph Bowman, were convicted of conspiring to smuggle laetrile. Bradford was fined $40,000, Richardson $20,000, and Salaman and Bowman $10,000 each.

Michael L. Culbert, CFCM's board chairman, is also vice-president and public relations director of American Biologics and editor of the committee's official publication, *The Choice*. A former newspaperman and freelance writer, Culbert has a bachelor of arts degree from the University of Wichita and an "honorary DSc degree" from Medicina Alternativa. His books include *Vitamin B17—Forbidden Weapon Against Cancer* (1974); *Freedom from Cancer— The Amazing Story of Laetrile* (1976); *Medical Revolution in America* (1981); *What the Medical Establishment Won't Tell You that Could Save Your Life* (1984); *AIDS: Terror, Truth and Triumph*; and *AIDS: Hope, Hoax and Hoopla* (1989); and several others co-authored with Bradford.

The Robert Bradford Research Institute (BRI), founded in 1979, is a private foundation that publishes reports and monographs said to be the results of research done by the institute. Its tax returns list income of $13,819 in 1987, $17,518 in 1988, and $1,549 in 1989.

The Robert W. Bradford Foundation is described as a nonprofit research and educational trust founded in 1978 to support private, independent scientific research into the metabolic management of degenerative disease and to provide a clearinghouse for educational materials to physicians, patients, medical students, health professionals, and institutions of higher learning. According to Culbert, the foundation's principal activity is publication of BRI research books and monographs.

*The Choice* began monthly publication in 1975 with Culbert as editor. Its assistant editor was Maureen Salaman, who later became president of the

National Health Federation. Since about 1980, *The Choice* has been published two to four times a year. A December 1981 report by the Committee for Freedom of Choice in Cancer Therapy to "committee chairmen and interested members" attributed the publication's decreased frequency to lack of funds. The articles invariably promote "alternative" treatment and criticize scientifically accepted treatment and government regulation of the health marketplace. Titles like "Herbal poultices demolish tumors at AB Hospital," "New research blasts 'standard' CA therapies," and "Fedstapo targeting our medical freedom" typify the organization's viewpoint.

American Biologics–Mexico, which opened in 1979, is described in its brochures as "North America's most advanced holistic medical center" and is claimed to offer "new hope for sufferers of cancer, heart disease, MS, allergies, all forms of metabolic dysfunction." The hospital is claimed to have treated more than fifteen thousand patients, most of them for cancer. It is advertised regularly in chiropractic and health-food publications. Treatments listed in the current brochure include cellular ("live cell") therapy, injectable laetrile, "oxidative therapies," "aggressive DMSO [dimethyl sulfoxide] therapy," "homeopathically refined herbal poultices," enzyme treatments, "bioelectrical therapy," Gerovital, vaccines and biologicals, large doses of vitamins and minerals, EDTA [ethylenediaminetetraacetic acid] chelation therapy, "natural interferons and interleukin-2," colonic therapy, and "detoxification." Some standard treatment modalities are also offered. Itemized statements to insurance companies have identified treatments as "chemother/inj" without indicating what substances were used. Dr. Richardson joined the American Biologics–Mexico staff in 1982, but later moved to Nevada to practice homeopathy.

American Biologics, a "metabolic pharmaceutical firm," has marketed products to health professionals and health-food stores. It is also the U.S. representative office for American Biologics–Mexico. During the early 1980s the company's "professional catalog" listed enzymes, digestive aids, emulsified vitamins, minerals, Gerovital, oral and injectable glandulars, and specialty products such as DMSO, benzaldehyde, apricot kernels, EDTA, and laetrile, as well as books, tapes, films, and lab test apparatus. In 1982, an article in *The Choice* stated that American Biologics was "the major amygdalin [laetrile] distributor in the world." In 1984, federal authorities in Texas seized a shipment of products that included injectable pangamic acid ("vitamin $B_{15}$") marketed by American Biologics; the shipment was destroyed under court order. In 1986, the FDA ordered American Biologics to stop making claims that a copper salicylate product (*Arthrinol*) was effective for "the temporary relief of minor aches and pains associated with arthritis, bursitis, neuritis, and rheumatism." In 1988, the

FDA ordered the company to stop selling calcium orotate, magnesium orotate, zinc orotate, evening primrose oil, and germanium products. In 1988, the company donated about $20,000 in money and laboratory equipment to Bastyr University, a naturopathy school in Seattle.

Choice Metabolics—said to be a representative of American Metabolics—sells a similar but smaller product line that is advertised in *The Choice*. It has also been described as a retail company providing metabolic products for patients upon their departure from American Biologics–Mexico.

CFCCT's membership is said to have peaked at about forty thousand members with 520 chapters nationwide. In 1989, Culbert stated that CFCCT had entered a "quiescent phase" in the early 1980s and "diminished in force . . . to a palace guard of a few dozen committees and about five thousand members." CFCM, however, does not appear to be organized in this manner. For several years, subscribers to *The Choice* were designated "members" of the committee even though, until recently, this was not disclosed to them.

CFCCT's tax returns filed with the California Registry of Trusts indicate that its gross income peaked at $155,916 in 1977 but had dropped to $11,148 in 1982. (The group's fiscal year runs from March 1 through the end of February.) None of its returns contained an entry for membership dues. The return for fiscal 1982 listed contributions of $1,014 and gross sales of $10,134. The next report is not due until 1993 unless gross revenues exceed $25,000.

At present, CFCM's income appears small. In 1988, Culbert attested that the organization's "mailing list" was between 2,000 and 2,500. Not all of these, however, were paid subscribers. In 1991, he said that ten thousand copies of *The Choice* were published quarterly, some four thousand of which were subscriptions. Although he has said that fifty chapters of the Committee are still active, no news of chapter activity has been reported in the newsletter for many years.

### The People's Medical Society (PMS)

PMS has been engaged in a wide variety of projects that may affect medical practice and consumer protection against quackery. Although some of its aims are laudable, PMS is rooted in deep antagonism to the medical profession and to medical science itself.

PMS was the brainchild of the late Robert Rodale, board chairman of Rodale Press and publisher of *Prevention* magazine. During 1982, he ran a series of editorials criticizing the medical establishment and promising "a grassroots campaign that will turn America's medical system on its head." PMS was officially launched on January 1, 1983, with a large initial loan from Rodale Press, but is now supported by dues payments ($15 per year) from about 80,000 members. The group's bimonthly newsletter occasionally contains valuable suggestions, but most of its information is slanted to undermine trust in conventional practitioners. The first issue stated the group's goals:

> Every part of the medical system is organized very effectively—except the customers. You and me. What we need is to create an umbrella of "civilian" control over the management of the medical system. Not a palace revolt, but a demand to get back to what is and ought to be rightfully ours.
> That's what the People's Medical Society is all about. That's why we exist: to plan a major drive against medical costs, to demand that the medical establishment be more accessible and more accountable. We are not anti-doctor, we are anti-abuse. And we are pro-knowledge.

Despite this "disclaimer," most articles in its newsletters imply that doctors cannot be trusted, and cartoons in every issue ridicule medical care as expensive, unnecessary, dangerous, or impersonal.

From time to time, PMS encourages its members to write letters to legislators or other government officials. Some campaigns have involved antiquackery legislation (opposed by PMS), funds for organic farming (favored), malpractice reform (opposed), licensing of nutritionists (opposed), and food irradiation (opposed).

PMS has published many books, booklets, and special reports. Some contain valuable information, while others promote unscientific methods and/or portray them as equivalent to scientific ones. The PMS booklet *Options in Health Care*, for example, uncritically promotes the theories and practices of acupuncture, acupressure, Chinese medicine, chiropractic, homeopathy, hydrotherapy, metabolic therapy, naturopathy, orthomolecular therapy, psychic healing, and reflexology. PMS's eight-page bulletin on cancer care options includes promoters of quack cancer methods in its list of sources of information. The bulletin on choosing doctors includes the ridiculous advice that obtaining a health-related degree through a correspondence course "does not in and of itself imply an inferior education." No one can become qualified as a health practitioner through this route, and *all* such programs teach health nonsense.

PMS's forty-eight-page report on high blood pressure contains sound advice but also suggests that practitioners of chiropractic, acupressure, homeopathy, herbal therapy, and megavitamin therapy may have something to offer:

> While many of these practitioners can't produce the years of studies and double-blind experimental results that the medical professionals can, they nonetheless provide treatment—often less invasive, less costly, and with fewer side effects than traditional medicine's—that has its adherents and success stories.

PMS's group's booklet on heart disease describes claims and criticisms of chelation therapy, concluding:

> Are chelation doctors all quacks? Not at all. Some are. But, then again, some establishment doctors are, too. Some see a trend or a fast buck and pounce. But most doctors who use EDTA chelation therapy are sincere, trying to help the ill and frightened, and do it because they see improvements in their patients and believe there is no better, safer, less painful and expensive way to treat the people they see. The dispute between doctors on both sides is one of methodology, not reputation; both sides are embarrassed by the quacks and charlatans in their own camps, and want them out.

This strikes me as a peculiar way to portray a method for which there is not the slightest documented evidence of benefit and which, if used instead of effective treatment for coronary artery disease, can result in the patient's death from a heart attack. Furthermore, as far as I can tell, the chelationists stick together like glue and never characterize a colleague as a quack or charlatan.

Another PMS booklet encourages members to start a People's Medical Library in their community. Along with such authoritative references as the *AMA Family Medical Guide, Cecil's Textbook of Medicine, JAMA,* and *The New England Journal of Medicine,* it recommends Rodale Press books on natural healing and natural home remedies and a few other highly questionable publications.

Another PMS booklet, *Deregulating Doctoring,* suggests that medical licensing laws be substantially limited in scope or even repealed. Written by Attorney Lori B. Andrews, vice-chairman of PMS's board of directors, the report suggests that everyone should be free to engage in "such nonhazardous, relatively innocuous activities like advising, giving tips on prevention, making recommendations and offering simple treatments." It recommends that "as a minimum, the definition of the practice of medicine should be restricted so that only inherently dangerous health care activities require a medical license." In other words, state governments should permit any quack whose methods won't kill you on the spot to market them to the public.

PMS also publishes bibliographies on various health topics. Like the People's Medical Library lists, however, these lists include unscientific publications as well as reputable ones. For example, the bibliography on arthritis includes a book which claims that food allergy is a major cause of arthritis; the cancer bibliography includes a book that boosts macrobiotics; and the diet and nutrition bibliography includes several unscientific books and refers readers to the Academy of Orthomolecular Psychiatry, a Canadian group that promotes megavitamin therapy for mental problems.

Several years ago, *Shape* magazine published a warning from me to be wary of any "nutritionist" who touts a degree, certificate, or other credential from any of fifteen nonaccredited schools. PMS's eight-page bulletin, "How to Choose a Nutritionist" contains the list, without mentioning its source, and advises that "other people . . . have found competent, legitimate practitioners with just such credentials." The bulletin also suggests that hair analysis can serve as the basis for nutritional advice. (The correct advice is that hair analysis is the hallmark of a quack.)

PMS's newsletter has referred readers to the Hearing and Tinnitus Help Association (HTHA), whose executive director, Paul Yanick, Jr., claimed to have helped thousands to overcome tinnitus (ringing in the ear) and other hearing and balance disorders through nutrition methods. Contributors to HTHA were eligible for a discount on the $200 price of "The Comprehensive Nutrient and Lifestyle Program," which Yanick helped design. According to a flyer distributed by HTHA, this is a computerized analysis that recommends nutrition supplements after analyzing information on dietary and exercise habits; "tissue mineral analysis"; tests on pH, urine, stool, and saliva; and "over 400 questions relating changes that take place in your body when a nutrient becomes deficient."

Several PMS books are equally misleading. *Take This Book to the Hospital With You: A Consumer Guide to Surviving Your Hospital Stay* (1985) mixes practical advice with medical and financial horror stories and advises people to be extremely distrustful of medical caregivers. *Medicine on Trial: The Appalling Story of Ineptitude, Malfeasance, Neglect, and Arrogance* (1988) cites some genuine problems in our medical-care system, but exaggerates their extent and oversimplifies their causes. *Getting the Most for Your Medical Dollar* (1990) contains some sensible advice but promotes many unscientific practices.

Publicity materials for one of its books describe PMS as "the largest consumer health organization in America" and state that it is run "by the people" and "for the people." However, its president and board of directors are not elected, and newsletters give no indication that its activities and policies are determined by anyone but the group's president.

In 1986, I received an interesting letter from a member of PMS's "Advisory Committee" who was appalled by the organization's activities. The advisory committee "is a farce," the letter said, "for it has never met, and I have not been apprised of the charge nor who the members are!" Soon afterward, the writer sent a set of the monthly reports that PMS's president, Charles Inlander, had sent to the group's board of directors from 1983 through 1986. A few weeks later, after *Medical Economics* reported on information from one of these reports, Inlander realized that PMS had a "security leak" and dissolved the advisory committee.

The most interesting "leaked" documents were memos from Vanguard Communications Corporation, a public relations firm. One outlined how PMS could capitalize on people's desire to exert more personal power and control over their life. Another (titled "AMA Scenario") proposed a "petition" campaign aimed at attracting new PMS members, promoting legislative reforms, and placing the AMA on the defensive:

> Our strategy is aggressive in style. It postures PMS as independent, feisty, willing and able to arouse a public outcry against the AMA.... It presents PMS as the thoughtful advocate of a series of common-sensical reforms that no one could oppose . . . except organized medicine. . . . PMS will portray the AMA as a guild determined to protect its own, even in the face of gross incompetence and abuse.

Properly directed, consumer groups can accomplish a great deal by educating their members and working constructively to reduce health-care costs and increase consumer protection. In my opinion, the People's Medical Society is doing neither and will do more harm than good in the long run.

## Overview

During the past century, scientists have developed rules for determining what methods are effective in preventing and treating disease. At the same time, laws have been developed to protect the public from methods that are ineffective, unproven, or promoted with misinformation.

NHF, FAIM, CFCM, and PMS are antagonistic to accepted scientific methods as well as to current consumer-protection laws. Instead of supporting the rules of science and law, they want to destroy them. They clamor for the right to market methods without ensuring that they are effective. The "freedom" they espouse would be nothing more than a hunting license for quacks. Despite their shortcomings, these groups can generate large letter-writing campaigns which create the illusion that they represent a large constituency. They have won some significant court and legislative battles and intend to win more.

Thwarting these groups will not be simple. A good first step would be a government crackdown on companies that are marketing illegally through their publications and on any leaders of these groups who are engaged in illegal activities or quack practices,

# 29

# The Mental Health Maze

## Stephen Barrett, M.D.

Although excellent help is available for emotional problems, selecting a suitable therapist or therapy can be a difficult task. There is a wide array of practitioners, many of whom are incompetent. This chapter outlines the various types of practitioners, discusses treatment methods, and provides guidelines for distinguishing between proper and improper treatment.

## Psychiatric Treatment

For purposes of discussion, psychiatric treatment may be divided into two types: "organic" and "psychodynamic." The organic model is basically an authoritarian one in which the patient is a passive recipient of the treatment. The assumption is often made, or at least implied, that the patient has a physical or biochemical abnormality that needs to be controlled or corrected. The organic therapist diagnoses a "mental illness" and prescribes a drug or other physical treatment for the patient. The psychodynamic model, on the other hand, assumes that the patient's mental state is not the result of biochemical factors but has been caused by past and present experiences and feelings. Using a primarily conversational approach, therapist and patient explore the patient's feelings and behavior, seeking ways to alter them by persuasion, environmental manipulation, or the development of new ways to react.

In actual practice, there is no sharp dividing line between the two philosophies, and most psychiatrists use both in their approach to patients.

## Drug Therapy

Drugs are commonly prescribed for the treatment of anxiety states, depression, psychosomatic disorders, and psychoses.

*Antipsychotic agents* (sometimes referred to as major tranquilizers) are used mainly to treat psychotic reactions (thought disorders manifested by hallucinations, delusions, or loss of contact with reality). Since the early 1950s these drugs have revolutionized the field of psychiatry. Many patients who otherwise would have required lengthy (even lifelong) hospital stays are now able to improve or recover quickly. In addition, large numbers of previously institutionalized patients have been able to return to their communities.

*Antianxiety agents* (sometimes referred to as minor tranquilizers) are used for the treatment of anxiety states and psychosomatic disorder. People in the United States have been accused (with some justification) of being a "drugged society" because of their high use of alcohol and antianxiety agents such as diazepam (*Valium*) and chlordiazepoxide (*Librium*). Although most people who receive antipsychotic medications probably need them, it is clear that physicians often prescribe antianxiety agents or antidepressants when it would be more appropriate to help patients identify and correct what is troubling them. However, physicians are not entirely to blame for this. Patients often press for instant and total relief.

The danger of addiction to *Valium* has been grossly exaggerated by the media, particularly the motion picture *I'm Running as Fast as I Can.* The central character in this film is an anxiety-ridden woman who takes huge doses of *Valium,* becomes addicted, suddenly stops the drug, and develops convulsions and other severe withdrawal symptoms. Although addiction develops occasionally with normally prescribed dosages of *Valium,* the ordinary precaution of tapering off dosage rather than stopping suddenly will prevent a withdrawal reaction from occurring.

*Antidepressants* are available to counteract severe depressions (those manifested by loss of appetite, weight loss, severe insomnia, feelings of hopelessness, or psychomotor retardation or agitation). These drugs usually require from three days to several weeks to take effect. They are not intended for use in countering the minor upsets that are part of ordinary living.

Antidepressants and antipsychotic drugs can often be prescribed as single bedtime doses. This method reduces the cost of the medication, usually aids sleep, and reduces the likelihood of annoying side effects.

All psychoactive drugs have the potential for adverse reactions, some serious and some not. In each case the value to the patient must be weighed against the nuisance or danger involved.

One complication of particular concern is tardive dyskinesia, an involuntary movement disorder characterized by twitching and tongue-thrusting, which can occur with prolonged high dosage of antipsychotic medications. Although uncommon, it is often irreversible. Since the dangers of psychosis far outweigh the risk of tardive dyskinesia there is no reason to withhold antipsychotic medication from individuals who are psychotic. However, it is poor medical practice to prescribe these drugs for nonpsychotic anxiety.

### Electroconvulsive Therapy

Electroconvulsive therapy, also referred to as ECT, EST (electroshock therapy), and "shock treatment," is a method of inducing a convulsion by giving a brief stimulus to the brain. To receive the treatment, the patient lies down and is rendered unconscious either by an electrical stimulus or by a short-acting barbiturate given intravenously. To protect against injury, a curare-like drug is also given so that the patient's muscles do not actually contract during the convulsion. Electrodes are then applied to one or both temples, and a small amount of current is transmitted to induce the convulsion. After the treatment the patient usually remains unconscious for about fifteen to thirty minutes. A series of treatments may cause memory difficulty, but this clears up in a few weeks. Although its mechanism of action is unknown, ECT can be dramatically successful in certain types of severe depression and is sometimes helpful in severe psychotic reactions. However, it is seldom appropriate unless medication alone fails to produce results.

### Psychosurgery

Psychosurgery is a method of diminishing a patient's reactions to unpleasant stimuli by severing various nerve pathways within the brain. Before the era of drug therapy, psychosurgery was widely used to reduce disturbed behavior in severely disturbed patients. Today, although still regarded as effective, it is appropriate for consideration only when all other treatments have failed.

### Psychotherapy

Psychotherapy may be defined as any type of persuasive or conversational approach that helps the patient. Although there are numerous schools of thought, most have in common a wish to understand the patient and help the patient alter emotional and/or behavioral patterns.

In *analytically oriented psychotherapy* patients are encouraged to say what comes to mind (free association) and are helped to understand their feelings, mental mechanisms, and relationships with people. Insights are used to help patients develop healthier ways of dealing with their feelings and life situation. This type of therapy typically involves one or two fifty-minute sessions per week. It is especially appropriate for people who communicate well and are motivated to change. *Psychoanalysis* is a more intensive form of psychotherapy that requires three to five sessions per week. Few people can afford its high cost.

*Behavioral therapy* (behavioral modification) is the systematic application of learning theory to the treatment of disorders of behavior. The therapist first conducts an analysis of the patient's maladaptive responses—the behaviors that cause stress, limit satisfaction, and affect important areas of the patient's life. Treatment techniques can include systematic desensitization (gradually facing stressful situations in order to master them), relaxation training, positive reinforcement (being rewarded for behaving more maturely), and aversive therapy (associating an unpleasant stimulus with undesirable behavior).

Aversive techniques have included verbal rebukes, imagined noxious scenes, unpleasant tastes, physical restraint, hitting, pinching, electric shocks, and drug-induced nausea and vomiting. The AMA Council on Scientific Affairs has reviewed use of these techniques for obesity, tobacco smoking, alcoholism, drug abuse, homosexuality, sexual offenses, thumbsucking, and dangerous behavior in mentally retarded individuals. The council's 1987 report concluded: (1) few well-designed studies have been performed; (2) the most positive results have been reported with rapid smoking for smoking cessation, induced vomiting for alcoholism, electric shock for self-injurious behavior in mentally retarded individuals, and covert sensitization for sexual offenders; (3) some studies have found non-aversive techniques equally effective; and (4) much more research should be done before definitive conclusions can be drawn.

*Biofeedback* is a relaxation technique that can help people learn to control certain body functions. The patient is connected to a machine that continuously signals the heartbeat, degree of muscle contraction, or other mechanisms. The patient is instructed to relax so that the signals decrease to a desirable level. The patient may ultimately learn to control the body function subconsciously without the machine. Biofeedback was popularized before it had scientific support, and it is still abused by fringe practitioners. Nevertheless, it has gained a measure of respectability. It has been utilized in helping patients control pain, anxiety, phobias, hypertension, sleep disorders, and some stomach and intestinal problems. Some specialized techniques have been used to treat abnormal heart rhythms, epilepsy, Tourette's syndrome (multiple tics), fecal incontinence, and Parkinson's disease. Most people who go through biofeedback training use it to acquire relaxation skills that could also be learned without electronic training. Most qualified practitioners are psychologists, but some have backgrounds in other health disciplines. Untrained individuals with or without a professional degree can easily obtain a biofeedback device and set up shop. Some promoters allege that "repatterning" of a person's brain waves can foster effortless learning, health, creativity, and prosperity; others claim to achieve similar effects by causing the left and right halves of the brain to function more synchronously. There is no scientific evidence to support such claims.

*Hypnosis* is a temporary condition of altered attention during which suggestibility is greatly enhanced. The trance state may be used to uncover repressed material or to increase the patient's control over a symptom or behavior. Hypnosis is not a treatment in itself but may accelerate the treatment process in properly selected cases. It has also been used for anesthesia during childbirth and dental procedures and for relief of headaches and other painful conditions. Because not everyone is amenable to hypnosis, the therapist must have adequate training in both the administration of the procedure and the selection of patients.

*Group therapy* is a method whereby several people, usually eight to ten, meet with a therapist for discussion. Groups may be homogeneous (composed of people with similar problems or backgrounds) or heterogeneous. The discussion may focus on specific topics or may deal with whatever comes up. Group discussions often help people feel less alone in their feelings and provide a "laboratory" for analysis of an individual's behavior in a group situation. Reticent individuals may find group sessions, in which they can simply sit and listen, preferable to individual sessions, which may be relatively silent.

*Marriage counseling* is a process whereby husband and wife meet, individually and/or together, with a therapist to help them identify current marital conflict. Acting as a referee, the therapist helps the couple communicate more effectively to negotiate solutions to their dispute. In *family therapy* the therapist meets with the family as a group to help resolve current conflicts. *Sexual therapy* is most appropriate for couples who basically get along well but who have a problem with sex. Couples with a sexual problem whose general relationship is poor will probably be better off with marital counseling or individual psychotherapy.

## Hospital Care

There are four basic situations in which psychiatric hospital care is indicated: (1) the patient is considered dangerous to himself because he is suicidal or is not eating enough to sustain life, (2) the patient is considered dangerous to others, (3) the patient has regressed to the point where he cannot care for himself in the community, or (4) specialized treatment that is available only on an inpatient basis is needed.

Many communities have day-care or "partial hospitalization" programs where patients spend six to eight hours per day in a therapeutic atmosphere. Some hospitals have night-care programs. In a number of communities, halfway houses are available to ease the transition from hospital to community living.

Patients who are judged sufficiently dangerous to themself or others can be committed involuntarily to either inpatient or outpatient treatment. Contrary to popular opinion, court decisions and state laws tend to define "dangerousness" rather narrowly. As a result, commitment against a person's will can be difficult to initiate or sustain.

## Treatment for Psychosomatic Problems

From time to time all individuals experience symptoms that are physical reactions to tension. Common examples are headaches, diarrhea, constipation, nausea, dizziness, muscle cramps, dry mouth, cold hands, indigestion, excessive sweating, and palpitations of the heart. Whether treatment is needed depends on the severity or frequency of the symptom. They may require no treatment, self-medication with an over-the-counter product, medical care, or psychiatric treatment. These so-called psychosomatic or psychophysiological reactions are mediated through the autonomic nervous system and are related to the action of adrenaline and related hormones on various parts of the body. Diarrhea before an examination, for example, is caused by increased intestinal motility. Tension headaches are caused by muscular tension in the back of the neck. Indigestion may be caused by excessive production of acid in the stomach. The symptoms of acute anxiety attacks—sweating, rapid heartbeat, palpitation, and a feeling of dread—are caused by release of adrenaline. On the more serious side, asthma, peptic ulcer, high blood pressure, backache, and ulcerative colitis can have significant emotional components.

Psychosomatic reactions may be treated with (1) drugs that prevent the hormones from affecting the target organs, (2) antianxiety drugs to reduce tension, (3) psychotherapy to attack the underlying causes of the tension, or (4) a combination of these. A large percentage of the ailments for which people seek medical attention are significantly related to tension.

Overdosage of caffeine is a common cause of symptoms that resemble those of chronic anxiety. Many people don't realize that in addition to being present in coffee, caffeine is also found in tea, some soft drinks, and certain pain-relievers and cold remedies. I have seen more than a hundred patients who suffered from insomnia and/or nervousness that—unknown to them— was caused by excess caffeine. The drug's effect can last up to eighteen hours in sensitive individuals. It is mildly addictive—withdrawal during the night can cause headaches and grogginess in the morning.

During the late 1970s, General Foods Corporation advertised heavily to doctors that millions of coffee drinkers with caffeine-related symptoms might benefit by switching to decaffeinated *Sanka*. Thinking that consumers deserved this information too, I petitioned the FDA to require that all food products that contain significant amounts of caffeine should be labeled with the amount and a list of the symptoms that excess amounts can cause. The FDA has neither granted nor denied my request.

## Mental Health Practitioners

There are many types of practitioners who profess to help people with mental, emotional, and personal problems. The training, professional standards, and legal status of the different types of practitioners vary considerably.

*Psychiatrists* are physicians (M.D. or D.O.) who have completed at least three years of specialized training in psychiatry after graduation from medical or osteopathic school. *Child psychiatrists* have a minimum of four years of psychiatric training, including two in adult psychiatry and two in child psychiatry.

*Psychoanalysts* are practitioners who have undergone personal psycho-analysis and completed an additional seven to ten years of part-time training in the theories and specialized techniques of psychoanalysis. Most are psychia-trists, but a few have background in psychology or another nonmedical discipline.

*Psychologists* are persons whose academic training has been the study of human behavior. Students of psychology study the mental, emotional, biologi-cal, and social bases for human behavior, as well as theories that account for individual differences and abnormal behavior. They are also instructed in research methodology, statistics, psychological testing, and a variety of skills applicable to their specialty if they intend to practice. The major recognized specialties are counseling, clinical psychology, school psychology, and industrial-organizational psychology. In most states, licensing or certification for independent practice as a psychologist requires as a minimum: (1) a doctoral degree from an accredited training program, (2) additional years of supervised clinical experience, and (3) passing of an examination. A few states allow persons with master's level training to work as psychological associates or assistants under the supervision of licensed or certified professionals.

*Clinical social workers* practice in private offices and under the auspices of public, voluntary, and proprietary agencies and institutions. They are licensed or regulated by most states. Certification by the Academy of Certified Social Workers (ACSW) requires: (1) a master's or doctoral degree from a school of social work that is recognized by the Council on Social Work Education, (2) two years or three thousand hours of postgraduate experience under supervision of a master's level social worker, and (3) passing a written examination given by the ACSW.

*Certified clinical mental health counselors* work in agencies, schools and colleges, and independent practice. They must have an appropriate master's degree (or equivalent) plus two years of counseling experience. They must pass a written examination conducted by the National Academy of Certified Clinical Mental Health Counselors. They are licensed or certified in thirty-five states. About twelve thousand clinical mental health counselors belong to the American Mental Health Counselors Association.

*Specialists in psychiatric nursing* are registered nurses (RNs) who usually hold a master's degree from a program that lasts one and a half to two years. However, the term "psychiatric nurse" may also be applied to any nurse who has worked in a psychiatric setting. The American Nurses' Association certifies psychiatric nurses on two levels. Certification as a psychiatric and mental health nurse requires two years of experience in a mental health setting, current clinical practice, and passage of an examination. Certification as a clinical specialist requires, in addition, a master's degree in psychiatric nursing (or equivalent training) and two years of postgraduate clinical experience. Some psychiatric nurses conduct their own groups or serve as co-therapists in mental hospitals and clinics. Master's level psychiatric nurses may function as primary psychotherapists in community mental health centers. Some have set up private practices, providing both individual and family therapy.

*Marital and family counselors* are licensed or certified in twenty-six states. The American Association for Marriage and Family Therapy (AAMFT) is a professional organization whose members must have an appropriate master's or doctoral level training plus two years of clinical experience with couples and families under the supervision of an AAMFT-approved supervisor. The AAMFT also accredits training programs.

*Sexual therapists* specialize in the treatment of sexual problems that can be helped by simple techniques and increased communication between sexual partners. They may or may not be able to deal with underlying emotional problems that require individual psychotherapy. Certification is available from the American Association of Sex Educators, Counselors, and Therapists (AASECT), an interdisciplinary interest group. Certification as a sex therapist requires a master's or doctoral degree, licensure or certification in an appropriate professional discipline, and about eight hundred hours of specialized training related to sex therapy. Certification as a sex counselor has similar requirements but can be obtained with a bachelor's degree.

Since sexual therapy is neither defined nor regulated by law, anyone can adopt the title of "sexual therapist" or "sexual counselor." For this reason, it is important to check the reputation of a prospective therapist. Those practicing at university-affiliated clinics can be presumed competent. Information about other therapists may be obtainable from your family physician, the local medical society, or the local family service agency.

There are many other types of mental health practitioners whose activities are not defined by law or regulated by licensure. Included in this category are caseworkers, social work aides, members of the clergy, school counselors, and a wide variety of self-proclaimed therapists. Some have sound training; others do not.

There are several reasons why finding a suitable therapist for a mental or emotional problem may be more difficult than finding one for a physical problem or for general medical care:

- There is a wide choice of types of practitioner.

- Some types of practitioners lack standardization of training and credentials.

- There may be many different approaches used by practitioners within each professional group.

- The person seeking help may have no idea which type of treatment approach might be most appropriate.

- Compatibility between patient and therapist is more important in psychological treatment than it is in the treatment of physical problems.

- A sizable number of practitioners use questionable practices, some of which may be difficult to recognize.

## *Selecting a Therapist*

People contemplating mental health treatment should consider the following basic questions: (1) What type of help do I want? (2) Which type of practitioner(s) can provide it? (3) Are they available in the community? (4) How much can I afford to pay?

If medication is desired, one must see a physician. Most nonpsychiatric physicians are competent to prescribe antianxiety agents for short periods. For antipsychotic drugs, antidepressants, or any type of long-range treatment, it is best to consult a psychiatrist.

If a conversational form of treatment is preferred, a recommendation may be obtained from a personal physician, clergyman, school counselor, or friend. Psychoanalytic institutes, which are located in some major cities, can provide names of psychiatrists who specialize in psychotherapy. So can the departments of psychiatry at most medical schools and large hospitals. Additional names of psychiatrists can be obtained from the local medical society and the yellow pages of the telephone directory. Information about the training and credentials of a prospective psychiatrist can be obtained from the biographical directory of the APA, from the local medical society, or from the psychiatrist directly. Those who have trained at university hospitals are more likely to be primarily interested in psychotherapy than those who have trained at state hospitals. "Do you do psychotherapy primarily?" is a good screening question.

Certification by the American Board of Psychiatry and Neurology is a good indication that a psychiatrist is qualified to administer organic forms of treatment, but is not as useful a guideline in selecting a psychotherapist. Some analytically oriented psychiatrists are not motivated to become certified because they believe the board is primarily oriented toward organic psychiatry.

Should one decide to consult a therapist who is not a psychiatrist, names may be obtained from a personal physician, clergyman, school counselor, friend, local professional society, or the yellow pages of the telephone directory. Most national professional organizations publish biographical membership directories, and most certifying organizations publish directories of the professionals they certify. Some of these publications are available at public, hospital, and medical school libraries. Credentials can also be checked by writing to the national professional organizations listed in Chapter 33.

Most private practitioners of psychotherapy charge $50 to $150 for a fifty-minute session. In 1992, the average fee for psychiatrists was about $100. For people who cannot afford these rates, most communities have mental health clinics whose fees are based on the ability to pay. Most psychotherapy at community clinics is done by psychologists and social workers. A limited amount of counseling is available without charge to students at most colleges and universities.

Psychiatrist Ronald Pies advises that consultation with a physician should be obtained whenever "mental" problems are associated with any of the following symptoms: blackouts; memory lapses (such as trouble recalling recent events); persistent headaches; significant unintentional weight loss; numbness, tingling, or other strange sensations; generalized weakness; dizzy spells; significant pain of any sort; difficulty walking; shortness of breath; seizures of any type; inability to control urination; unduly rapid and/or forceful heartbeats; frequent, heavy sweating; tremor; or slurred speech.

## Self-Help Groups

Self-help groups, the goal of which is to encourage the emotional growth of their members, are growing throughout the nation. Participants believe that by sharing their problems with others and by receiving the support of an interested group, they can gain more control over their emotional problem.

Recovery, Inc., is a self-help group that tries to prevent recurrences of mental illness of former mental patients. Individuals are taught how to recognize symptoms of approaching difficulties and to head them off. Alcoholics Anonymous (AA) and Secular Organizations for Sobriety (SOS) assist people with drinking problems. Neurotics Anonymous has a program similar to that of AA but is suitable for people with many different types of problems.

## Questionable "Self-Help" Products

Thousands of videotapes and audiotapes containing repeated messages are being marketed with claims that they can help people lose weight, stop smoking, enhance athletic performance, quit drinking, think creatively, raise I.Q., make friends, reduce pain, improve vision, restore hearing, cure acne, conquer fears, read faster, speak effectively, handle criticism, relieve depression, enlarge breasts, and do many other things. At least one company sells subliminal tapes for children, including a toilet-training tape for toddlers. Many tapes contain music said to promote relaxation. Most tapes are said to contain messages that are inaudible, but some contain messages that are fully audible. Videotapes may combine images that are supposed to be relaxing with repeated messages shown so briefly that they cannot be seen at normal playing speed.

Many researchers have found that subliminal tapes provide no benefit to the user. For example, Philip Merickle, a psychology professor at the University of Waterloo (in Canada), used computerized equipment to analyze several samples. He found no evidence of hidden speech, either above or below the range of human hearing. (In other words, there was no reason to believe that the user's brain could detect any message on these tapes.) A research team tested volunteers for a study of tapes said to improve memory and self-esteem—but switched the tapes for half of the participants. Regardless of the tape used, about half claimed to achieve the results they were told to expect—but objective tests of memory and self-esteem showed no change. A National Research Council committee has concluded that, although many people claim that subliminal self-help tapes contribute to self-improvement, there is no scientific evidence to support such claims. Thus there is no reason to believe that musical tapes with "subliminal" messages can do anything more for physical or mental well-being than listening to one's favorite music. Nor is there evidence that inaudible messages are unconsciously or subconsciously perceived or can influence behavior.

Many audiotapes, videotapes, and self-help books have been marketed to the public with claims that they inspire people to function better mentally, improve relationships with others, relieve anxiety or depression, or achieve other desirable emotionally-related goals. Gerald Rosen, Ph.D., former chairman of the American Psychological Association's Task Force on Self-Help Therapies, has noted the following:

- Although some of these materials may be helpful, most have not been tested to see if they are valid.

- Many self-help materials are promoted with extravagant and ethically questionable claims.

- The fact that a technique is useful when included as part of a therapy program does not mean the technique will work as a self-help measure. Self-help books are more likely to be helpful during periods of therapy than at other times.

- Few do-it-yourself books have provisions to protect readers against failing to comply with instructions. Should treatment failure occur, the readers may inappropriately blame themselves, become skeptical that they can be helped, and fail to seek professional help.

Battery-operated skin temperature monitors and devices that measure muscle or brain-wave activity have been marketed through the mail for home use. The *Harvard Health Letter* has warned that such devices have not been systematically evaluated and are likely to "have a short working life before they wind up in a closet or attic, gathering dust." Tests on home biofeedback devices claimed to help people manipulate their alpha waves have shown that the devices were actually signaling in response to the user's eye movements or to interference from household electrical currents.

Ellon USA, Inc., of Lynbrook, New York, markets the Bach Flower Remedies, a line of thirty-eight products said to alleviate "negative" emotions. These remedies were developed about sixty years ago by Edward Bach, a British bacteriologist and homeopath, who—according to the company's literature—"believed that the only way to cure illness was to address the underlying emotional causes of disease." Remedies can be selected according to responses to a 116-item questionnaire published by Ellon USA. Someone who feels overwhelmed with work, for example, is advised to take the product called *Elm,* while someone who has strong opinions and is easily incensed by injustices is advised to use *Vervain.* In a recent mailing to retailers, the company stated:

> Spring is in the air. . . . Many of [your customers] will be embarking on diet regimens and strenuous exercise routines. So, while you are advising them on nutritional supplements and low fat foods, keep in mind that their emotions play a large part in their ultimate success or failure to lose weight or get in shape.
>
> All too often, negative feelings about themselves and outside pressures drive them to strive for unrealistic goals and they set themselves up for failure from the beginning.
>
> To help them, introduce them to the remedies. . . .
>
> *Crab Apple* is a good choice to help them accept their physical being. *Larch* is a good boost for self-esteem. *Hornbeam* is excellent for overcoming mental fatigue and *Impatiens* is good for those customers who can never achieve their goals fast enough.

## Questionable Practices

A wide variety of questionable practices exists among practitioners who profess to treat mental, emotional, and personal problems. Since terms such as "therapist," "psychotherapist," and "counselor" are not defined by law, anyone may use these words to represent himself. The fields of sensitivity training, sexual counseling, marriage counseling, hypnosis, and encounter groups contain many self-proclaimed therapists who have little or no training. Other types of unqualified practitioners masquerade under such titles as metaphysician, astrolotherapist, autohypnotist, palmist, reader-adviser, graphologist (handwriting analyst), and character analyst. Some have certificates from diploma mills or brief correspondence courses, while others do not even have these.

Some practitioners with reputable training and credentials use methods that are not based on scientific evidence of their efficacy. Some have personal problems that interfere with proper care of their patients; and some deliberately exploit their patients.

The trouble with questionable mental health treatment is not merely lack of efficacy. A disillusioning experience can cause the patient to abandon further effort to obtain help, or can even trigger a personal disaster such as suicide. Let's look at some of the common types of questionable mental health practices.

## Sensitivity Training

Sensitivity training began in the 1950s with training groups (T-groups) whose purpose was to help community leaders ease social tensions in their communities. This was accomplished by an intense small-group experience that encouraged self-disclosure and expression of strong feeling while focusing on the attitudes and interactions of group members. The process was never intended for the treatment of emotionally disturbed individuals. Over the years, these groups have proliferated under such names as marathon groups, growth centers, encounter groups, and human relations laboratories. Unfortunately, many leaders of such groups are incompetent.

The stated purpose of encounter groups is to help people experience personal growth by learning to express their feelings more openly. The groups may take a variety of forms. Participants usually talk under the guidance of a group leader. Some groups involve physical comfort or contact such as touching. Some have supportive and/or aggressive confrontations.

The following factors should be considered before participating in a sensitivity group: (1) the psychological condition and motivation of the individual, (2) the reputation and accountability of the sponsoring organization, (3) the qualifications of the group leaders and consultants, (4) the methods used to prescreen participants, and (5) the stated agenda and goals of the program.

Sensitivity training can be very upsetting to individuals who are not self-confident enough to handle the confrontation and emotional expression that can take place at such meetings. Depression, psychosis, major personality disorganization, panic reactions, and physical injuries have resulted from improperly conducted meetings.

## Meditation

Meditation is generally defined as a class of techniques intended to influence an individual's consciousness through the regulation of attention. It may involve lying quietly or sitting in a particular position, attending to one's breathing (yoga), adopting a passive attitude, attempting to be at ease, or repeating a word aloud or to oneself (transcendental meditation). A National Research Council committee has concluded that people who meditate regularly may have a more restful lifestyle and that a variety of relaxation techniques might be appropriate for stress-reduction. However, the committee found no scientific evidence that meditation reduces stress more than does simply resting quietly or that meditation alone provides lasting benefits such as reducing high blood pressure or other unhealthful responses to stress.

## Megavitamin Therapy

During the early 1950s, a few psychiatrists began adding massive doses of nutrients to their treatment of severe mental problems. The original substance used was vitamin $B_3$, (nicotinic acid or nicotinamide), and the therapy was termed "megavitamin therapy." Since that time the treatment regimen has been expanded to include other vitamins, minerals, hormones, and diets, any of which may be combined with conventional drug therapy and/or ECT.

Today the treatment is called "orthomolecular psychiatry," a term meaning "the treatment of mental disease by the provision of optimum molecular environment for the mind, especially substances normally present in the human body." Proponents suggest that abnormal behavior is caused by molecular imbalances correctable by administration of the "right" nutrient molecules at the right time (*ortho* is Greek for "right"). The orthomolecular approach is now used to treat many other diseases. It is described in such books as *Orthomolecular Psychiatry: A Treatment Approach*, by Linus Pauling and David Hawkins, M.D.; *Mega-Nutrition*, by Richard Kunin, M.D.; and *Dr. Pfeiffer's Total Nutrition,* by Carl C. Pfeiffer, M.D., Ph.D. Dr. Kunin's book claims that a balanced diet is a practical impossibility and that "the nutrition-prescription movement is . . . a new direction toward which all of medicine is moving." Both he and Dr. Hawkins are psychiatrists who have served as president of the Orthomolecular Medical Society.

Dr. Pfeiffer, who died in 1989, was director of the Princeton Brain Bio Center (now called the Princeton Bio Center), Skillman, New Jersey, a facility that offers "nutritional" treatment for:

> the schizophrenias and biochemical deficiencies associated with aging, alcoholism (must be in AA and not drinking), allergies, arthritis, autism, epilepsy, hypertension, hypoglycemia, migraine, depression, learning disability, retardation, mental and metabolic disorders, skin problems, and hyperactivity.

Its fee for an initial evaluation has been about $300, including $100 for consultation with a doctor and the rest for laboratory tests that most physicians would not consider necessary or useful for diagnosing the above disorders. (Nor would most doctors agree that the disorders are associated with biochemical deficiencies.) The evaluation fee does not include the ten or more nutrients typically prescribed.

A special task force of the American Psychiatric Association has investigated the claims of the megavitamin and orthomolecular therapists. Its 1973 report notes that orthomolecular psychiatrists use unconventional methods not only in treatment, but also in diagnosis. The report's conclusion, perhaps the most strongly worded statement ever published by a scientific review body, states:

> This review and critique has carefully examined the literature produced by megavitamin proponents and by those who have attempted to replicate their basic and clinical work. It concludes in this regard that the credibility of the megavitamin proponents is low. Their credibility is further diminished by a consistent refusal over the past decade to perform controlled experiments and to report their new results in a scientifically acceptable fashion.
>
> Under these circumstances this Task Force considers the massive publicity which they promulgate via radio, the lay press and popular books, using catch phrases which are really misnomers like "megavitamin therapy" and "orthomolecular treatment," to be deplorable.

The Research Advisory Committee of the National Institute of Mental Health reviewed pertinent scientific data through 1979 and agreed that megavitamin therapy is ineffective and may be harmful. After the U.S. Defense Subcommittee looked into this therapy, it was removed as a treatment covered under the CHAMPUS insurance program for military dependents.

Various claims that megavitamins and megaminerals are effective against psychosis, learning disorders, and mental retardation in children were debunked in reports by the nutrition committees of the American Academy of Pediatrics in 1976 and 1981 and the Canadian Academy of Pediatrics in 1990. Both groups have warned that there is no proven benefit in any of these conditions and that megadoses can cause serious toxic effects. The 1976 report concluded that a "cult" had developed among followers of megavitamin therapy.

### The Feingold Diet

Many school-age children have been labeled "hyperactive" or "hyperkinetic." In 1973, Dr. Benjamin Feingold, a pediatric allergist from California, proposed that salicylates, artificial colors, and artificial flavors were causes of hyperactivity. To treat or prevent this condition, he suggested a diet that was free of these chemicals. Feingold's followers now claim that asthma, bedwetting, ear infections, eye-muscle disorders, seizures, sleep disorders, and stomach aches may respond to the Feingold program and that sensitivity to synthetic additives and/or salicylates may be a factor in antisocial traits, compulsive aggression, self-mutilation, difficulty in reasoning, stuttering, and exceptional clumsiness.

Adherence to the Feingold diet requires a drastic change in family lifestyle and eating patterns. Homemade foods prepared "from scratch" are necessary for many meals. Feingold strongly recommended that the hyperactive child help prepare the special foods and encouraged the entire family to participate in the dietary program. *The Feingold Cookbook* states: "A successful response to the diet depends on 100 percent compliance. The slightest infraction can lead to failure: a single bite or drink can cause an undesirable response that may persist for seventy-two hours or more."

Many parents who have followed Feingold's recommendations have reported improvement in their children's behavior. In fact, many families have banded together into local groups and a national association to promote the dietary program. But carefully designed experiments have failed to support the idea that additives cause hyperactivity.

Because the Feingold diet does no physical harm, it might appear to be helpful therapy in some instances. However, the potential benefits should be weighed against the potential harm of teaching children that behavior is related to what they eat rather than what they feel. There is additional potential for harm in creating situations in which a child's eating behavior is regarded as peculiar by other children. I will never forget the youngster who announced on a Phil Donahue TV show that he had misbehaved because he had "slipped" off his diet and eaten a candy bar!

Additional Feingold-related mischief may loom on the horizon. The September 1992 issue of the Feingold Association's newsletter, *Pure Facts,* claimed that teachers and children have been noted to suffer from the effects of chemicals used in construction, furnishing, housekeeping, maintenance, renovation, pest control, food service, and classroom activities at their schools. An article titled "The Sick Building Syndrome" stated that one child was repeatedly disciplined for reacting to his teacher's perfume, another child became abusive toward his mother because of the school's newly-painted lunchroom, and that yet another child required tutoring because of a very bad reaction to a leak in the school's oil furnace. Claims like these are similar to those made by clinical ecologists (see Chapter 10).

## Questionable Treatments for Learning Disabilities

Several other treatment approaches to learning disabilities and mental retardation have been identified as unproven and controversial:

• *Dolman-Delacato treatment*, also known as "patterning," is an approach developed during the mid-1950s and offered at the Institutes for Human Potential in Philadelphia, Pennsylvania. Its proponents claim that the great majority of cases of mental retardation, learning problems, and behavior disorders are caused by brain damage or "poor neurological organization." The treatment is based on the idea that high levels of motor and sensory stimulation can train the nervous system and lessen or overcome handicaps caused by brain damage. Parents following the program may be advised to exercise the child's limbs repeatedly and use other measures said to increase blood flow to the brain and decrease brain irritability. In 1982, the American Academy of Pediatrics issued a position paper concluding that "patterning" has no special merit, that its proponents' claims are unproven, and that the demands on families are so great that in some cases there may be actual harm in its use.

• *Optometric visual training* is based on the idea that learning can be improved by exercises that improve coordination of the eye muscles and/or improve hand-eye coordination. Its proponents assume that the basic problem that leads to reading disability is some deficit in the visual system. The American Academy of Pediatrics and the American Academy of Ophthalmology have criticized this approach and cautioned that no eye-muscle defects can produce the learning disabilities associated with dyslexia. (Dyslexia is a reading disorder—not due to mental retardation, lack of schooling, or brain damage—characterized by omissions, faulty word substitutions, and impaired comprehension.) This condition is described further in Chapter 25.

• *Neural Organization Technique (NOT)* is based on the idea that learning disorders, childhood psychoses, mental retardation, cerebral palsy, bedwetting, and color-blindness are related to muscle imbalances caused by misplaced bones of the skull. This method, a chiropractic variant of cranial osteopathy (see Chapter 22), was developed by New York chiropractor Carl Ferreri and has been taught to hundreds of others. Its proponents claim that "blocked neural pathways" can be corrected by "adjusting" the bones of the skull by applying pressure to various parts of the head. NOT came to public attention in 1988 when chiropractors subjected children to it in a "research" project sponsored by school officials in Del Norte County, California. A lurid report in the November/December 1988 issue of *Hippocrates* magazine described how children from ages four to sixteen with epilepsy, Down's syndrome, cerebral palsy, dyslexia, and various other learning disorders had their skull compressed with viselike hand pressure and were forced to endure painful thumb pressure against the roof of the mouth and finger pressure against their eyes. One parent even complained that pressure against her son's eye sockets had caused him to have a seizure. In 1991, a jury ordered Ferreri to pay $565,000 in damages to seven children and their parents who had filed suit for physical and emotional pain related to the treatment. Two other chiropractors involved in the case settled out of court for a total of $207,000.

### Stimulation of False Memories

Patients who are suggestible and/or eager to please their therapist may "remember" past events that did not actually take place. Usually it is the therapist who stimulates this process, either deliberately or unwittingly. Occasionally, however, the patient (possibly inspired by a book or television talk show) initiates the problem and the therapist fails to help sort out fact from fantasy. Critics are using the term "false memory syndrome" (FMS) to describe the mental state generated in these situations.

"Past-life therapy" is based on the idea that psychological disorders arise from the influence of traumas and personality traits from previous lives intruding on the subconscious. Proponents of this approach use hypnosis, meditation, or guided imagery to "regress" the patient to earlier incarnations ("past lives") which, when brought to consciousness, lead to resolution of the patient's problems. There is, however, no scientific evidence that these notions are valid.

Experiments conducted by Nicholas P. Spanos, a psychology professor at Carlton University, Ottawa, Canada, have shown that "past-life" reports during hypnotic trances are related to the subject's suggestibility and proneness to fantasize. In one experiment, 35 out of 110 subjects who were asked to regress to times before their birth enacted "past lives." In most of these cases, their past-life personalities were the same age and race as themselves. In another experiment, half of the subjects were informed by researchers that previous incarnations were often a different sex or race and had lived in exotic cultures. Those who received this advice were significantly more likely to incorporate one or more of the suggested characteristics into their past-life descriptions. In a third experiment, the researchers found that subjects who gave information specific enough to be checked were much more often incorrect than correct. Dr. Spanos believes that past-life reports obtained from hypnotically regressed subjects are fantasy constructions of imaginative persons absorbed in make-believe situations and responding to regression suggestions--and that those who believe in reincarnation are the most likely to believe that such fantasies are related to an actual past life.

During the past several years, hundreds of poorly trained therapists—many of them calling themselves "traumatists"—have been encouraging patients to recall childhood traumas that supposedly had been repressed for decades. In response, many patients have developed vivid and detailed "memories" of such events and become very angry with a once-loved relative. As the anger crystallizes, these therapists encourage confronting and possibly even suing the alleged perpetrator.

In March 1992, a number of parents and mental health professionals founded the FMS Foundation to deal with the problem of adults who mistakenly believe that they were victims of incest or child abuse. Within fifteen months, more than 4,200 distressed families contacted the foundation for advice on how to cope with sudden attacks by angry daughters who accused them of misdeeds that may not have taken place.

Martin Gardner, a prominent science writer, has noted that FMS can take other forms as well. In the Summer 1993 issue of *Skeptical Inquirer,* he states that thousands of suggestible patients have been induced to "remember" childhood participation in satanic cults and abduction by aliens from faraway planets. He refers to the burgeoning number of FMS cases as "the mental health crisis of the 1990s."

### *Simplistic Advice*

A deep understanding of the dynamics of a case may enable a therapist to give good advice that appears to be simple in content. But sometimes therapists give advice without taking into consideration the complexity of the patient's situation. Such ill-conceived action may be the result of inadequate training, an emotional problem of the therapist, or both. The following composite cases illustrate this point:

- A sixty-year-old business man complained of insomnia and depression. Worry about his business was keeping him awake. The physician advised him to take a vacation to "get away from it all so you can stop worrying." The man went to a seaside resort but found he could not relax. He thought that his business would suffer from his absence, and idleness merely served to intensify his worry.

- A thirty-five-year-old junior executive sought treatment for headaches and abdominal fullness. The physician correctly diagnosed that these were bodily reactions to tension, which was generated primarily at work. The patient believed he was being asked to do more than his share but was afraid to speak up about it. The physician encouraged the man to express his resentment, but failed to discuss how to do this in a constructive manner. The patient "told off" his boss and quit in a huff, a decision he later regretted.

• A middle-aged couple who consulted a counselor spent the entire first two sessions berating each other for one thing after another. Seeing only the hostility in the relationship, the counselor advised them to get a divorce. A more qualified therapist would have realized that they could not have remained together for many years without a positive side to their relationship. The therapist should have terminated the verbal slugfest, explored the positive aspects of the relationship, identified the issues in conflict, and tried to help the couple resolve them.

• A thirty-year-old housewife sought help in understanding why she became angry with important people in her life, particularly her husband. The therapist encouraged discussion of her childhood and "analyzed" the similarities between her father and her husband. The connection was made that "you get angry with your husband when he reminds you of your father." Feeling that this information "justified" her resentment, the patient acted more nastily toward her husband, and their relationship deteriorated. Actually, the marital situation had been far more complex than the therapist realized. He should have explored the patient's contribution to the marital friction and helped her learn better ways to handle her feelings.

## Mismanagement of Psychotherapy

Psychotherapy should not only help patients solve problems but should also (with rare exceptions) help them become independent of the therapist. Just as children must learn to handle situations without always running to their mother, patients must learn to handle upset feelings between sessions without the direct help of the therapist. A therapist who permits or encourages frequent telephone calls is also encouraging overdependence. Therapists who receive many such calls from many patients are likely to have an unconscious problem, a neurotic need to have people depend on them, which interferes with treatment of the patients.

A more subtle example of this problem is the therapist who cannot adhere to a schedule. Patients are scheduled for particular times, but sessions are allowed to run considerably overtime when patients are upset or appear to be talking about particularly meaningful material. Although an occasional brief extension may be justified, a general policy of this type encourages patients to manipulate the therapist to gain more attention.

A more malignant type of therapist behavior is that of exploiting patients. Although it is not unusual for therapist and patient to feel a personal or physical attraction toward each other, acting on such feelings is not therapeutic. A composite case history illustrates what can happen:

• An unmarried twenty-seven-year-old woman entered therapy to over-come shyness, feelings of inadequacy, and fear of involvement with men. Few men had seemed interested in her, and she had rarely dated. As therapy proceeded, she developed an intense fondness for the therapist, based largely on the fact that he was the first man who ever spent time with her on a regular basis. At this point, instead of helping her learn how to attract suitable dates, the therapist suggested that sex with him would help her become more comfortable with men. She consented, hoping that marriage to the therapist would result. Her eventual disillusionment was a shattering experience that led to suicide.

Almost all psychiatrists believe that sexual contact with a patient is inappropriate and is usually harmful. In some states it is a criminal offense, while in others it is malpractice and can lead to loss of license. In 1990, a California jury awarded $1.5 million to a woman who claimed that a psychiatrist had exploited her. Testimony during the trial indicated that following almost two years of treatment, they began dating. The patient said that although she was extremely happy during the beginning of their affair, she became severely depressed when it ended. I believe that therapists who make passes at their patients should be prosecuted as criminals.

**Navigating the Mental Health Maze**

Although excellent help is available for the treatment of mental and emotional problems, selecting a suitable therapist can be difficult. Some people respond best to a conversational approach, some to medication, and some to both. Before seeking treatment, it is advisable to understand the types of help available and the training that various types of practitioners undergo. Although most practitioners with accredited training are competent, some engage in practices that are unscientific or reflect underlying problems of their own. For this reason, it is important to be able to recognize the common signs of inappropriate therapy.

# 30

# The Mind Robbers

### John G. Clark, Jr., M.D.

Cults can be very dangerous to the health and welfare of their converts and menacing to their critics. At one time or another, millions of Americans have been involved with one or more of the thousands of cult groups that range in size from two or three members to many thousands who obey a guru.

Most studies of deviant cults have found them composed primarily of middle-class or upper middle-class converts. Whether political or religious, their belief systems are uniformly absolutist, intolerant, polarized, provocative, simplistic, and unwavering. However, it is not the private beliefs of the members of these groups that matter—cult doctrines vary enormously. It is the behavior of the cultists toward those outside their worlds and the effects on the health of both the involved persons and their families that deserve our attention.

## Goals of Cults

The destructive cults are usually first-generation entities with living leaders. Their primary goals are expansion through rapid, aggressive conversion and the amassing of money. Most are self-styled as religions for tax advantages and other first amendment privileges. Cult members are expected to bend their will and yield control of their mind to the group and its leaders; failure to do so is punished or corrected. Banishment is the ultimate sanction in some groups, while in others it may be death.

Cults rarely launch truly charitable projects as they claim, largely because needy persons outside their groups are seen as different and undeserving. It is not unusual for cult members to raise hundreds of dollars per day by begging or soliciting for nonexistent charities. Nor is it unusual for cults to extract large sums of money from their converts.

## Susceptibility to Conversion

A great mix of persons from early teens to their mid-fifties, with a wide variety of personality strengths and weaknesses, have entered these groups. The cults themselves select a segment of the marketplace and, as with any new enterprise, thrive only if they develop the technical skills to build a core group and maintain internal congruity. Although many observers have tried to identify personality traits that make individuals susceptible to conversion, the fact is that most people can be vulnerable under the right circumstances.

My studies of persons in various stages of cult involvement show that more than half of them were substantially disturbed and unhappy for many years. Many of these people had sought conversions actively and repeatedly; the rest, however, were essentially normal, maturing persons. Their susceptibility to conversion was the result either of aggressive manipulation by a proselytizer or of a normal, painful crisis of maturation. Similar findings have been reported by other experts.

## The Conversion Process

An individual's involvement with a cult typically begins with an invitation to attend a lecture, a course, or a social gathering. Further invitations will then be issued to attend a weekend seminar, a workshop, or a spiritual retreat. Recruiters, who generally misrepresent their intentions, may not reveal their organizational ties. They may display false affection and radiate spiritual fulfillment that can have considerable impact on the potential recruit.

"I didn't know who they were until I had signed up for the twenty-one-day workshop—and by then I didn't care," a nineteen-year-old former cult member told me. "From the first moment, she was all over me—touching, flattering, questioning. Even when I went to the bathroom. I had been kind of depressed. My girl had told me to get lost, and the first friendly voice was so welcome that I accepted her invitation to the center."

Once contact is established, highly programmed behavioral techniques are used to narrow the subject's attention to the point of trance. Loss of privacy, lack of sleep, a new vocabulary, and continuous control of excitement level amount to an onslaught of information that sustains the trance-like state. Throughout this period of focused attention, new information is absorbed at an accelerated rate and rapidly becomes integral to the available mechanisms of the mind. As a result, the convert becomes dependent on this new environment for definitions of reality.

"When I was given knowledge, I gave up my mind," said a twenty-two-year-old engineering student. "That's the kind of logic we all accepted. . . . I was ready to believe everything I'd known was crazy all my life. They could tell me anything, or ask me to do any stupid thing and I'd jump and feel great."

At this stage, the group controls not only behavior but also thought content by means of confessions, training, and conditioning. To think wrongly is "satanic" and punishable by psychosomatic reactions such as headaches, gastrointestinal symptoms, depressions, and panic states.

## The Effects of Conversion

The nervous system may be so profoundly affected by the conversion process that menstrual periods may stop and beard growth may slow down considerably. While in this state, personality changes drastically, a fact that often terrifies parents. Converts often seem drab and dreamy outside the group, robot-like and somewhat expressionless when discussing anything other than their new experience. They lack humor and richness of vocabulary. The devices of expression—irony, metaphor, and delight in the use of abstraction—are gone. Many converts report hallucinations and experience group-validated delusions as well as nightmares. The sense of current history is quickly lost. If challenged, converts may become excited or even violent, but at best will answer difficult questions with memorized clichés.

Rapid conversion, brought about by a skillful and determined group or individual, results in a sustained state of "dissociation" in which a large share of one's lifetime of memories is switched off and quickly replaced by the overwhelming presence of the cult itself. Because the guiding lessons of past experience are no longer available, the personality is drastically and rapidly remade. The resultant mental state, rigid and obedient, is close to chaos.

Most converts are used for recruiting and begging. They work extremely long hours to meet impossible goals. Some have reported sleeping less than four hours nightly for many years. They are often aware of their prior personalities through dreams or shadowy memories.

Almost all cults embrace many forms of magic and reject scientific linear thinking. Many also reject modern medicine and consider physicians to be enemies. Faith healing is not uncommon. (The Reverend Jim Jones, who led more than nine hundred people to death in Guyana, practiced faith healing in Indianapolis before moving to northern California with many of his faithful flock.) Even cultists who occasionally use medical facilities may be extremely reluctant to seek this help or pay for it. Many emergency room physicians have observed severe cases of physical neglect, including malnutrition, untreated diabetes, broken bones that had been prayed over, and infectious diseases that were the result of communal living. Therapeutic compliance and follow-up are often poor. Small children—as well as adults—have died from medical neglect.

Many former cult members illustrate the dire effects of living in a prolonged dissociative state. They may appear mentally preoccupied ("floating") and may remain very suggestible. Depressions, loneliness, and indecisiveness may seriously interfere with a return to ordinary living. A simple decision such as choosing a pair of socks may take an inordinate amount of time and energy. Ex-cult members are often aware of a double personality. They may feel painfully guilty, both for hurting their parents and for leaving their "loving" cult family. They may also have frequent illnesses.

A few cults resort to blackmail. One former member, who had been assured that conversations with cult leaders would be confidential, "had told everything, including every fantasy I could recall or invent. . . . When I left, I found that they were willing to use all of this against me in order to prevent me from hurting them."

**Danger to Society**

Cults of various sorts have been useful to society as agents of change. As antagonists to the status quo, they may very well serve as leavening in a stagnant culture. There is no question of their right to stand against other opinions; nor should there be any question of the right of others to stand against them. It is through this kind of confrontation that change may be negotiated safely. But in groups organized as I have described, there is an inherent danger, from their techniques and their deviant doctrines, that they can become destructive for destruction's own sake or intolerant beyond the capacity to negotiate. At that stage cultists are willing to injure other human beings without scruple. Among the burned-out rejects of these groups, some have apparently disappeared, leaving their family unable to determine whether they are alive or dead. Others are simply unable to use their mind as tools of survival. They are supremely difficult to treat; they are mutilated.

Professionals who have studied the wide range of dangerous cults are not surprised by the slaughter of Jim Jones's followers, the recent Branch Davidian tragedy, or the violence of other groups. Political manipulations, amassing of firearms, and other menacing cult behavior have been reported in other countries as well. It is clear that the destructiveness of cults should be taken seriously and not condoned.

# 31

# Quackery and the Media

## Stephen Barrett, M.D.

Publicity is obviously a major factor—if not the major factor—in the success of quackery. Freelance writer Max Gunther has observed:

> The media have four main functions: to entertain, to inform, to carry advertisements, and to make money for their stockholders. Because of the ways in which these are carried out . . . an appalling amount of misinformation—ranging from the faintly biased to the downright wrong—is fed every day to an unfortunately gullible public. Hardly anywhere is this more evident than in the fields of medicine and its unwanted cousin—quackery!

## The Handling of News

Information that will attract a wide audience is considered "newsworthy." It may be new, startling, alarming, or amusing; or it can have any other quality that an editor or producer believes will interest the particular audience toward which the material is directed. Sensational claims tend to be regarded as more newsworthy than what J.I. Rodale called the "unvarnished truths" of medical science. People who make such claims may be equally regarded as newsworthy.

If you were a writer, would you try not to arouse false hopes in your readers? Several years ago, I asked twenty editors and reporters from Eastern Pennsylvania newspapers to fill out a questionnaire about the news coverage of controversial health topics. One question was:

Dr. John Banks, President of the National Nutrition Research Association, is the speaker at the local women's club which you often cover. He claims that a certain nutrient has great healing powers not yet sufficiently appreciated by scientists. He does not seem to be far-fetched, but his ideas are completely new to you. Would you be more likely to report this as a straight news event or to evaluate his claims by seeking another opinion?

Fifteen of the twenty said they would report this as a straight news event. Seven out of those fifteen said that even if they consulted a physician who called the claims utter nonsense, they would still report the event without including any criticism. When questioned further, they said that reporters of news events should report them as they happen, without making judgments. If critics of "Dr. Banks" (a fictitious name) want their say, they should create their own news events to get coverage.

"Nonjudgmental" attitudes of this sort, which are common among reporters, help explain why sensational health-related claims frequently appear without challenge in the media. Other factors contributing to the spread of misinformation through the media include:

- Time works to quackery's advantage. It is much easier to report a health claim as a straight news event than it is to investigate whether it can be substantiated.

- Journalists with strong beliefs in quack methods cannot write accurately about them.

- Many promoters of misinformation often are regarded as "underdogs" in a struggle against the "establishment." As such, they tend to be treated much more sympathetically than they deserve. Most editors insist that attacks on false ideas be "balanced" so that the apparent "underdog" gets a "fair" hearing. Even science editors who know a promoter is selling the public a bill of goods rarely feel a duty to issue an effective public warning.

- Many more people are actively promoting health misinformation than are actively opposing it. The sheer force of numbers works against the truth.

- Many publications are unwilling to risk offending their advertisers. A blatant example occurred in 1980 when *Self* magazine published an article by a freelance writer listing money-saving tips from my consumer health textbook. A tip about not wasting money on vitamins was deleted from the writer's manuscript by the magazine's editors.

- Many publications pander to advertisers by using articles that promote their products and/or services. This policy is more prevalent among smaller, low-quality magazines and newspapers with small editorial budgets, but many large publications do this also. "Health-food" publications and some women's magazines are consistent offenders in this category.

- Many publications use sensational claims to generate sales. Tabloid newspapers and women's magazines, for example, frequently carry articles on "quickie" reducing diets or "superfoods." Marilynn Larkin, a freelance writer in New York city, has noted that topic selection is commonly based on sales appeal rather than scientific merit.

- Many editors fear that attacks on quackery will stir up trouble from people who believe in the method being attacked. Editors may also fear that attacking a promoter's credibility will provoke a libel suit. After NBC's *Dateline* did its superb exposé of dubious homeopathic methods (see Chapter 13), homeopathic groups urged their members to complain to network executives and reported that their effort generated thousands of protest messages. As far as I know, the campaign did not persuade NBC to air a rebuttal program, but the vigor of the protest might discourage the production of similar programs in the future.

During the past few years, mindless articles on "alternative" methods have been published by *Time, Newsweek, U.S. News & World Report, Shape, Redbook*, and *Kiplinger's Personal Finance Magazine*. (A "mindless" article is one that repeats claims by proponents without attempting to indicate whether they are true.) *Newsweek* has also published irresponsible attacks on fluoridation and mercury fillings. The most popular health magazines—*Health, Prevention,* and *American Health*—have been inconsistent. While *Health* has done some excellent investigative reports on quackery-related topics, it has published others that were misleading. Most articles in *Prevention* are accurate, but its editorials and research news tend to promote inappropriate use of vitamin supplements. In addition, it appears to have a policy against criticizing quack methods. *American Health* recently changed editors. Its new medical editor, Larry Katzenstein, was for many years the principal medical writer for *Consumer Reports*. His work is outstanding. However, some quackery-related articles produced by less experienced writers have been filled with overgeneralizations, unsubstantiatable statements, and doubletalk that provide no guidance for the reader. If Katzenstein is given more editorial control, *American Health* will tower above the rest.

At a press conference I gave about quackery, a reporter asked how he could be sure that I was telling the truth. I replied: "The real question is 'Do you *want* to know the truth?' If you do, find out what 'truth' is and seek out information sources you can trust."

C. Eugene Emery, Jr., science writer for the *Providence Journal,* is an expert at ferreting out the truth. He believes that "most hoaxes aren't exposed because too many news organizations make no attempt to really investigate supernatural or quack claims. Even if editors are interested, many reporters lack the background to evaluate such claims." He advises journalists to rely on three questions to determine whether something is fact or fancy, breakthrough or quackery:

1. *Where's the evidence?* Ask whether the proponent's work has been published in a peer-reviewed scientific journal.

2. *How good is the evidence?* Don't be swayed by nifty anecdotes and testimonials. Those who have the evidence want to talk about the evidence. Those who don't have evidence want to talk about testimonials. Those who have neither, just talk.

3. *What do the critics say?* Don't simply pick a quote from an interview with a critic that says, in effect, "I don't believe it." I see that all the time. Similarly, too many writers simply drop generic clauses in a pseudoscience story and figure they've given the other side their say. Such clauses include "although scientists dispute it," or the ever-popular "this theory is controversial." Ask *why* they have reason to doubt a claim. The answers can be *very* revealing and may suggest a way to test a claim yourself.

Often the best way to investigate an "alternative" method is to observe practitioners doing their work. Among other things, Emery has followed the course of people treated by faith-healers (see Chapter 24), visited chiropractors for check-ups, and asked iridologists to evaluate his health status.

In January 1993, the *New England Journal of Medicine* published "Unconventional Medicine in the United States." Based on a telephone survey of 1,539 individuals, the authors estimated that in 1990, Americans had made 425 million visits to "providers of unconventional therapy" at a cost of approximately $13.7 billion. The media gave massive publicity to the study as evidence that "alternative therapies" were very popular. This interpretation was incorrect, however, because the survey was improperly designed. The study's authors defined "unconventional therapies" as "medical intervention not taught widely at U.S. medical schools or generally available at U.S. hospitals"—a definition much broader than the usual definition of "alternative therapies." Moreover, the survey included some approaches that are medically appropriate (self-help groups such as Alcoholics Anonymous and Weight Watchers, for example) and some that may or may not be appropriate, depending on the circumstances (relaxation therapy, biofeedback, hypnosis, massage, and commercial weight-loss clinics). Thus the reported totals were meaningless.

## The Electronic Soap-Box

The biggest factors in the spread of health misinformation are television talk shows and tabloid news programs. The typical talk-show guest has written a popular book, is promoted by a professional public relations firm, and can afford to spend lots of time publicizing his claims because book sales will repay him for the time. Opponents of quackery are rarely in this position. Some opponents are willing to appear on talk shows in their home community and in other cities when they attend professional meetings. But virtually all of them have other professional duties (teaching, research, or patient care) that limit their availability for public appearances.

All the major television talk shows have given tremendous publicity to promoters of quackery. Critics rarely appear on these shows, and when they do, they are almost always outnumbered by proponents and by members of the audience who give testimonials. The most dangerous example I have seen was Sally Jesse Raphael's 1988 program in which four patients stated that an unconventional method had cured them of cancer when conventional methods had failed. Although a token rebuttal expert was permitted to comment briefly, she could not evaluate these claims because she was unable to investigate them before the show. Subsequent investigation by "Inside Edition" found that three of the four had not been cured and the fourth, who had been treated conventionally, had a good prognosis (see Chapter 6). "Inside Edition" has great interest in protecting the public against health frauds and quackery and has produced a steady flow of excellent reports.

Among television tabloids, CBS's "60 Minutes" is by far the worst offender. In 1990, for example, it aired a half-hour program called "Poison in Your Mouth," which suggested that mercury-amalgam fillings were dangerous. Although this allegation was false (see Chapter 22), the broadcast induced many viewers to seek replacement of their fillings with other materials.

After the program was broadcast, I wrote to executive producer Don Hewitt, explaining why I thought the program was irresponsible. I also asked, "How come you have never aired a program on the most serious danger of them all: cigarette smoking? Is it a policy of your program to attack only nonexistent health risks?" CBS's director of audience services replied: "Our aim was not to condemn dentists or their use of silver amalgam fillings. . . . Rather, the *60 MINUTES* staff made every effort to ensure that our report was balanced in presenting arguments from both sides of the issue."

A few months later, the harmfulness of the program was demonstrated by a letter published in *Consumer Reports*:

> My mother, who was diagnosed with Lou Gehrig's disease more than two years ago, had her mercury fillings removed immediately after the show aired. After she had spent $10,000 and endured more than 18 hours of dental work so painful she once fainted in the waiting room, her condition did not improve. The pain was outweighed only by the monumental disappointment she and the whole family experienced as we lived through one false hope.

In the spring of 1993, "60 Minutes" struck again with a program called "Sharks Don't Get Cancer," narrated by Mike Wallace and focusing on the theories of biochemist William I. Lane, Ph.D., author of *Sharks Don't Get Cancer*. Wallace began by calling attention to the book and stating that Lane says that sharks don't get cancer. The program focused on a study in Cuba of twenty-nine "terminal" cancer patients who were given shark-cartilage preparations. Although the program contained many disclaimers, it was clearly promotional. Wallace visited the site of the experiment, filmed several of the patients doing exercise, and reported that most of patients felt better several weeks after the treatment had begun. (The fact that "feeling better" does not indicate whether a cancer treatment is effective was not mentioned.) Two American cancer specialists then described the results as intriguing. One, who is aligned with the health-food industry, said that three of the patients appeared to have improved. The other, who appeared to be solidly scientific, noted that evaluation was difficult because many of the x-ray films were of poor quality, but he thought that a few tumors had gotten smaller. (The reasons why this might not be significant were not mentioned.) After noting that shark cartilage was sold in health-food stores, Wallace remarked on the inadvisability of "going to the nearest health-food store" and was seconded by the radiation therapist who said it would be foolish to do so unless all else had failed.

About two weeks before the program aired, a leading manufacturer of shark-cartilage capsules telephoned health-food retailers about the program and advised them to stock up on their product. Following the program, other manufacturers began marketing shark-cartilage products and referring to the program in their advertising. The leading distributor of books to health food stores has advertised *Sharks Don't Get Cancer* with the headline: "As featured on 60 Minutes. Finally, What The World Has Been Waiting For . . . A Major

Cancer Breakthrough." Meanwhile, a review by the National Cancer Institute concluded that the data from the Cuban study were scanty and unimpressive.

Curiously, Mike Wallace neglected to mention an important fact. Like all animals, sharks *do* get cancer. Lane's book actually says so, although it claims that the number is "insignificant." The preface notes that "while *ALMOST No Sharks Get Cancer* might have been a bit more accurate, it would have been a rotten title." The Smithsonian Institute's *Registry of Tumors in Lower Animals* indicates that sharks even get cancers of their cartilage.

## Tabloid Newspapers

Tabloid newspapers are another steady source of health misinformation. In 1987, I analyzed 322 articles on health, nutrition, and psychology appearing during a three-month period in *National Enquirer, Globe, National Examiner, Sun,* and *Weekly World News* and concluded that only 135 (42 percent) were reliable. Nutrition articles scored especially poorly, because many of them were based on the views of promoters of nutrition misinformation.

One article in the *National Examiner,* for example, claimed that "a miraculous diet pill will flatten your tummy . . . and you can do it fast without a complicated diet program." The article discussed the Optifast system of weight control, a reputable, medically supervised program. However, the program is not simple, the results are not instant, and the pills involved do not cause weight loss but simply add nutrients to the low-calorie program. "How to Use Vitamins and Minerals to Beat Stress," which appeared in the *National Enquirer,* claimed that "some 50 million Americans may suffer stress and stress-related problems due to vitamin and mineral deficiencies," which is complete nonsense. Articles like these can cause harm by inducing people to waste money on worthless or overblown products.

I also examined 247 articles involving supernatural beliefs, faith healers, psychics, alleged kidnappings by space aliens, and similar topics. All but eight presented occult events as factual. Few of the articles contained skeptical comments, and fewer still suggested that their writers did much investigating. When asked about this, *Weekly World News* editor Eddie Clontz replied, "We don't question ourselves out of a story. We think people enjoy reading about these things whether they believe them or not. . . . We'll publish things if we know the writer and we believe the information was presented in good faith." *Globe's* editorial director Mike Nevard said his policy was "to publish only stories that we can verify—except in areas of the occult—where such verification is impossible." Articles on occult topics tend to reinforce false beliefs in supernatural forces, which I believe is harmful to our society.

## The Media As Label

Under federal law, all products (except devices) intended for the cure, mitigation, treatment, or prevention of disease are regulated as drugs. Drug products cannot be legally marketed unless they are (1) recognized by experts as safe and effective, and (2) adequately labeled for their intended use. Labeling includes any written, printed, or graphic material that accompanies a product. Intended use is determined by the facts at hand.

Suppose a manufacturer wishes to market a vitamin concoction for the treatment of cancer. Under federal law, the product would be a drug. Since no vitamin concoction has been proven effective as a cancer remedy, no such product could be legally marketed for that purpose. Thus it would be illegal for the label to state that the product is useful against cancer. It would also be illegal for the manufacturer to publish or distribute literature making such a claim. Placing the claim on the label or in product literature would invite seizure of the product by the FDA.

To evade the law's intent, the "health food" industry is organized to promote the ingredients in their products through books, magazines, newsletters, booklets, lectures, and radio and television broadcasts. As long as there is no direct collusion between manufacturers and publicists, the claims appearing in these media are legal under the doctrines of freedom of speech and freedom of the press. Publishers of magazines aligned with the industry know that as long as they promote the industry's products, they will attract advertising revenue. Manufacturers aligned with the industry know that as long as they advertise, they can count on articles that will generate sales of their products. Some "health food" magazines even place ads for the products adjacent to articles promoting their ingredients. Some trade magazines offer reprintable "consumer education" materials and sell reprints of their articles to retailers.

Book publishers know that health-food stores are interested in carrying books that promote the products sold in their stores. In fact, many publishers use this as a selling point. A few years ago, for example, Health Plus Publishers, of Scottsdale, Arizona, encouraged retailers to stock up on *How to Get Well,* by naturopath Paavo Airola:

> That book recommends vitamins, minerals and other supplements, herbs, juices, and natural foods for more than 60 common ailments, as well as equipment such as juicers, seed grinders, and flour mills.
>
> For example: for osteoporosis . . . you have the potential of selling: 14 vitamins and supplements, modestly estimated at $5.00/product; 5 herbal products @ $3.00 each; groceries . . . $20; possibly a piece or two of equipment such as a juicer or seed grinder ($200). TOTAL:

$305.00 . . . And your customer will most likely return for replenishment of supplements and foods.

These figures might not be accurate, but you get the picture. Now multiply these figures times hundreds of customers and 60+ ailments, and you can see what far-reaching effects one book such as *How to Get Well* can have on your overall sales volume.

Nutri-Books, of Denver, Colorado, describes itself as the world's largest supplier of health-related books and magazines. Its merchandising manual for retailers states:

Books and magazines are your "silent sales force." . . . They tell your customers what your products will do for them. They explain the ways your products can be used. Very often this is information you may not be able to give—or may not be permitted to discuss."

The box below lists periodicals that are aligned with the health-food industry in one way or another. Most encourage unnecessary or unproven use of "dietary supplements" and other "alternative" health methods. Most are unfairly critical of scientific medical care, the food industry, and/or government consumer-protection agencies.

---

**Publications Philosophically Aligned with the Health-Food Industry**

*Magazines*
Better Nutrition for Today's Living; Body, Mind & Spirit; The Choice; Choices; Delicious!; Energy Times; FACT; Flex; Forefront; Health Consciousness; Health Counselor; Health Freedom News; Health Science; Health World; Healthier Times; Herbalgram; Holistic Medicine; The Human Ecologist; Innovation; Let's Live; Longevity; Muscle & Fitness; Natural Health (formerly East West); New Age Journal; New Body; Nutrition & Fitness; Nutritional Perspectives; Penthouse (Gary Null's articles); Prevention (editorials); Search for Health; Senior Health; Total Health; Townsend Letter for Doctors; Vegetarian Times; Your Health

*Newsletters*
Alternative Health Issues; Alternatives (published by David Williams; D.C.); Antha; Cancer Chronicles; Dr. Atkins' Health Revelations; Forefront; Fountain; Health & Healing; Health Alert; Health Resource Newsletter; HealthFacts; Men's Health Newsletter; Nutrition News (published by Siri Khalsa); People's Medical Society Newsletter; Pure Facts; Second Opinion

*Newspapers*
Health News & Review; Health Store News; Nutrition Health Review

**Lack of Peer Review**

Chapter 32 of this book describes how scientists are eager to point out the deficiencies in each other's theories and experimental techniques. This process of "peer review" is basic to scientific growth and the establishment of "scientific truth." The comparable goal of journalism is (or ought to be) to report accurate information. Yet journalists almost never publicly criticize each other's work—particularly when health topics are involved.

While the media seem to feel free to criticize whatever they please, and to demand that all sorts of officials and institutions be accountable, there is no visible accountability within the media itself. Have you ever seen a letter to the editor from a reporter who charged that his own newspaper or magazine misled the public in an article or advertisement about health? Have you ever heard a radio or TV commentator state that misinformation about health was broadcast on his station? Have you ever seen an editorial in print which charged that a health topic was mishandled by another publication? Have you ever seen an expression of editorial outrage directed against poor reporting that could cause thousands of unsuspecting people to become victims of quackery? Have you ever encountered a warning that the "miracle" claims found frequently in the tabloid newspapers are not worth the paper they are printed on? Except for *Consumer Reports* and a few other publications listed in the Appendix of this book, there seems to be an unwritten rule that reporters and editors never criticize each other's health-related errors in public.

Another thing I have observed is that major media almost never retract misinformation even when faced with indisputable evidence that they have erred. This point was brought home following the recent uproar over an NBC "Dateline" program in which a General Motors Corporation (GMC) truck exploded in flames after a car crashed into its side. When GMC protested, NBC officials dismissed the protests as unwarranted—until GMC filed suit and announced proof that the truck had been rigged with small rockets that had exploded seconds before the crash. NBC quickly issued an apology, and many media outlets criticized NBC's misconduct. *As far as I know, no comparable retraction or criticism has ever taken place following a botched quackery-related story, even one that was capable of killing someone.*

# 32

# Why Quackery Persists

James Harvey Young, Ph.D.

Americans, generally being an optimistic people, have believed that problems are for solving. Early in this century, when quackery came to be recognized as a major problem in the health field, many observers predicted its certain death. Common sense, increasing education, the truths of science, and laws aimed at securing honest labeling would drive quackery from the marketplace. Especially as modern medicine developed and conquered one disease after another, anything so outmoded and unneeded as quackery would shortly wither away.

But this has not happened. Quite the contrary! Health quackery today is a multibillion-dollar business, and its future prospects look brighter still. Why does quackery persist in our modern scientific era? Let's seek an explanation for this disturbing fact by examining the roles of four parties involved: the patient, the scientific practitioner, the quack, and the regulator who enforces antiquackery laws.

## The Patient

The field of health is extremely complicated. The common man—whom we shall call John Doe—has absorbed a great mass of information about it. What he knows, however, is likely a jumble of chance facts learned from a variety of sources, sound and unsound, including the folklore of family tradition and the self-serving pitch of current advertising. Statistically, perhaps, most people may be nearer right than wrong, but few people escape blind spots and areas of error that make them vulnerable to deception under suitable circumstances.

This goes even for some John Does of mighty intellect with various degrees after their name.

When an episode of ill health looms, John Doe faces it by self-reliance, by seeking help from a health authority, or by doing both. If he chooses self-treatment, he tries some remedy from folk tradition or from recent reading or television viewing. He may try garlic from the garden, a huge dose of vitamin C, or a trade-named tonic. He tends to judge results by the same rule-of-thumb common sense by which he judges everyday cause-and-effect sequences: Did the axe cut? Did the suit fit? Did the motor run? He asks: Did the symptoms go away? Did my digestion settle down? Did my nerves calm? Did my sniffles stop?

John Doe does not usually realize that most ailments are self-limiting and improve with time *regardless of treatment.* When a symptom goes away after he doses himself with a remedy, he is likely to credit the remedy with curing him. He does not realize that he would have gotten better just as quickly if he had done nothing! He may also fail to distinguish between cure and temporary symptom relief. Thousands of well-meaning John and Jane Does have boosted the fame of folk remedies and have signed sincere testimonials for patent medicines, crediting them, instead of the body's recuperative powers, for a return to well-being.

Nor does John Doe take the "placebo" effect into account when he judges remedies. Worry has a great effect upon how we feel when we are ill. The more we are worried about being sick, the more uncomfortable our symptoms will seem. Conversely, the less we are worried, the better we may feel. When John Doe takes a remedy that he thinks will help, he will often feel less pain or discomfort. Feeling better when the doctor walks into the room is another example of this mechanism. The placebo effect can work in a second way. Some ailments that are bodily reactions to tension subside when the feeling that a person is taking an effective treatment lessens the tension.

A considerable element in the success of the legitimate proprietary remedies purchased at the drugstore undoubtedly resides in the placebo effect. Spokespersons for the proprietary industry have occasionally acknowledged this. Exaggerated claims made in advertising may build up consumers' expectations even more and so enhance the placebo effect. Yet such a slim benefit does not justify exaggeration. Overuse of occasionally useful drugs poses health hazards. Youth's readiness to experiment with dangerous drugs may owe something to the attitude, conditioned by constant advertising, that a drug exists to banish almost any problem. A good deal of advertising implies that common remedies are somehow able to do more than relieve simple symptoms, that they can make a person socially desirable or can solve undesirable behavior like "snapping at your wife." Moreover, too much or too long a reliance on self-dosage, in violation of label warnings, may lead people to delay getting more appropriate treatment for serious ailments before it is too late. Outright quackery, of course, operates without any of the restraints under which the proprietary industry abides and hence poses a danger far greater.

The John Doe whom I have been describing so far turns to self-treatment occasionally when his normally healthy life is disrupted. Some of his unhappy cousins, however, live in constant fear of imminent health disaster. They seem governed by an all-consuming anxiety that leads to continuous self-treatment, often with bizarre "preventive" programs. An example might be taking twenty-five food supplement pills per day. Some beleaguered patients go so far as to follow all-inclusive systems that mix diet practices, exercises, gadgetry, and mystical philosophies. Such life-style combination approaches, indeed, represent a growing segment of unscientific therapy. Such troubled people provide an important reservoir for quack exploitation.

Often, of course, these worriers abandon self-treatment and join a guru-led group—just as less extreme John and Jane Does might give up self-reliance and seek help from someone touted as an "expert" in the media. A great deal of public confusion exists about who is a competent health authority.

Some patients have an authority problem and tend to reject the orthodox merely because it is orthodox. Others turn to unscientific practitioners under a miss-no-bets philosophy. They believe in family doctors as treaters of physical ailments and prescribers of drugs; however, they also believe in chiropractors as manipulators of bones and perhaps as operators of "healing" machines. They likewise follow the gospel of food faddists. And they sense nothing wrong with using several such forms of treatment at the same time, science and pseudoscience having equal validity in their minds.

One last point about the patient: When his health is seriously threatened, he obviously hopes something may be done to cure him. His desires may outrun what responsible orthodoxy can accomplish, however. Confronted with the possibility of chronic suffering or death, many people who never before strayed from orthodox treatment are not able to accept orthodoxy's grim verdict and so turn elsewhere. Such desperation has fattened quackery related to cancer and to AIDS.

## The Scientific Practitioner

The medical profession has always believed its current knowledge valid and has sometimes exhibited a tendency toward smugness. On occasion—though rarely in recent years—true scientific breakthroughs have been regarded as quackery. Conversely, many treatments that were once highly regarded have been abandoned as worthless. As medical science improves, of course, it becomes easier to draw the line between orthodoxy and quackery. Ignoring this fact, quacks parade medicine's old mistakes and portray themselves as scientists ahead of their time who are being suppressed by a greedy establishment.

Many people have suffered side effects from modern "miracle" drugs. This circumstance, added to the overprescribing of antibiotics, tranquilizers, and stimulants, has helped foster a stereotype of our nation being "drugged," thereby giving "natural" healers a promotional boost. In the early nineteenth century, quacks termed the doctor a butcher; today they call him a poisoner.

Scientific physicians, moreover, have a problem because of their power and status. Many laypersons feel ill at ease in the presence of an expert. The patient is upset because he is sick and worried. Perceiving the physician as busy and under pressure, the patient may feel like an intruder. Doctors may be brusque, fail to take the time to listen, or neglect to explain; their prognoses may be discouraging, their therapy prolonged and unpleasant. They charge hefty fees, earn more money, and live better than the patient, perhaps causing irritation and envy. Some patients are just plain frightened away from reputable doctors whose amiability falls below that which quacks are able to muster. Even patients who think well of their own doctors may think ill of doctors as a group. The power side of establishment medicine has alienated many people. Organized medicine, they have felt, works for its own economic and political self-interest more than for the common good. Such an image in the popular mind aids and abets quackery. Indeed, throughout history, any criticism of the power or the science of orthodox medicine has been pounced upon by the quack, magnified, and loudly trumpeted abroad.

## The Quack

The unscientific healer does not need to observe the restraints of reputable medicine. Where true medical science is complex, the quack can oversimplify. All diseases are "imbalances," and whatever the quack does restores "balance." Where ailments are self-limiting, the quack makes nature his secret ally, crediting his tonic with curing tuberculosis when in fact nature has alleviated the patient's postnasal drip. Where the placebo effect may operate, the quack prescribes it adeptly. It may be something for arthritis as ancient as a copper bracelet or as modern as "moon dust."

The quack pays more attention to the person than to the ailment, seeking to convince the patient that the treatment is necessary. A dose of fright can be an effective persuader. Ralph Lee Smith, in his book *At Your Own Risk,* tells of infiltrating a school run by a Texas chiropractor aimed at teaching other chiropractors how to increase their incomes. "If *the patient has a pain in his left shoulder,*" the professor said, his pupils should ask, "*Has the pain started in your right shoulder yet?*" [The so-called "Yet Disease."]

Along with fright go tenderness and self-confidence. Most quacks manage a superb "bedside manner." Since they can't really provide a cure if major disease is present, they specialize in promises, sympathy, consideration, concern, and reassurance. The patient responds to such attention. This helps explain one of the odd paradoxes relating to quackery—that failure seldom diminishes patient loyalty. When regulatory agencies seek to prosecute quacks, the agencies have a difficult task getting hapless patients to testify in court. Partly this results from the desire to avoid public exposure as a dupe; but often this objection to testifying rests on an inability to realize that deception has taken place. Many quacks do such a good job of exuding sincerity that their explanations seem all too plausible. Even patients faced with death believe in the "kindly" person who says the special remedy would have worked if treatment had only begun a little sooner.

Some points I have made suggest that doctors might improve their human relationships. Other aspects of vulnerability may be so inherent in human nature that they can never be eliminated. While physicians seek to help their patients if they can, they must sometimes confess that they cannot. Quacks need make no such confession, for honesty is not contained in their code of ethics. This gives charlatans a great advantage in competing with physicians for the kind of patient I have described. For quacks can promise anything—tailoring their appeals to all the susceptibilities, vulnerabilities, and curiosities which human nature reveals.

## The Regulator

A fabric of laws aimed at circumscribing the quack has been created during this century. Regulators wielding these laws have won significant victories. The Federal Trade Commission has quashed much deceptive advertising. The Food and Drug Administration and the Postal Service have driven many fraudulent drugs and devices from the marketplace and have put some charlatans in jail. The Kefauver-Harris Act of 1962 requires that new drugs be proven effective as well as safe before they can be marketed. As a result of this law, many quack ventures have failed to see the light of day or have been quickly suppressed.

But regulation has not stifled quackery. In order to act against a deceptive health promotion, the regulator must first learn of its existence and then determine whether regulatory action is practical. Some forms of quackery escape detection and others evade prosecution because the overall budget of regulators is insufficient to attack all of the illegal activities they observe. Matters of major public concern other than quackery clamor for their attention. Frauds that threaten only the purse, not the health, of the victims get low priority on the regulatory scale. Though some quack promotions are quickly stopped, others can result in lengthy court battles while the promotions continue.

Many times the regulator must compromise, allowing a wrongdoer to escape severe penalty because full prosecution would overtax the limited resources of the regulator. At other times, the regulator must suffer the leniency of the courts. While the average judge may become duly outraged when a victim of quackery is seriously harmed, in the majority of cases, no such victim is in sight. The con artist who peddles phony "reducing belts" for $9.95 is unlikely to be sent to prison even if his total take amounts to millions of dollars. For small sums of money, the courts seem to feel, fools must be allowed to suffer the consequences of their folly.

The regulator's task would be eased greatly if victims of quackery would rally to his support. But an opposite trend is evident: many victims are so thoroughly deceived that they engage in political activities that oppose regulation. During the 1970s, when the FDA tried to limit false claims and dangerously high doses of vitamins, a coalition of vitamin sellers and their brainwashed customers persuaded both Congress and the courts to limit FDA jurisdiction over this matter (see Chapter 28). When the FTC considered banning commercial use of the words "natural" and "organic," another avalanche of protest persuaded the agency to back down. The health-food industry continues to lobby fiercely to prevent the FDA from strengthening labeling regulations to curb the industry's deceptions.

In some instances the regulator has been so cleverly labeled a villain in the quack's promotion that the very existence of regulation has been made to enhance quackery's appeal. Events like Vietnam and Watergate created widespread disillusionment with government. Inflation, the filling-out of tedious forms, and other irritating circumstances evoked widespread assertions of overregulation. Quacks profit from such distrust. It makes them sound credible when they charge that health regulators are not interested in the welfare of the individual but are conspiring selfishly with the medical profession, the drug industry, or the food industry.

Antigovernment feeling certainly helped the promoters of laetrile, an unproven and ultimately discredited cancer remedy, to generate the greatest public furor over an unorthodox remedy in our nation's history. Crying "freedom of choice," supporters of this quack remedy pressed mightily to persuade state legislators and the courts to legalize its use. Half the states passed laws giving laetrile special status, and one federal judge authorized its importation by "terminal" cancer patients, a ruling that lasted for a dozen years until higher courts forced its reversal.

Close inspection of the "freedom of choice" slogan is in order. Freedom, one of the glorious words in our lexicon, can arouse powerful sympathy. But freedom of choice cannot operate in a vacuum; the easier it is to market unproven health products, the easier it will be to mislead people into trying them. What quacks really wants is freedom from government interference with their promotions. Laws that require proof of efficacy before marketing make it too easy, as the shady promoter sees it, to remove their products from the marketplace. The National Health Federation, an alliance of quackery promoters and their followers, has for years tried to persuade Congress to repeal the 1962 law. Repeal of the efficacy requirement would put back on the regulator's shoulders the burden of proving that each worthless product lacked value—a task far more demanding than the present law requires. The resultant "freedom" would benefit only quacks whose chicanery is too sophisticated for the average citizen to recognize.

There is another aspect of the freedom theme to consider. Desperate victims and their families, having just heard a diagnosis of cancer or AIDS, may soon find themselves pressed by zealous promoters to try an unorthodox remedy for which glowing promises are made. Under the double stress of fear and salesmanship, many sick persons are unable to exercise sensible freedom of choice. Such sufferers especially need the protection of experts who can evaluate alleged remedies honestly.

A special case has been made that patients with "terminal" disease should have ready access to quack remedies. The argument is appealing but specious. Should swindlers be allowed to "comfort" terminal patients by selling them phony stock—telling them it will make them rich before they die—on the theory that they don't need their money anyway? Moreover, even if it were possible to pinpoint the terminal state (which it usually is not), there is no way to open the door for one group of patients without opening it for others. The Supreme Court recognized this fact when it ruled unanimously in 1979 in a laetrile case that no exception to the 1962 efficacy law should be made for so-called terminal cancer patients. Congress, the high court ruled, had not intended to protect only those suffering from curable diseases.

"Freedom of choice" in this context turns out to be a way of manipulating a cherished symbol so as to free quacks from the law's restraints. We need strong antiquackery laws enforced by dedicated regulators.

**What of the Future?**

Efforts to educate against the dangers of quackery have met with modest success. But the future of quackery remains bright because many people have attitudes that make them highly vulnerable. Fears of dread diseases hold high priority on the list of our citizens' worries. They have, moreover, become skeptical of gigantic institutions, including big science, and many look askance at reason as a way for seeking truth. Whatever merit may lie in suspecting reason's inadequacies, the reaction has often gone to an extreme of deliberate flirtation, if not open liaison, with wild varieties of unreason. The acceptance of astrology has soared, not merely as a pastime but as a legitimate "science," even in high places. Publishing houses have made millions from it. During the 1960s, almost every college campus had a peripheral course in "reading the stars." Spiritualism made a comeback, with "spiritual churches" blossoming in almost every city. Tarot cards, palmistry, and numerology flourished. Witchcraft and devil worship made an appearance. Paperbacks on these themes were among the hottest items in university bookstores. Many among the young turned their backs on civilization and its discontents, displaying a new primitivism, sometimes retreating into communes remotely located, sometimes merely buying "organic" foods at the nearest health-food store.

The decade of the 1970s witnessed an enormous boom in the self-help search for health. Though wholesome in many ways—if, for example, exercise and dieting are governed by prudence—a passionate dedication to self-help can be wasteful of money and harmful to health if guided by wrong counsel. With respect to eating, wrong counsel abounded—and still does— much of it aimed at selling books or special dietary wares. During the 1980s, "channeling" and the "New Age" became household words, dubious weight-loss ventures boomed, bogus "immune boosters" and "ergogenic aids" found a ready market, and the health-food industry continued to exploit public concern about "chemicalization" of our society. In the 1990s, the promotion of "alternative" methods has appealed to a public hungry for choices and control over its destiny.

One may strongly sympathize, I hope, with criticisms of the disorders of our world. But those who embrace irrational creeds fervently, who throw themselves headlong into self-help regimens, furnish a fertile recruiting ground for unscientific health wares. For, as we have seen, quacks are agile. They sense quickly and rush in to exploit people's real concerns. Thus, for many timeless reasons, and for current reasons too, quackery may be expected to continue, to expand, and to remain a challenge to scientific health care.

Quacks never sleep. But education and regulation can reduce the toll they take in wasted resources and human suffering.

# 33

# The Truth-Seekers

### Stephen Barrett, M.D.

One way to avoid being robbed of cash and health is to get good information when you need it. Most of this book tells about people who can cheat you because they are confused or dishonest. In this chapter, let's talk about where you can get honest, true, and accurate answers to your health questions.

First, what is meant by "truth" in medical science and how is it determined? Humans have always been curious about disease and what causes it. The more we understand, of course, the better we can control illness. Down through the centuries, countless people have shared their observations and ideas. Thousands of theories have been formulated to explain the reasons behind various phenomena. During the past century, however, mere theorizing has been supplanted by sound knowledge based on experimentation and sound clinical experience. Armed with this new knowledge, doctors have been able to prevent and cure many diseases in a way that seems almost miraculous.

As part of the process of scientific development, good methods have developed to test whether theories are logical. The sum of these methods is known as the "experimental" or "scientific" method, which is used to answer questions like: "If two things happen, are they related or coincidental?" For example, suppose you take a pill when you have a headache and the headache goes away. How can we tell whether the pill relieved you or whether the headache would have gone away by itself without medication? Throughout the world, hundreds of thousands of scientists work continuously to determine the boundaries of scientific thought.

As mountains of information are collected, how can we tell which evidence is valid? "Valid" means honestly collected and properly interpreted—

using good techniques of statistical analysis. One hallmark of a good experiment is that others can repeat it and get the same results.

This brings us to the question of who can interpret experimental findings. Scientists are judging each other all the time. People with equal or superior training look for loopholes in experimental techniques and design other experiments to test conclusions. Skilled reviewers also gather in groups whose collective level of ability far exceeds that of the average scientist. Such experts are not likely to be misled by poorly designed experiments. Among the reviewers are editors and editorial boards of scientific journals; these people carefully screen out invalid findings and enable significant ones to be published. As good ideas are put to use, more reports are generated. When controversies arise, further research can be devised to settle them. Gradually a shared set of beliefs is developed that is felt to be scientifically accurate. Expert panels convened by government agencies, professional groups, voluntary health agencies, and other organizations also contribute to this effort. When we speak of the "scientific community," we refer to this overall process of separating what is scientific fact from what is not.

Quacks, of course, operate outside of the scientific community. They do not use the scientific method to evaluate what they see. In fact, they seldom bother to experiment at all. (Nor do they report their failures.) Quacks try to cover up their inadequacies by pointing out that the scientific community has made mistakes in the past. This, of course, is true; but in recent years, the chances of major error by the scientific community have decreased greatly. So if you find someone referred to as a "scientist ahead of his time," he is probably a quack!

## How to Get Help

Where should you go if you want advice about a health problem? The best source is probably your own doctor. Chapters 9 and 35 of this book should help you find a doctor who is trustworthy. If your doctor can't provide what you need, he or she should be able to help you find the answer.

What if your doctor can't help you? Or what if you want supplementary reading material or general information? There are many places you can contact. If you write for information, be sure to keep in mind that the person who receives your letter may be extremely busy. You will most likely receive a helpful response if you do the following:

• Type your letter. Make sure your return address is on the letter as well as the envelope, and include your telephone number.

• Ask your question as specifically as possible.

• Tell something about yourself and why you need the information. Indicate briefly what you already know or have read.

• Enclose a stamped, self-addressed envelope large enough to accommodate what might be sent.

• If writing to a voluntary organization, consider making a small donation if you can afford one.

Here are the names of organizations that offer reliable health information and sometimes free services. Most of them are nonprofit and noncommercial. Use them in good health!

## Federal Government Agencies

U.S. Department of Agriculture, Washington, DC 20250
    Food and Nutrition Information Center: 301-504-5414 (for consumer questions)
    Food and Nutrition Service: 3101 Park Center Dr., Alexandria, VA 22302
    Human Nutrition Information Service: 6505 Belcrest Rd., Hyattsville, MD 20782
       (primarily a research agency)
    Cooperative Extension Services are located in many cities (see telephone directory
       blue pages)
Centers for Disease Control and Prevention, Office of Public Inquiries, 1600 Clifton Road,
    N.E., Atlanta, GA 30333
Clearinghouse on Child Abuse and Neglect Information, P.O. Box 1182, Washington, DC
    20013
Consumer Information Center, P.O. Box 100, Pueblo CO 81002 (free and low-cost
    publications)
Consumer Product Safety Commission, 5401 Westbard Ave., Bethesda, MD 20207
Environmental Protection Agency (EPA), 401 M St., S.W., Washington, DC 20460
Food and Drug Administration, 5600 Fishers Lane, Rockville, MD 20857
    Consumer Affairs Offices:
    201 E. Indianola, Phoenix AZ 85012
    1521 W. Pico Blvd., Los Angeles, CA 90015, 213-252-7597
    50 United Nations Plaza, San Francisco, CA 94102, 415-556-1458
    P.O. Box 25087, Denver, CO 80225, 303-236-3018
    6601 N.W. 25th St., Miami, FL 33159, 305-526-2919
    7200 Lake Ellenor Drive, Orlando, FL 32809, 407-648-6922
    60-8th St., N.E., Atlanta, GA 30309, 404-347-7355
    300 S. Riverside Plaza, Chicago, IL 60606, 312-353-7126
    101 W. Ohio St., Indianapolis, IN 46204, 317-226-6500
    4298 Elysian Fields Ave., New Orleans, LA 70122, 504-589-2420
    One Montvale Ave., Stoneham, MA 02180, 617-279-1479
    900 Madison Ave., Baltimore, MD 21201, 301-962-3731
    1560 E. Jefferson Ave., Detroit, MI 48207, 313-226-6260

240 Hennepin Ave., Minneapolis, MN 55401, 612-334-4103
1009 Cherry St., Kansas City, MO 63106, 816-374-6086
808 N. Collins Alley, St. Louis, MO 63102, 314-425-5021
200 S. 16th St., Omaha, NE 68102, 402-221-4675
61 Main St., West Orange, NJ 07052, 201-645-6365
850 Third Ave., Brooklyn, NY 11232, 718-965-5043
599 Delaware Ave., Buffalo, NY 14202, 716-846-4483
320 Central Ave., Brunswick, OH 44212, 216-273-1038
1141 Central Parkway, Cincinnati, OH 45202, 513-684-3501
Room 900 U.S. Customhouse, 2nd & Chestnut Sts., Philadelphia, PA 19106,
    215-597-0837
P.O. Box 5719, Puerto de Tierra Sta., San Juan, PR 00906, 809-729-6852
297 Plus Park Blvd., Nashville, TN 37217, 615-781-5372
3032 Bryan St., Dallas, TX 75204, 214-655-5315
1445 North Loop West, Houston, TX 77008, 713-220-2322
10127 Morocco, San Antonio, TX 78216, 512-229-4531
1110 N. Glebe Rd., Arlington, VA 22201, 703-285-2578
22201 23rd Drive, S.E., Bothell, WA 98021, 206-483-4953
U.S. Court House Rm. 5-B-06, 517 E. Wisconsin Ave., Milwaukee, WI 53202,
    414-297-3097
Federal Trade Commission, 6th & Pennsylvania Ave., N.W., Washington, DC 20580
Health Care Financing Administration (HCFA), 200 Independence Ave., S.W.,
    Washington, DC 20201
National AIDS Information Clearinghouse, P.O. Box 6003, Bethesda, MD 20850
National Cholesterol Information Education Program Information Center, 4733 Bethesda
    Ave., Room 530, Bethesda, MD 20814.
National Health Information Clearinghouse, P.O. Box 1133, Washington, DC 20013
National Information Center for Rare Diseases and Orphan Drugs, 450 5th St., Washington,
    DC 20001
National Institutes of Health, 9000 Rockville Pike, Bethesda, MD 20892
    National Cancer Institute
    National Eye Institute
    National Heart, Lung, and Blood Institute
    National Institute of Allergy and Infectious Diseases
    National Institute of Arthritis and Musculoskeletal and Skin Diseases
    National Institute of Diabetes and Digestive and Kidney Diseases
    National Institute of Child Health and Human Development
    National Institute of Dental Research
    National Institute of Mental Health
    National Institute of Neurological Disorders and Stroke
    National Institute on Aging
    National Institute on Alcohol Abuse and Alcoholism
    National Institute on Drug Abuse
National Maternal and Child Health Clearinghouse, 38th & R St., N.W., Washington, DC
    20057
Office of Technology Assessment, U.S. Congress, Washington, DC 20510
Office on Smoking and Health, 5600 Fishers Lane, Rockville, MD 20857
U.S. Postal Service, 475 L'Enfant Plaza, Washington, DC 20260
President's Council on Physical Fitness and Sports, 450 E. 5th St., Washington, DC 20201

## Voluntary and Professional Organizations

Most of the organizations listed below are voluntary groups that draw support and members from the general public as well as from professionals. Some have a single national office, while others have chapters in various cities. Most of these organizations provide educational materials on request. Some raise and distribute funds for research. Some conduct educational programs for the public and encourage and develop local support groups. Some offer individual counseling.

Business and professional groups are composed exclusively or primarily of health professionals or other professionally trained individuals. Most of these groups publish a scientific journal and hold educational meetings for their members. Most of them also help the public by setting professional standards, disseminating information through the news media, and responding to inquiries from individual consumers.

Action on Smoking and Health, 2013 H St., N.W., Washington, DC 20006 (nonsmokers' rights)
Al-Anon Family Group Headquarters, P.O. Box 862, Midtown Station, New York, NY 10018
Alcoholics Anonymous, P.O. Box 459, Grand Central Station, New York, NY 10163
Alexander Graham Bell Institute for the Deaf, 3417 Volta Pl., N.W., Washington, DC 20007
Amyotrophic Lateral Sclerosis Association, 21021 Ventura Blvd., Woodland Hills, CA 91364
Alzheimer's Disease and Related Disorders Association, 70 E. Lake St., Chicago, IL 60601
American Academy of Allergy and Immunology, 611 E. Wells St., Milwaukee, WI 53202
American Academy of Family Physicians, 8880 Ward Parkway, Kansas City, MO 64114
American Academy of Ophthalmology, 655 Beach St., P.O. Box 7424, San Francisco, CA 94109
American Academy of Otolaryngology-Head and Neck Surgery, 1 Prince St., Alexandria, VA 22314
American Academy of Pediatrics, 141 Northwest Point Blvd., Elk Grove Village, IL 60009
American Alliance for Health, Physical Education, Recreation and Dance, 1900 Association Drive, Reston, VA 22091
American Association for Counseling and Development, 5999 Stevenson Ave., Alexandria, VA 22304
American Association for the History of Medicine, Boston Univ. School of Medicine, 80 E. Concord St., Boston, MA 02118
American Association for Marriage and Family Therapy, 1100 17th St., N.W., Washington, DC 20036
American Association for Partial Hospitalization, 1411 K St., N.W., Washington, DC 20005
American Association for the Study of Headache, 875 Kings Highway, West Deptford, NJ 08096
American Association of Blood Banks, 1117 N. 19th St., Arlington, VA 22209

American Association of Homes for the Aging, 1129 20th St., NW, Suite 400, Washington, DC 20036

American Association of Kidney Patients, 1 Davis Blvd., Tampa, FL 33306

American Association of Pastoral Counselors, 9508A Lee Highway., Fairfax, VA 22031

American Association of Plastic Surgeons, 10666 N. Torrey Pines Rd., La Jolla, CA 92037

American Association of Retired Persons, 601 E St., N.W., Washington, DC 20049

American Association of Sex Educators, Counselors, and Therapists, 435 N. Michigan Ave., Chicago, IL 60611

American Association of Suicidology, 2459 S. Ash, Denver, CO 80222

American Association on Mental Retardation, 1719 Kalorama Rd., N.W., Washington, DC 20009

American Board of Medical Specialties, 1 Rotary Center, Evanston, IL 60201

American Burn Association, Francis Scott Key Hospital, 4940 Eastern Ave., Baltimore, MD 21224

American Cancer Society, 1599 Clifton Road, N.E., Atlanta, GA 30329

American Celiac Society, 58 Musano Ct., West Orange, NJ 07052 (dietary guidance for celiac disease)

American Cleft Palate Association, 1218 Grandview Ave., Pittsburgh, PA 15211

American College Health Association, 1300 Piccard Dr., Suite 200, Rockville, MD 20850

American College of Cardiology, 9111 Old Georgetown Road, Bethesda, MD 20814

American College of Health Care Administrators, 325 S. Patrick St., Alexandria, VA 22314 (nursing homes)

American College of Obstetricians and Gynecologists, 409 12th St., S.W., Washington, DC 20024

American College of Physicians, Independence Mall W., 6th St. at Race, Philadelphia, PA 19106

American College of Radiology, 1891 Preston White Dr., Reston, VA 22091

American College of Sports Medicine, P.O. Box 1440, Indianapolis, IN 46206

American College of Surgeons, 55 E. Erie St., Chicago, IL 60611

American Council on Science and Health, 1995 Broadway, 2nd Floor, New York, NY 10023

American Dental Association, 211 E. Chicago, Ave., Chicago, IL 60611

American Diabetes Association, 1660 Duke St., Alexandria, VA 22314

American Dietetic Association, 216 W. Jackson Blvd., Chicago, IL 60606

American Epilepsy Society, 638 Prospect Ave., Hartford, CT 06105

American Family Foundation, P.O. Box 2265, Bonita Springs, FL 33959 (news and advice about cults)

American Federation of Home Health Agencies, 1320 Fenwick Lane, Silver Spring, MD 20910

American Fertility Society, 2140 11th Ave., Suite 200, Birmingham, AL 35205

American Foundation for AIDS Research, 5900 Wilshire Blvd., Los Angeles, CA 90036

American Foundation for the Blind, 15 W. 16th St., New York, NY 10011

American Geriatrics Society, 770 Lexington Ave., New York, NY 10021

American Group Psychotherapy Association, 25 E. 21st St., New York, NY 10010

American Health Care Association, 1201 L St., N.W., Washington, DC 20005 (nursing home standards)

American Heart Association, 7320 Greenville Ave., Dallas, TX 75231

American Hospital Association, 840 N. Lake Shore Drive, Chicago, IL 60611

American Industrial Hygiene Association, 345 White Pond Dr., Akron, OH 44320

American Institute of Nutrition, 9650 Rockville Pike, Bethesda, MD 20814
American Kidney Fund, 6110 Executive Blvd., Rockville, MD 20852
American Liver Foundation, 1425 Pompton Ave., Cedar Grove, NJ 07009
American Lung Association, 1740 Broadway, New York, NY 10019
American Medical Association, 515 N. State St., Chicago, IL 60610
American Medical Women's Association, 801 N. Fairfax St., Alexandria, VA 22314
American Medical Writers Association, 9650 Rockville Pike, Bethesda, MD 20814
American Mental Health Counselors Association, 5999 Stevenson Ave., Alexandria, VA
    22304
American Narcolepsy Association, P.O. Box 1187, San Carlos, CA 94070
American Nurses' Association, 2420 Pershing Rd., Kansas City, MO 64108
American Occupational Therapy Association, 1383 Piccard Dr., Rockville, MD 20850
American Ophthalmological Society, Duke University Eye Center, Durham, NC 27710
American Optometric Association, 243 N. Lindbergh Blvd., St. Louis, MO 63141
American Osteopathic Association, 142 East Ontario St., Chicago, IL 60611
American Parkinson Disease Association, 60 Bay St., Suite 401, Staten Island , NY 10301
American Pharmaceutical Association, 2215 Constitution Ave., N.W., Washington, DC
    20037
American Physical Therapy Association, 1111 N. Fairfax St., Alexandria, VA 22314
American Podiatric Medical Association, 9312 Old Georgetown Road, Bethesda, MD
    20814
American Psychiatric Association, 1400 K St., N.W., Washington, DC 20005
American Psychoanalytic Association, 309 E. 49th St., New York, NY 10022
American Psychological Association, 1200 17th St., N.W., Washington, DC 20036
American Public Health Association, 1015 15th St., Washington, DC 20005
American Red Cross, 17th & D Sts., N.W., Washington, DC 20006
American School Health Association, P.O. Box 708, Kent, OH 44240
American Sleep Disorders Association, 604 Second St., S.W., Rochester, MN 55902
American Social Health Association, P.O. Box 13827, Research Triangle Park, NC 27709
    (venereal disease)
American Society for Artificial Internal Organs, P.O. Box C, Boca Raton, FL 33429
American Society for Clinical Nutrition, 9650 Rockville Pike, Bethesda, MD 20814
American Society of Clinical Hypnosis, 2200 E. Devon Ave., Des Plaines, IL 60018
American Society of Clinical Oncology, 435 N. Michigan Ave., Chicago, IL 60611
American Society of Hematology, 6900 Grove Rd., Thorofare, NJ 08086
American Society of Internal Medicine, 1101 Vermont Ave., Washington, DC 20005
American Society of Law and Medicine, 765 Commonwealth Ave., Boston, MA 02215
American Society of Plastic and Reconstructive Surgeons, 444 E. Algonquin Rd.,
    Arlington Heights, IL 60005
American Speech-Language-Hearing Association, 10801 Rockville Pike, Rockville, MD
    20852
American Tinnitus Association, P.O. Box 5, Portland, OR 97207
American Urological Association, 1120 N. Charles St., Baltimore, MD 21201
American Transplant Association, P.O. Box 822123, Dallas, TX 75382
American Venereal Disease Association, P.O. Box 1753, Baltimore, MD 21203
American Veterinary Medical Association, 930 N. Mecham Rd., Schaumburg, IL 60196
Americans for Nonsmokers' Rights, 2530 San Pablo Ave., Berkeley, CA 94702
Arthritis Foundation, 1314 Spring St., N.W., Atlanta, GA 30309
Association for Retarded Citizens, P.O. Box 6109, Arlington, TX 76005

Association for the Advancement of Health Education, 1900 Association Dr., Reston, VA 22091

Association for the Care of Children's Health, 7910 Woodmont Ave., Bethesda, MD 20814

Association for Macular Diseases, 210 E. 64 St., New York, NY 10021

Association for Voluntary Sterilization, 122 42nd St., New York, NY 10168

Asthma and Allergy Foundation of America, 1125 15th St., NW, Washington, DC 20005

Autism Society of America, 8601 Georgia Ave., Silver Spring, MD 20910

Bald-Headed Men of America, 3819 Bridges St., Morehead City, NC 28557

Better Hearing Institute, Box 1840, Washington, DC 20013

Better Vision Institute, 1800 N. Kent St., Rosslyn, VA 22209

Blue Cross and Blue Shield Association of America, 676 N. St. Clair St., Chicago, IL 60611

Braille Institute of America, 741 N. Vermont Ave., Los Angeles, CA 90029

Cancer Care, Inc., 1180 Avenue of the Americas, New York, NY 10036

Candlelighters Childhood Cancer Foundation, 1312 18th St., N.W., Washington, DC 20006

Children of Aging Parents, 2761 Trenton Road, Levittown, PA 19056

Children's Healthcare Is a Legal Duty (CHILD), P.O. Box 2604, Sioux City, IA 51106

Children's Hearing Education and Research, 928 McLean Ave., Yonkers, NY 10704

Child Welfare League of America, 440 1st St., NW, Washington, DC 20001

Choice in Dying, 200 Varick St., New York, NY 10014 (death with dignity)

Committee for the Scientific Investigation of Claims of the Paranormal (CSICOP), P.O. Box 703, Amherst, NY 14226

Consumer Federation of America, 1424 16th St., N.W., Washington, DC 20036

Consumer Health Information Research Institute (CHIRI), 3521 Broadway, Kansas City, MO 64111.

Consumers Union, 101 Truman Ave., Yonkers, NY 10703

Cooley's Anemia Foundation, 105 E. 22nd St., New York, NY 10010

Council for Agricultural Science and Technology (CAST), 137 Lynn Ave., Ames, IA 50010 (nutrition, food science, and agriculture)

Council of Better Business Bureaus
   Headquarters Office: 1515 Wilson Blvd., Arlington, VA 22209
   National Advertising Division: 845 Third Ave., New York, NY 10017

Crohn's & Colitis Foundation, 444 Park Ave. South, New York, NY 10016

Cystic Fibrosis Foundation, 6931 Arlington Rd., 200, Bethesda, MD 20814

Deafness Research Foundation, 9 E. 38th St., New York, NY 10016

Delta Dental Plans Association, 211 E. Chicago Ave., Chicago, IL 60611 (dental insurance)

Doctors Ought to Care (DOC), 5510 Greenbriar, Suite 235, Houston, TX 77005 (tobacco and other preventive health issues)

Dysautonomia Foundation, 20 E. 46th St., New York, NY 10017

Dystonia Medical Research Foundation, 8383 Wilshire Blvd., Beverly Hills, CA 90211

ECRI, 5200 Butler Pike, Plymouth Meeting, PA 19462 (medical devices)

Emphysema Anonymous, P.O. Box 3224, Seminole, FL 34642

Endometriosis Association, 8585 N. 76th Pl., Milwaukee, WI 53223

Epilepsy Foundation of America, 4351 Garden City Dr., Landover, MD 20785

Eye Bank Association of America, 1725 I St., NW, Washington, DC 20006

Family Service America, 11700 W. Lake Park Dr., Milwaukee, WI 53224

Federated Ambulatory Surgery Association, 700 N. Fairfax St., Alexandria, VA 22314

Federation of Societies for Experimental Biology, 9650 Rockville Pike, Bethesda, MD 20814

FMS Foundation, 3401 Market St., Philadelphia, PA 19104 (false memory syndrome)
Food and Nutrition Board, National Academy of Sciences, 2101 Constitution Blvd., N.W.,
    Washington, DC 20418
Foundation for Hospice and Home Care (see National Homecaring Council for address)
Gamblers Anonymous, 3255 Wilshire Blvd., Los Angeles, CA 90015
Gerontological Society, 1275 K St., N.W., Washington, DC 20005
Group Against Smoking Pollution (GASP), P.O. Box 632, College Park, MD 20740
Group Health Association of America, 1129 20th St., NW, Washington, DC 20036
Guide Dog Users, c/o Kim Charlson, 57 Grandview Ave., Watertown, MA 02172
Health Insurance Association of America, 1025 Connecticut Ave., N.W., Washington, DC
    20036
Help for Incontinent People, P.O. Box 544, Union, SC 29379
Huntington's Disease Society of America, 140 W. 22nd St., New York, NY 10011
Information Exchange on Young Adult Chronic Patients, 151 S. Main St., New York, NY
    10956 (mental illness)
Institute for Aerobics Research, 12330 Preston Road, Dallas, TX 75230
Institute of Food Technologists, 221 N. LaSalle St., Chicago, IL 60601
International Association for Medical Assistance to Travelers (IAMAT), 417 Center St.,
    Lewiston, NY 14092
International Association of Laryngectomees, c/o American Cancer Society
International Health Society, 1001 E. Oxford Lane, Englewood, CO 80110 (public health)
International Life Sciences Institute, 1126 16th St., N.W., Washington, DC 20036
    (nutrition, toxicology, technology risk assessment)
Interstitial Cystitis Association, P.O. Box 1553, Madison Sq. Station, New York, NY
    10159
Jewish Guild for the Blind, 15 W. 65th St., New York, NY 10023
Joint Commission on Accreditation of Healthcare Organizations, One Renaissance Blvd.,
    Oakbrook Terrace, IL 60181
Juvenile Diabetes Foundation, 432 Park Ave. S., New York, NY 10016
La Leche League International, 9616 Minneapolis Ave., Franklin Park, IL 60131
    (breastfeeding)
Learning Disabilities Association of America, 4156 Library Rd., Pittsburgh, PA 15234
Lehigh Valley Committee Against Health Fraud, P.O. Box 1747, Allentown, PA 18105
Leukemia Society of America, 733 Third Ave., New York, NY 10017
Little People of America, 7238 Piedmont Drive, Dallas, TX 75227 (dwarfism)
Living Bank, P.O. Box 6725, Houston TX 77265 (organ donor registry)
Lupus Foundation of America, 1717 Massachusetts Ave., N.W., Washington, DC 20036
Make Today Count, 101½ S. Union St., Alexandria, VA 22314 (support groups for cancer
    patients)
March of Dimes Birth Defects Foundation, 1275 Mamaroneck Ave., White Plains, NY
    10605
Maternity Center Association, 48 E. 92nd St., New York, NY 10128
Medic Alert Foundation International, 2353 Colorado Ave., Turlock, CA 95380 (warning
    bracelets, organ donor registry)
Medical Library Association, 6 N. Michigan Ave., Chicago, IL 60602
Mended Hearts, c/o American Heart Association (support group for cardiac surgery
    patients)
Mental Health Association, 1021 Prince St., Alexandria, VA 22314
Muscular Dystrophy Association, 810 7th Ave., New York, NY 10019

Myasthenia Gravis Foundation, 53 W. Jackson Blvd., Chicago, IL 60604

Narcotics Anonymous, P.O. Box 9999, Van Nuys, CA 91409

National Alliance for the Mentally Ill, 2101 Wilson Blvd., Arlington, VA 22201

National Amputation Foundation, 12-45 150th St., Whitestone, NY 11357

National Association for Ambulatory Care, 21 Michigan St., Grand Rapids, MI 49503

National Association for Chiropractic Medicine, P.O. Box 794, Middleton, WI 53562.

National Association for Hearing and Speech Action, 10801 Rockville Pike, Rockville, MD 20852

National Association for Home Care, 519 C St., N.E., Washington, DC 20002

National Association for Sickle Cell Disease, 3345 Wilshire Blvd., Los Angeles, CA 90010

National Association of Anorexia Nervosa and Associated Disorders, P.O. Box 7, Highland Park, IL 60035

National Association of Area Agencies on Aging, 600 Maryland Ave., Washington, DC 20024.

National Association of Attorneys General, 444 N. Capitol St., Washington, DC 20001

National Association of the Deaf, 814 Thayer Ave., Silver Spring, MD 20910

National Association of the Physically Handicapped, Bethesda Scarlet Oaks, 440 Lafayette Ave., Cincinnati, OH 45220

National Association of Social Workers, 750 First St., Washington, DC 20002

National Ataxia Foundation, 600 Twelve Oaks Center, 15500 Wayzata Blvd., Wayzata, MN 55391 (loss of muscle coordination and balance)

National Center for Nutrition and Dietetics, 216 W. Jackson Blvd., Chicago, IL 60606

National CFS Association, 3251 Broadway, Kansas City, MO 64111 (chronic fatigue syndrome)

National Committee for the Prevention of Child Abuse, 332 S. Michigan Ave., Chicago, IL 60604

National Consumers League, 815 15th St., N.W., Washington, DC 20005

National Council Against Health Fraud
    Headquarters: P.O. Box 1276, Loma Linda, CA 92354
    Resource Center: 2800 Main St., Kansas City, MO 64108
    Task Force on Victim Redress: P.O. Box 1747, Allentown, PA 18105

National Council on Alcoholism and Drug Dependence, 12 W. 21st St., New York, NY 10010

National Council on Family Relations, 3939 Central Ave., St. Paul, MN 55421

National Council on the Aging, 600 Maryland Ave., S.W., Washington, DC 20024

National Council on Patient Information and Education, 666 11th St., N.W., Washington, DC 20001

National Dairy Council, 6300 North River Road, Rosemont, IL 60018

National Easter Seal Society, 70 E. Lake St., Chicago, IL 60601 (handicapped children and adults)

National Family Planning and Reproductive Health Association, 122 C St., NW, Washington, DC 20001

National Federation of the Blind, 1800 Johnson St., Baltimore, MD 21230

National Foundation for Asthma, P.O. Box 30069, Tucson, AZ 85751

National Genetics Foundation, 180 W. 58th St., New York, NY 10019

National Headache Foundation, 5252 N. Western Ave., Chicago, IL 60625

National Head Injury Foundation, 333 Turnpike Rd., Southborough, MA 01772

National Health Council, 1730 M St., N.W., Washington, DC 20036

National Hearing Aid Society, 20361 Middlebelt Rd., Livonia, MI 48152
National Hemophilia Foundation, 110 Green St., New York, NY 10012
National Homecaring Council, 519 C St., N.E., Washington, DC 20002
National Hospice Organization, 1901 N. Moore St., Arlington, VA 22209
National Kidney Foundation, 30 E. 33rd St., New York, NY 10016
National League for Nursing, 350 Hudson St., New York, NY 10014
National Leukemia Foundation, 585 Stewart Ave., Garden City, NY 11530
National Lupus Erythematosus Foundation, 2635 N. 1st St., San Jose, CA 95134
National Mental Health Association, 1021 Prince St., Alexandria, VA 22314
National Multiple Sclerosis Society, 205 E. 42nd St., New York, NY 10017
National Neurofibromatosis Foundation, 141 Fifth Ave., New York, NY 10010
National Organization for Rare Disorders (NORD), 4960 Sentinel Drive, Bethesda, MD
    20816
National Organization on Disability, 910 16th St., NW, Washington, DC 20006
National Osteoporosis Foundation, 2100 M St., Washington, DC 20037
National Parkinson Foundation, 1501 N.W. Ninth Ave., Miami, FL 33136 (Parkinson's
    disease and related neurological disorders)
National Psoriasis Foundation, 6443 S.W. Beaverton Highway, Portland, OR 97221
National Rehabilitation Association, 633 S. Washington St., Alexandria, VA 22314
National Resource Center for Worksite Health Promotion, 777 N. Capitol St., N.E.,
    Washington, DC 20002.
National Safety Council, 444 W. Michigan Ave., Chicago, IL 60611
National Self-Help Clearinghouse, 25 W. 43rd St., Room 620, New York, NY 10036
National Society of Patient Representatives, c/o American Hospital Association, 840 N.
    Lake Shore Dr., Chicago, IL 60611
National Society to Prevent Blindness, 500 E. Remington Rd., Schaumburg, IL 60173
National Spinal Cord Injury Association, 600 W. Cummings Park, Woburn, MA 01801
National Sudden Infant Death Syndrome Foundation, 10500 Little Patuxent Parkway,
    Columbia, MD 21044
National Tay-Sachs and Allied Diseases Association, 385 Eliot St., Newton, MA 02164
National Tuberous Sclerosis Association, 8000 Corporate Drive, Landover, MD 20785
National Wheelchair Athletic Association, 3595 E. Fountain Blvd., Colorado Springs, CO
    80910
Neurotics Anonymous International Liaison, 11140 Bainbridge Dr., Little Rock, AR 72212
Orton Dyslexia Society, 724 York Rd., Baltimore, MD 21204
Osteogenesis Imperfecta Foundation, P.O. Box 14807, Clearwater, FL 34629
Overeaters Anonymous, 4025 Spencer St., Torrance, CA 90503
Paget's Disease Foundation, P.O. Box 2772, Brooklyn, NY 11202
Parents Anonymous, 6733 S. Sepulveda, Los Angeles, CA 90045 (child abuse)
People-to-People Committee for the Handicapped, P.O. Box 18131, Washington, DC
    20036
Phoenix Society, 11 Rust Hill Rd., Levittown, PA 19056 (burn injuries)
Planned Parenthood—World Population, 902 Broadway, 10th Floor, New York, NY 10010
Psoriasis Research Institute, P.O. Box V, Stanford, CA 94305
Public Citizen Health Research Group, 2000 P St., NW, Washington, DC 20036
RAND Corporation, P.O. Box 2138, Santa Monica, CA 90407.
Reach to Recovery, c/o American Cancer Society (mastectomy support group)
Recovery, 802 N. Dearborn St., Chicago, IL 60610 (mental illness)

Resolve, 5 Water St., Arlington, MA 02174 (infertility)
RP Foundation Fighting Blindness, 1401 Mt. Royal Ave., Baltimore, MD 21217 (retinitis
    pigmentosa and similar degenerative diseases)
Secular Organizations for Sobriety (SOS), Box 5, Buffalo, NY 14215
Self-Help Center, 1600 Dodge Ave., Evanston, IL 60201
Scoliosis Association, P.O. Box 51353, Raleigh, NC 27609
Sister Kenny Institute, 800 E. 28th St., at Chicago Ave., Minneapolis, MN 55407
    (rehabilitative care)
Society for Clinical and Experimental Hypnosis, 128-A Kings Park Drive, Liverpool, NY
    13090
Society for Computer Medicine, 1901 Fort Meyer Drive, Arlington, VA 22208
Spina Bifida Association of America, 1700 Rockville Pike, Rockville, MD 20852
Stroke Club International, 805 12th St., Galveston, TX 77550
Suicide Prevention Center of Los Angeles, 626 S. Kingsley Dr., Los Angeles, CA 90005
Take Off Pounds Sensibly (TOPS), P.O. Box 07360, Milwaukee, WI 53207
Tourette Syndrome Association, 42-40 Bell Blvd., Bayside, NY 11361
United Cerebral Palsy Associations, 7 Penn Plaza, New York, NY 10001
United Network for Organ Sharing (UNOS), P.O. Box 13770, Richmond, VA 23225.
United Ostomy Association, 36 Executive Park, Irvine, CA 92714
United Parkinson Foundation, 360 W. Superior St., Chicago, IL 60610
United Scleroderma Foundation, P.O. Box 350, Watsonville, CA 95077
United States Pharmacopeial Convention, Inc., 12601 Twinbrook Parkway, Rockville, MD
    20852 (drug publications)
Victims of Chiropractic, P.O. Box 956, Watkinsville, GA 30677
Weight Watchers International, Jericho Atrium, 500 N. Broadway, Jericho, NY 11753
Wellness and Health Activation Networks, P.O. Box 923, Vienna, VA 22182 (self-help and
    healthy lifestyles)

Additional information on most of these organizations can be obtained from the *Encyclopedia of Medical Organizations and Agencies* or the *Encyclopedia of Associations*. Both are updated periodically by Gale Research Company and are available in the reference department of most public and college libraries.

The Appendix to this volume includes information about books, newsletters, and magazines that offer reliable advice on health matters.

# 34

# Strengths and Weaknesses of Our Laws

### Stephen Barrett, M.D.

Three federal agencies and various state and local agencies are responsible for enforcing the laws that pertain to quackery and health frauds. The Postal Service has jurisdiction over products sold by mail. It has a vigorous program but is hampered by loopholes in its law. The Federal Trade Commission (FTC) can regulate the advertising of nonprescription products and health-related services. It has a powerful law but insufficient manpower. The Food and Drug Administration (FDA) presides over the labeling of products marketed with therapeutic claims. It has a powerful law but an inconsistent enforcement program. State enforcement activities are administered by the state attorney general, local district attorneys, and state licensing boards. State laws and their enforcement priority vary considerably from state to state. Courts also play an important role in regulating quackery and health frauds.

Most people overestimate the extent to which laws can protect our society against quackery and health frauds. As should be apparent from this book, the amount of wrongdoing exceeds the resources of law enforcement agencies and the courts.

## FTC Regulation

The FTC has jurisdiction over the advertising of foods, nonprescription drugs, cosmetics, devices, and services that are marketed in interstate commerce. Section 12 of the Wheeler-Lea Act (1938) allows the agency to attack false advertising.

The FTC has broad powers to investigate complaints. If it concludes that the law has been violated, it may attempt to obtain voluntary compliance by entering into a consent order with the violator. Signers of a consent order need not admit that they have violated the law, but they must agree to stop the practices described in an accompanying complaint. If a consent agreement cannot be reached, the FTC may issue an administrative complaint or—if a problem is considered serious enough—seek a court order (injunction) to stop the improper practices.

When an administrative complaint is disputed, an administrative law judge holds a formal hearing similar to a court trial. Evidence is submitted, testimony is heard, and witnesses are examined and cross-examined. If the judge finds that the law has been violated, a cease-and-desist order or other appropriate relief can be issued. Initial decisions by administrative law judges can be appealed to the five-member commission, which acts like a court of appeal. Respondents who are dissatisfied with the commission's decision can appeal their case through the federal court system. FTC actions often result in restitution to consumers and/or a financial penalty against the advertiser.

Cease-and-desist orders set forth findings and prohibit respondents from engaging in practices determined to be illegal. When final, these orders act as permanent injunctions. Penalties for violating consent agreements or cease-and-desist orders can be very heavy—including prison sentences, corrective advertising, and fines of up to $10,000 per day for continued violations.

When the FTC believes that a problem affects an entire industry, it may promulgate an industry guide or trade regulation rule. Guides are interpretive statements without the force of law; rules represent the conclusions of the commission about what it considers unlawful. Before guides and rules are established, interested parties are given the opportunity to comment. Once a rule is established, the commission can take enforcement action without lengthy explanations about why a particular ad is unfair or deceptive. A reference to the rule is enough. In health matters, problems are almost always handled on a case-by-case basis rather than through rulemaking.

The FTC's activities are reported in the weekly *FTC News Notes* and an annual report, both of which are available free of charge to interested parties.

Although the FTC has a very effective law, the agency can handle only a small percentage of the violations it detects. The situation could be greatly improved if Congress passed a law enabling state attorneys general to enter federal court so that the results of their regulatory actions would apply nationwide.

## FDA Regulation

The FDA traces its roots to just after the turn of this century, when consumers needed all the protection they could get. Patent medicines, which were worthless but not always harmless, were widely promoted with cure-all claims. The country was plagued by unsanitary conditions in meat-packing plants. Harmful chemicals were being added to foods, and labels rarely told what their products contained.

The Pure Food and Drug Act, passed in 1906, has been strengthened by many subsequent amendments and related acts. Together, these various laws are concerned with assuring the safety and effectiveness of all products intended for use in the diagnosis, prevention, and treatment of disease. The 1938 Food, Drug, and Cosmetic Act bans false and misleading statements from the labeling of foods, drugs, medical devices, and cosmetics. Drugs must have their active ingredients listed and be proven safe before marketing. The Kefauver-Harris Drug Amendments, passed in 1962 in the wake of the Thalidomide tragedy, require that drugs must also be proven effective before marketing. Other amendments extend this requirement to devices.

Under the law, "labeling" is not limited to what is on a product's container. It also includes claims made by any written or graphic matter which explains a product's use and is physically or contextually connected with its sale. Thus promotional material used to sell a product or to explain its use can be construed as labeling whether it is used before or after a sale.

The FDA's jurisdiction covers all intended uses of a product, whether they are contained in labeling or not. Section 502(f)(1) of the Food, Drug and Cosmetic Act requires that all drugs and devices bear adequate directions for all intended uses, whether promotion is done by oral claims, advertising, or otherwise.

Complaints about quack remedies are usually received from consumers, members of Congress, FDA field inspectors, and various government agencies. Significant complaints may be followed up by FDA field inspectors and evaluated by physicians and other scientists. If an investigation shows that a product is a "new drug," it must have FDA approval for movement in interstate commerce. Violation of this provision can lead to seizure of the product and a court injunction against its sale. To be classified as a "new drug," a product does not actually have to be new; it can also be a familiar substance proposed for a therapeutic use that is "not generally recognized by experts as safe and effective." For example, a claim that wheat germ oil "prevents heart stress" would make the oil a new drug with respect to that claim. The oil would also be misbranded because—since the product doesn't work—it is impossible to provide adequate directions to achieve the intended effect. (A product is misbranded if its labeling lacks required information or contains false or misleading information.)

It is a criminal offense to market a drug or device that is unapproved or is misbranded. A first offender may be imprisoned for up to one year. Any offense committed after a first conviction is a felony punishable by up to three years in prison. Because misbranding and marketing an unapproved new product are separate offenses, a repeat offender could be sentenced to as much as six years in jail. The 1984 Criminal Fines Enhancement Act amended all federal criminal laws to allow fines of up to $100,000 (or $250,000 if death results) per offense for up to two offenses. To obtain a conviction, intent to mislead need not be proven. Even a single shipment of one product is sufficient grounds for conviction.

When products are marketed improperly, the FDA may issue a warning letter specifying the violations and demanding to know how the problem will be corrected. If a warning is ignored, or if the FDA decides to begin with more forceful action, the agency can initiate court proceedings for a seizure, injunction, or criminal prosecution. If an injunction is violated, the court has considerable discretion in determining the punishment and can order imprisonment or a large fine. The FDA has concentrated its efforts against health frauds on products that are inherently unsafe or are illegally marketed for the treatment of serious diseases. Worthless yet harmless articles promoted to improve health, athletic ability, or appearance—which the agency classifies as "economic frauds"—have been given little regulatory attention.

Examples of FDA regulatory actions are reported in the weekly *FDA Enforcement Report* and monthly magazine *FDA Consumer,* both of which are available by subscription.

Many observers believe that FDA enforcement would be much more effective if it emphasized criminal cases rather than civil ones. If this were done, wrongdoers might hesitate to commit acts that could land them in jail. Within the past three years, the FDA has created an Office of Criminal Investigations and increased the number of agents doing undercover criminal investigation. However, it is not yet apparent how much priority the new program will give to quackery-related products.

Civil action, which carries no financial penalty, stops some schemes but does not usually prevent them from being profitable. This problem could be solved by a law enabling the FDA to generate civil penalties in the same manner as the FTC. About two years ago, when Congress began considering such legislation, the health-food industry reacted with great alarm and began a vigorous campaign to stop its passage.

FDA officials have said that their agency has been hampered by unwillingness of the Justice Department to handle criminal prosecutions. If this is true, the law should be changed so that FDA attorneys can prosecute in federal court when the Justice Department won't do so.

FDA Commissioner David Kessler, M.D., J.D., who assumed office in 1990, is by far the most effective leader the FDA has had in modern times. Under his direction, agency function has been streamlined and enforcement activities have increased greatly. The health-food industry is very alarmed about this and has introduced legislation that would greatly hamper regulation of dietary supplements (see Chapter 2).

**Postal Regulation**

The Postal Service has jurisdiction over situations where the mail is used to transfer money for products or services. Postal inspectors look for misleading advertisements in magazines and newspapers and on radio or television. They also receive complaints from the public and from other government agencies. From the thousands of complaints it receives each year, the Postal Service selects those that it feels are most significant—particularly cases that might generate a large amount of mail or pose physical danger to the public.

Title 39, Section 3005, of the United States Code can be used to block promoters of misleading schemes from receiving money through the mail. If sufficient health hazard or economic detriment exists, an immediate court order to impound mail may be sought under Section 3007 of the Code. Title 18, Section 1341, provides for criminal prosecution. The maximum penalties are five years in prison and a fine for each instance proved. The 1984 Criminal Fines Enhancement Act allows fines of up to $100,000 (or $250,000 if death results) per offense for up to two offenses. Under Section 1341, intent to deceive must be proved—a task which can be difficult and time-consuming. Although Section 1341 is seldom used in health-related cases, almost all cases actually brought to trial result in convictions.

The Postal Service does not usually assert jurisdiction when companies solicit only credit card orders by telephone and deliver through private carriers such as United Parcel Service. However, the Justice Department may seek an injunction under Section 1345, which allows federal district courts to enjoin acts of mail and wire fraud.

Most mail-order health schemes attempt to exploit people's fear of being unattractive. Their promoters are usually "hit-and-run" artists who hope to make a profit before the Postal Service stops their false ads. Common products include "miracle weight-loss" plans, fitness and bodybuilding products, spot-reducing devices (claimed to reduce specific parts of the body), anti-aging products, and supposed sex aids. When a scheme is detected, postal inspectors can file a complaint or seek an agreement with the perpetrator. When a complaint is contested, a hearing is held by an administrative law judge. If the evidence is sufficient, this judge will issue a False Representation Order (FRO) enabling the Postal Service to block and return money sent through the mail in response to the misleading ads. Although the order can be appealed to the courts, very few companies do this. Each voluntary agreement and FRO is accompanied by a cease-and-desist order that forbids both the challenged acts and similar acts. Under the Mail Order Consumer Protection Amendments of 1983, if this order is violated, the agency can seek a civil penalty in federal court of up to $10,000 per day for each violation.

Criminal cases, consent agreements, and FROs are noted in the quarterly *Law Enforcement Report,* which is issued free of charge to interested media and consumer protection agencies. The agency probably handles between twenty and forty health-related cases per year, but exact figures are not available. Most of these cases are handled with voluntary agreements or FROs, which impose no financial penalty. The agency's effectiveness would be greatly increased by passage of a law enabling it to generate financial penalties larger than the amount of money collected by the perpetrator of a fraudulent scheme. It would also help if laws were passed to make it simple for the Postal Service to initiate criminal prosecution in cases where health products are involved. Current mail-fraud laws require that intent to deceive be proven, which is difficult to do if a perpetrator professes a sincere belief in his product. As noted above, the Food, Drug, and Cosmetic Act has no such requirement.

Postal officials have said that their agency has been hampered by unwillingness on the part of the Justice Department to handle more of their cases. If this is true, the law should be changed so that Postal Service attorneys can pursue cases in federal court when the Justice Department refuses.

## State Regulation

State efforts against health frauds and quackery are carried out under licensing and consumer protection laws. The grounds for disciplinary action and the effectiveness in policing the marketplace vary considerably from state to state and from one agency to another.

State licensing boards can take action against practitioners who appear to be unfit or who engage in various quack or unethical practices. Some physicians and dentists have been disciplined for departing from accepted standards of scientific care, but actions of this type are not common.

The situation is even worse where clinical standards are minimal or don't exist. State boards that regulate chiropractors, acupuncturists, naturopaths, and homeopaths appear to be doing little or nothing to protect the public from unscientific and unethical practices. A study by the U.S. Office of the Inspector General concluded that in 1985, only twelve out of about thirty thousand chiropractors were disciplined for matters involving clinical competence. As far as I know, no comparable evaluation has been made of the boards that regulate acupuncturists, naturopaths, or homeopaths—virtually all of whom claim to heal by manipulating the body's "vital force." Do you think that board members who believe in this notion can judge the clinical competence of their colleagues?

State attorneys general and local district attorneys may have jurisdiction in cases that involve false advertising, theft by deception, practicing without a license, marketing of unapproved drugs, and various other types of consumer fraud. Again, both the nature of the laws and the vigor with which they are enforced vary considerably from state to state.

In most cases where a state attorney general stops a dubious promotion, the action will not stop the promotion in other states. To address this problem, state attorneys general have begun to team up for multistate actions and their national organization has formed a health care task force that will deal with frauds. The FDA is helping to coordinate this effort.

## The Role of the Court System

Our court system also plays an important role in regulating quackery, because judges and sometimes juries must decide how to interpret the laws and penalize lawbreakers. Several types of situations undermine efforts to control quackery:

- Court delays often work to the advantage of lawbreakers, especially in the appeals process. Companies under fire from the FDA, for example, may be permitted to continue selling bogus products until all appeals have been exhausted. Practitioners facing revocation of their license sometimes remain in practice for years while appealing their case through the courts.

- In some cases, courts have ordered insurance companies to pay for unproven treatment. In others, courts have refused to order parents to see to it that their children receive proven treatment; several deaths have been reported among children with cancer whose parents discontinued or failed to utilize conventional treatment.

• In quackery-related cases where criminal convictions are obtained, sentencing tends to be light.

## More Accountability Would Help

Consumer protection would probably be improved if the FTC, FDA, the Postal Service, and state regulatory agencies were forced to be more accountable. As far as I know, none of them has ever revealed meaningful statistics about the number of health frauds they have detected and what percentage they have acted against. Statistics of this type would enable legislators and the public to see the scope of the problem and what might be done about it.

I believe that all agencies charged with protecting the public from health frauds and quackery should be required to make meaningful data available on what they are doing about them. This could be accomplished by maintaining a list of prosecutions, both in progress and completed, that is accessible year-round through each agency's public information office and is published at least once a year in a report to Congress (or, in the case of state agencies, to the state legislature). The report should include tabulations of the number of health-related complaints received, the number judged valid, and the number subjected to regulatory action. The agencies should also be required to recommend improvements in the law that might enable them to work more effectively.

To encourage the reporting of health frauds, a share of any penalties assessed could be given to the complainant and/or nonprofit groups involved in fighting health frauds.

Ultimately, your best protection will be your own good sense. If the majority of American physicians wouldn't use a particular product or service or recommend it to their loved ones, you shouldn't either. A reasonable level of caution plus guidance from reliable sources should protect you from being victimized.

# 35

# Getting the Most from Your Doctor

### Philip R. Alper, M.D.

Medical science may not be able to answer all your questions or solve all your health problems. Doctors, like anybody else, can get tired or irritable and be rushed or preoccupied. They may keep you waiting. And sometimes they make mistakes.

But don't despair. In most parts of this country, good medical care can be yours if you work at two things—finding a doctor you can trust and learning to communicate effectively.

## Your Doctor's Personality

Some years ago, an eloquent Texan named Max Scheid told a medical audience what he expected from his physician:

- Honesty
- Care for himself and his family in sickness and in health
- Treatment as an individual with dignity from the doctor and the doctor's staff
- Availability when needed
- Concern for soul as well as body
- Treatment on the adult level
- A charge of a customary fee
- Use of an accredited hospital
- Personal concern with the patient's health
- Referral to a competent specialist when necessary

• The ability to listen as well as trust
• Ordering only the necessary laboratory tests
• A nondefensive practice of medicine.

After Mr. Scheid had finished, his doctor spoke. A warm and personal relationship existed between the two, and the doctor acknowledged this with visible pleasure.

Contrast this with auto-magnate Henry Ford II's expectation of medical care as reported in *Medical Economics* magazine. Mr. Ford wanted top-flight doctors who worked in top-flight institutions; he wasn't interested in personalities, but just in getting the job done quickly and efficiently. His expectations were all *technical* rather than *personal* or even a mixture of both. In fact, they bore a startling resemblance to automobile repair!

Obviously, these two gentlemen looked at medical care differently. Mr. Scheid saw his physician as a part of his life. Mr. Ford viewed his as a periodic and barely tolerable intruder into his busy schedule.

## Primary Care

For first-rate care to occur, your personality and your doctor's personality must fit one another. This is especially true for so-called *primary care*—ongoing care by a doctor who knows you and is the first one you turn to for help.

Some people are more comfortable with an *institution* than with a particular physician. They may be perfectly content to be seen episodically on an outpatient basis or in emergency rooms by any number of different doctors. This is far from ideal care, but it is common in county hospitals and in some group practices. I call this *compromise care*. With luck, a strong constitution, and a basically good medical staff, it may work out.

It is far better to choose a *personal physician*. He or she may be in either solo or group private practice or in a multidoctor clinic. Even in a group, a personal physician ally can help steer you through the medical maze while looking out for your welfare. Most groups, including the large ones, allow patients to pick a physician from their roster.

## Choosing a Doctor

Your best bet is a specialist who is board-certified in internal medicine or family practice. Such a physician is sure to have taken advanced training in the diagnosis and treatment of general medical problems. Staff affiliation with a hospital connected with a medical school indicates that a physician is working with colleagues who keep abreast of the latest medical developments and that the physician keeps up, too. Affiliation with a hospital that trains interns and residents is also favorable. Less certain is affiliation with only proprietary hospitals— especially small ones—unless they are the only ones in the area. Lack of any hospital affiliation should be suspect.

Consumer-oriented directories that list a doctor's affiliations and credentials have been appearing lately. But much, if not all, of the information they contain can be obtained by calling the doctor's office, a local hospital, or the county medical society.

Other positive indicators include membership in the American College of Physicians or the American College of Surgeons (though a surgeon is not a usual choice for a primary physician). Teaching appointments in a medical school are also a good sign.

Some consumer advocates favor physicians who practice in a group rather than alone. Their theory is that in a group, since doctors can watch each other, blatant incompetence is less likely to occur. Although this theory has considerable merit, membership in a group is no guarantee against mediocrity. Besides, there are many outstanding solo physicians. Several years ago, when the American Board of Internal Medicine offered a voluntary "recertification" exam, it expected that physicians practicing in universities would rank highest, followed by doctors in group practice and with solo doctors trailing badly. However, the results showed little difference among the three physician categories.

My own bias is toward a well-credentialed, well-affiliated, solo physician or one practicing in a group *in the same specialty*. Should you need referral to a specialist, a first-class primary physician is likely to select a specialist of equal caliber. The defect of multispecialty groups is lack of free choice of consultants. Then again, some of these specialty groups are outstanding across the board from specialty to specialty; the Palo Alto Medical Clinic and the Mayo Clinic are examples. Some people use multispecialty groups for some of their medical care and go outside them for particular problems.

Asking a neighbor, fellow worker, or relative for the name of a doctor is an exceedingly common practice, but is often criticized as unreliable. If people do it, though, there has to be a reason. Perhaps they don't know any better way. If so, the suggestions given above should help. Nonetheless, laypersons are not entirely lacking in judgment when it comes to evaluating physicians. It doesn't take an expert to evaluate courtesy, attentiveness, thoroughness, whether an office is efficiently run, or whether the doctor is personable and likely to get along with you. So personal recommendations *do* have a place—albeit a limited one.

Don't be surprised if you are given the name of a woman physician. Between a third and a half of medical students are female, and the percentage of female practitioners has been rising steadily. Some patients have reasons for preferring a doctor of either one sex or the other; others have discovered—sometimes to their own surprise—that it usually makes no difference.

People who enroll in a health maintenance organization (HMO), preferred provider organization (PPO), or other managed-care program may be faced with choosing their primary physician from a list without benefit of background information. Switching of insurance plans by employers coupled with restricted lists of available physicians may create additional problems. The above recommendations still apply, but may be more difficult to carry out. I hope that health-reform efforts will result in greater freedom to choose one's physician and in more continuity of care than we have now.

## Be Prepared

Medical diagnoses are based on the history of the patient's problem, the physical findings, and laboratory tests. Of these, the history is usually most important. For this reason, whenever you consult a doctor, you should try to present a detailed and well-organized account of your present symptoms and relevant past history. Before contacting the doctor, think about them carefully and draw up a list to guide your presentation. If you have more than one problem, start with the one that is most important. If you are taking medications, either write down their names and dosages or bring the medications to the appointment.

## Meeting Your Doctor

An excellent way to begin your relationship with a new doctor is a thorough physical examination when you are not ill. Such an examination will give your doctor a "baseline"—a personal health profile against which changes in future years can be compared. This may be a big help in making a diagnosis and planning treatment later on.

A "get-acquainted" physical exam is also an ideal time to bring up any health questions that have been troubling you. "My father had diabetes. What are my chances of getting it?" Or perhaps, "What do you think of vasectomies?" Questions like these are important, but tend to be put aside during the treatment of an acute illness.

If you don't wish to have a complete physical exam, it still may pay to schedule a brief visit with your prospective doctor. This should help you decide whether he or she is the person you wish to consult in the future. During this visit you can also sign a release form so that your past medical records can be obtained.

Advance "registration" has an additional advantage. Some doctors will not accept new patients under emergency conditions, particularly outside of regular office hours. Once a doctor has accepted you as a patient, however, there is a *legal* obligation either to treat you or to provide a substitute.

Having chosen a primary physician, examine the doctor's policies. Some doctors have printed instruction sheets for this purpose. If yours does not, ask questions: When is the office open? Who covers during the doctor's absence? Does the doctor make house calls? Which hospital(s) does the doctor use? This last bit of information is especially important. Few physicians are on the staff of every hospital in town. In an emergency, ambulance drivers usually take patients to the nearest hospital—unless they are told differently. If you go to the wrong hospital, your doctor may not be able to take care of you.

**Telephone Manners**

Proper use of the telephone can do a lot to make your doctor's life easier while at the same time helping you to receive better service. Before calling the doctor's office, take a moment to organize your thoughts. What is bothering you? When did it begin? If you have a pain, does it come and go or is it steady? Does anything bring it on or relieve it? If you have an infection or any other reason to suspect you might have a fever, take your temperature.

Try to decide whether your problem is urgent or not. You are not expected to know all the answers, but often you will have a good idea. For example, a cold lingering for five days is not an emergency, but squeezing chest pain may be. If in doubt, simply say, "I am not sure if this is urgent, but . . ."

It is not unusual for a busy physician to receive fifty to a hundred telephone calls per day—many more than one person could handle alone. So when you call, don't start out by asking to speak with the doctor. The receptionist or nurse is trained to assemble the information needed for a preliminary evaluation of your situation. Staff members are an *extension* of your doctor and will usually know which matters they can handle by themselves and which ones the doctor must handle personally. After dealing with the staff member, if you still feel you must speak with the doctor, that is the time to ask.

Memory is notoriously faulty; when you telephone, have a pad and pencil handy to write down any instructions you receive. Call as early in the day as possible. That way your doctor can handle your case most efficiently—while assistants are on duty to help, and while hospitals and laboratories are able to give their best services. Above all, avoid waiting until Friday afternoon for a problem that has troubled you all week!

When you call to ask for a prescription refill, know the phone number of your drugstore. Make your request during the doctor's office hours and before you get down to the last pill. That way the doctor can review your office record to see whether you still need the medication, whether the dosage should be changed, and so on. Such a review will make your medical care safer. If you telephone outside of office hours, many physicians (especially those covering another doctor's practice) will order only enough medication for a few days. That is the safest way in the absence of your medical records, but it does increase the cost of your medication.

In an emergency, try to telephone your doctor immediately. Don't simply show up in a hospital emergency room. Advance notice will enable the doctor to alert emergency room personnel to begin treatment or arrange for necessary tests. Also, doctors find it very exasperating to have a patient arrive at an emergency room moments after they have finished treating another patient and left the hospital.

**Voice Your Concerns!**

Although good communication is essential to good medical care, speaking with a doctor is not always easy. You may be afraid (*What will the doctor tell me? Maybe the worst is true?*), or embarrassed (*I can't admit that. What will she think?*), or even resentful (*Who does he think he is? He probably won't even be able to help me.*).

Try not to let feelings like these create a barrier between you and your physician. Instead, put the feelings to work *for you* by sharing them. State your prejudices and concerns such as "I don't like to take medicines." Or "I don't want to take anything that might do me more harm than good." Or perhaps "I had some bad reactions to medication in the past." You may have heard or read something or seen something on TV that strikes you as relevant to your condition. If any of these—or other concerns—are on your mind, be sure to mention them.

Suppose you have doubts about a recommended treatment. Voice them. Don't play a waiting game and end up with a misunderstanding that could have been avoided. Relating to a physician should not mean taking a back seat.

Doctors know that how a patient feels about treatment may influence its outcome. If you find a treatment particularly objectionable, your doctor may suggest a more acceptable alternative. Even if you are slated to disagree (let's say you think your heart condition would best be treated by vitamins rather than digitalis), you still owe it to yourself to hear the doctor's point of view. Approached properly, a compromise satisfactory to both you and your doctor may be possible.

## Ask Questions

Doctors may sometimes be authoritarian and even patronizing. It is an occupational hazard—the result of years of counseling and treating others. Don't accept this! Ask your physician to explain why you are having your symptoms: why, for example, your ulcer hurts, and why it hurts less if you drink milk. Ask what the suggested medication is supposed to do. What will happen if the condition remains untreated. Whether there are alternative treatments. The key word is *ask*. The more you know, the more you can help yourself and help the doctor to help you.

Make sure your doctor's explanations make sense to you. Even very technical concepts can be phrased in words that are easy for laypersons to understand. For example, why does a "spastic stomach" hurt? There are a number of explanations, but a simple analogy can make the point. Clench your fist as tightly as you can for five or ten minutes. Not only will your hand hurt, but it will get stiff and difficult to open; in other words, the muscles go into spasm. The logic of using a drug to reduce the spasm is then obvious. Similarly, if you are tense, you can actually feel the tension in the muscles of your face or arms. It is not difficult to imagine the same thing happening inside of you. Perhaps a medication to relieve tension is in order, or perhaps only a change in your routine. Knowing the cause of your problem is sometimes enough to relieve it.

Learn the names and dosages of your medications. Ask about their side effects and whether treatment should be stopped or continued when you feel better. Long-term medication is especially important in painless but potentially serious conditions such as high blood pressure. Untreated, hypertension can lead to heart attacks and strokes. Patients who don't understand why they need long-term treatment often discontinue their medications and then develop complications. Lack of understanding may not be the only problem, however. Unpleasant side effects (dry mouth, stuffy nose, or other uncomfortable effects of the drugs apart from their basic treatment function) may occur. If you suffer side effects, don't simply stop your medicine—discuss them with your doctor. Often a change of dosage or a different drug is the best solution.

## If You Have A Grievance

As in any human relationship, miscommunications between doctor and patient are inevitable from time to time. Not long ago, I heard about a patient who left another physician "because he was cold." I was astonished, since this particular physician cared very much about his patients and I knew him to be a very warm human being. What actually had happened? The woman had presented a lengthy list of puzzling complaints. The doctor was concentrating intently on what she was saying, trying to organize her symptoms into a pattern that would lead to a diagnosis. His effort must have shown on his face—but the *meaning* of his expression was misinterpreted as coldness.

The lesson is clear. Don't be too hasty to judge. If you have a grievance, *voice* it. "You don't seem to care, doctor." Or, "I am not sure you are listening to me." Perhaps the doctor really is listening; or maybe he or she is tired or preoccupied with another patient's problem—or even a personal one. A good doctor should appreciate being told that you are displeased because this provides an opportunity to either straighten out your misconception or apologize if there is reason to. (A doctor who can't take such criticism may not be right for you.) Don't suffer in silence or leave the doctor's care without telling him why.

Language can cause problems, too. Physicians often choose their words poorly when trying to reassure patients about minor but irritating symptoms. When doctors say, "It's nothing," they probably mean, "I think it isn't serious and should clear up by itself with time." When doctors say, "It's your nerves," they are probably trying to say "It's your body's reaction to tension." But to some patients, such remarks may sound like an accusation that they are imagining or exaggerating their symptoms. Medical school does not turn doctors into great communicators (quite the contrary). If a doctor's clumsy shorthand remarks bother you, say so and ask for a fuller explanation. I would caution, however, that not every ailment warrants a lengthy explanation or an intensive series of diagnostic tests right away. Most illnesses are self-limiting. So be prepared to accept an answer like, "If your problem does not clear up in the near future, we can explore it further."

While preparing this chapter, I took an informal poll among physician colleagues. The need for patients to voice their grievances was a recurrent theme. A typical comment was: "If you have a problem with a doctor— his office, his bills, *or him*—let him know. He'll appreciate it and try to help." Resolving disagreements and dissatisfactions can do much to build bonds between human beings. Consultation or a change of doctors will always be possible. You'd be surprised, however, how often a strong mutual understanding can develop in spite of some initial friction. Two quick illustrations will show how this works.

Dr. X was attending a man who had to undergo a third operation to salvage a knee badly damaged by arthritis. One day, as the doctor was about to leave the hospital room, the patient asked him to sit down. "I wouldn't tell you this if I didn't like you and feel that you would want to know," said the patient with masterful tact. "But you are in and out of here like a flash. Some patients would get the idea that you are only interested in rushing around to make more money."

Dr. X was shocked. There were many excuses—emergency calls, hospital committee work, and the like. But as he thought about it, the doctor realized that although he himself handled only the patient's nonsurgical care, the man's bad luck with surgery frustrated and bothered the doctor so much that he cut his visits short. Instead of offering excuses, Dr. X told the truth. The exchange cleared the air and solved the problem.

The other incident involved a healthy woman who had been checked routinely by Dr. Y for many years. He knew her and her family well. On the morning of her appointment, three unscheduled patients arrived one after another with urgent problems. Normally, Dr. Y was able to adhere to his schedule, so the woman waited patiently. When the third emergency patient was taken, the doctor's nurse told her that there would be an additional delay. Rather than wait any longer, the patient scheduled a new appointment. But instead of keeping it, she sent a request to Dr. Y to transfer her records to another physician.

Dr. Y might simply have complied, but the incident didn't sit right with him. So he telephoned the patient's husband. The patient was upset about both having to relieve her daughter who was covering the patient's job and "seeing three people who came in after me go in first—especially after ten years as a patient." After explaining the circumstances to the husband, Dr. Y added his hope that the relationship would not end on a sour note. "I would be happy to speak to your wife if she would like to call," he concluded.

Shortly afterward, the patient did call. She had a point. The nurse could have told her earlier about the additional delay. But the doctor had a point, too: "You have been lucky never to have had an emergency yourself," he said, "but if you had, you would have bumped the schedule and someone else would have been unhappy." The conversation ended pleasantly, and the appointment was rescheduled.

Remember, good medical care should be a partnership, with open two-way communication between you and your doctor. Like most things in life, it is available to those who work for it.

# 36

# Fighting Quackery:
# Tips for Activists

## Stephen Barrett, M.D.

Many people concerned about quackery wonder what they can do about it. The crucial first step is to overcome any negative feelings about becoming involved. So before discussing techniques, let's look at the concerns faced by would-be activists.

Almost everyone who thinks about fighting quackery experiences some fear of being sued for *libel* or *slander*. The fact is, however, that no one who understands the law and follows commonsense rules faces any significant risk. To be libelous, a statement must be *defamatory, malicious,* and *false,* and must be *published.* Slander is similar but applies to oral claims and requires proof of actual damages. A defamatory statement is one that accuses someone of being dishonest, criminal, or professionally incompetent. One that is malicious is done for an improper reason, either with knowledge that the statement is false or with reckless disregard for the truth. It is possible for a statement to be false but not defamatory. In any case, truth is a complete defense against libel and slander. A published statement is one that a third party sees or hears in a letter, article, book, tape recording, or other fixed medium. It is possible to defame an individual, a small group of individuals, or an organization. But one cannot defame a large class of individuals (such as "all doctors") or an entire industry.

## Avoid Name-Calling

It is never libelous to criticize an idea. Therefore, it is safe to attack ideas or to list ideas characteristic of quackery. It is legal to mention adverse facts—such as criminal convictions or dubious credentials—about people who place themselves in the public spotlight by claiming to have expert knowledge. But avoid statements about motivation (such as "He's only in it for the money") because they may be impossible to prove. The appearance of malice can usually be avoided by investigating carefully and citing reliable sources of information. Also avoid name-calling; above all, never call anyone a name (such as "quack," "crook," or "fraud") unless you are willing to defend this claim in court.

It should be apparent from the above discussion that antiquackery actions based on facts and done for legitimate reasons cannot provide the grounds for a successful libel suit. But what about suits whose purpose is intimidation? The National Nutritional Foods Association (NNFA) and some of its leaders tried this approach with Fredrick J. Stare, M.D., Ph.D., emeritus professor of nutrition at Harvard's School of Public Health, and Elizabeth M. Whelan, Sc.D., M.P.H., executive director of the American Council on Science and Health. Filed in 1979, NNFA's suit charged them with "recklessly, maliciously, and knowingly disseminating false and defamatory remarks with respect to plaintiffs and the health food industry" through books and published articles.

It was obvious that the plaintiffs would lose in court. Their names had not even been mentioned in the publications to which they objected. In 1980, the suit was dismissed by a federal judge who warned that "any further suit by plaintiffs against critics of the health food industry should be scrutinized carefully to determine whether it was brought in good faith." (In other words, if plaintiffs filed another spurious suit, they would be held responsible for defendants' legal bills.)

The suit was actually part of an announced effort to silence critics of the health-food industry. Very few such suits have been filed, and all have been against leading critics. As far as I know, none has ever been filed against a critic who was not nationally prominent unless the critic called someone a quack. Thus it is very unlikely that anyone who sticks to facts and does not engage in name-calling will be unjustly sued for libel.

Of course, if it makes you more comfortable, you can avoid criticisms of individuals altogether. Just criticize ideas with which you disagree, and provide the correct information. For additional safety, you can use the word "questionable" (e.g., "That idea is certainly questionable"), which is not defamatory.

Some people fear that taking a stand against quackery will embroil them in unpleasant public controversy. While that certainly can happen, many effective actions require no public exposure at all. For example, you can: (1) offer background information to a reporter with a request that you not be quoted; (2) send letters to the media marked "not for publication"; (3) complain about false advertising to appropriate agencies; (4) encourage victims of quackery to file lawsuits; (5) contact legislators and encourage others to do this, too; and (6) contribute time and/or money to an antiquackery organization. All these things can be done privately and without risk.

Lack of confidence may also interfere with taking action. Non-experts often feel that only experts can be effective. Even experts may hesitate when they aren't sure what action would be most effective. However, although expert knowledge is helpful, the number of people taking action is often more important than the nature of what they do. Moreover, many antiquackery actions require no expertise.

Fighting quackery can be very time-consuming. But keep in mind that many actions (such as reporting illegal ads) take only a few minutes.

## Dealing with the Media

Much can be done to counter the spread of misinformation through talk shows and publications.

If you object to a broadcast, make your objections known by writing or phoning its producer or the station manager. Persist until you learn how those you contact feel about your request. If you encounter resistance, get as many people as you can to make similar contacts. Don't be discouraged if no immediate corrective action is taken; expressions of protest may still influence what happens in the future.

If you object to a newspaper or magazine article, write a letter to the editor and get others to do the same. If the publication is local, phone calls can also be useful because they ensure that the person you are contacting really thinks about your complaint. Contacting the writer may also help prevent future difficulty. If you have expert knowledge and would like to be interviewed or used as a consultant, make your interest known and send story ideas and pertinent background literature to reporters or editors. When accurate information is published, expressions of support will encourage more of the same.

Objections to advertising can be made to advertising managers, editors, publishers, and/or station managers. Although advertising revenue may count more than your opinion, protests are sometimes effective. If you report a misleading ad to an enforcement agency, tell your local media. Reporters who value the credibility of the press may relish an opportunity to embarrass their own advertising department by publicizing what you did.

The National Advertising Division (NAD) of the Council of Better Business Bureaus can exert pressure against misleading messages in national advertising. NAD's director, Ronald Smithies, Ph.D., J.D., appears to favor supplement industry viewpoints, but complaints to NAD are sometimes effective. Its address is 845 Third Avenue, New York, NY 10022.

## Reporting Illegal Activities

Suspicious activities can be reported to government agencies. Some people hesitate to do this for fear they will become embroiled in legal controversy. This fear is unfounded, however. Enforcement agencies conduct their own investigations and obtain outside experts as needed. Anyone has the right to complain to any regulatory agency.

The U.S. Food and Drug Administration (FDA) has jurisdiction over the labeling of products that enter interstate commerce. Labeling includes not only the actual words on the label, but also any claims made through literature or oral claims involved in the sales process. Supplement products or questionable devices claimed to be effective against disease should be reported. Complaints made through FDA regional offices sometimes get more attention than those made to the agency's central office.

The Federal Trade Commission (FTC) has jurisdiction over advertising of products or services involving interstate commerce. However, the FTC almost never gets involved with the claims made by practitioners who are licensed by the states. Trouble of this kind should be reported to state licensing boards. The Postal Service maintains jurisdiction over products sold through the mails.

When making a complaint, include as much information as possible. If you can, spell out what is wrong, point out why it may be harmful, and suggest what can be done to correct the problem. Where more than one agency may have jurisdiction, complain separately to all of them. Federal violations should also be reported to Congressional representatives with a request that they ask the appropriate federal agency to take action and let you know the outcome. When a state agency has jurisdiction over a problem, state legislators may be interested in getting involved. Complaints from lawmakers often get greater attention than those from individuals.

If you complain to an agency, please send a copy to me at P.O. Box 1747, Allentown, PA 18105. I may be able to investigate and write about the situation. All complaints should be typewritten.

Unscrupulous practitioners may be prosecuted by state agencies, but a lawsuit by an injured victim may be more effective. The trick is to find an attorney interested in fighting quackery who will file suit on a contingency basis. Under this arrangement, the attorney gets paid a percentage of the winnings but charges no fee if the case is lost. The National Council Against Health Fraud's Task Force on Victim Redress may be able to help locate a suitable attorney.

## Where to Complain or Seek Help*

| Problem | Agencies to contact |
|---|---|
| False advertising | FTC Bureau of Consumer Protection<br>Regional FTC office<br>National Advertising Division, Council of Better Business Bureaus<br>Editor or station manager of media outlet where ad appeared |
| Product marketed with false or misleading claims | National or regional FDA office<br>State attorney general<br>State health department<br>Local Better Business Bureau<br>Congressional representatives |
| Bogus mail-order promotion | Chief Postal Inspector, U.S. Postal Service<br>Regional Postal Inspector<br>State attorney general<br>Editor or station manager of media outlet where ad appeared |
| Improper treatment by licensed practitioner | Local or state professional society (if practitioner is a member)<br>Local hospital (if practitioner is a staff member)<br>State professional licensing board<br>National Council Against Health Fraud Task Force on Victim Redress |
| Improper treatment by unlicensed individual | Local district attorney<br>State attorney general<br>National Council Against Health Fraud Task Force on Victim Redress |
| Advice needed about questionable product or service | National Council Against Health Fraud<br>Consumer Health Information Research Institute<br>Local, state, or national professional or voluntary health groups |

*If more than one agency appears appropriate, complain to each one. See Chapter 33 for addresses. Dr. William T. Jarvis can be contacted at 909-824-4690. Dr. Stephen Barrett can be reached at 215-437-1795 (610-437-1795 after January 1, 1994).

## Linking with Others

Individual efforts against quackery can be greatly multiplied when coordinated with those of others. The National Council Against Health Fraud (NCAHF) now has more than one thousand members and has chapters in thirteen states. Organized in 1977 as the Southern California Council Against Health Fraud, the group became national in 1984. Its purposes are to: (1) conduct studies and investigations to evaluate claims made for health products and services; (2) educate the public, professionals, legislators, business people, organizations, and agencies about untruths and deceptions; (3) provide a center for communication between individuals and organizations concerned about health misinformation, fraud, and quackery; (4) support sound consumer health laws and oppose legislation which undermines consumer rights; and (5) encourage and aid in legal actions against law violators.

NCAHF's current activities include a speaker's bureau, a media clearinghouse, consumer complaint referral services, legislative advisement, expert testimony, law enforcement assistance, research on unproven methods of health care, and seminars for professionals and the general public. The council also appoints task forces that conduct extensive investigations and issue position papers.

Membership in NCAHF is open to anyone who supports its beliefs and purposes. Regular membership costs $20, and professional membership is $30. Donations are tax-deductible. Members receive a bimonthly newsletter, ready access to printed information on hundreds of topics, and discounts on anti-quackery publications. The group has chapters in Arizona, Florida, Illinois, Iowa, Kentucky, Michigan, Minnesota, New York, Ohio, Oregon, Texas, Washington, and Wisconsin.

Other groups that give high priority to fighting quackery are the Committee for the Scientific Investigation of Claims of the Paranormal (CSICOP), which deals with occult practices, and the American Council on Science and Health, which emphasizes food and chemical issues.

Remember that in matters of health there should be no tolerance for deception. Your effort in opposing quackery may save many people from being hurt—and may even save a life!

# Recommended Reading

The following publications can help you deepen and keep current your knowledge of health information and misinformation. Most of the books can be obtained from bookstores, either directly or by special order. Out-of-print books not available at your local public library may be obtainable through interlibrary loan. Back issues of newsletters and magazines may be available at libraries or from the publisher.

## Contemporary Quackery

Arthritis Foundation. *Unproven Remedies Resource Manual.* Atlanta: Arthritis Foundation, 1991.

S. Barrett (ed.). *The Health Robbers: How to Protect Your Money and Your Life.* Philadelphia: George F. Stickley Co., 1980. A comprehensive exposé of health frauds and quackery.

S. Barrett and the editors of Consumer Reports. *Health Schemes, Scams, and Frauds.* Yonkers, N.Y.: Consumer Reports Books, 1990.

S. Barrett and B.R. Cassileth (eds.). *Dubious Cancer Treatment: A Report on "Alternative" Methods and the Practitioners Who Use Them.* Tampa: American Cancer Society, Florida Division, 1991.

A. Bender. *Health or Hoax: The Truth about Health Foods and Diets.* Buffalo: Prometheus Books, 1986. An analysis of the "health food" industry and many of its products.

L. Bennion. *Hypoglycemia: Fact or Fad?* New York: Crown Publishers, 1985. A lucid analysis of the fad diagnosis versus the real disease.

R.J. Brenneman. *Deadly Blessings: Faith Healing on Trial.* Buffalo: Prometheus Books, 1990.

502    *The Health Robbers*

C.C. Cook-Fuller and S. Barrett (eds.). *Nutrition 93/94*. Guilford, Conn.: Dushkin Publishing, 1993. A sourcebook containing more than sixty well-written articles from magazines, newsletters, and journals. Updated about once a year.

H. Cornacchia and S. Barrett. *Consumer Health: A Guide to Intelligent Decisions, Fifth Edition*. St. Louis: Mosby Year Book, 1993. A referenced textbook covering all aspects of health care.

R.P. Doyle. *The Medical Wars*. Buffalo: Prometheus Books, 1985. A lucid analysis of the scientific method and its application to sixteen medical controversies.

The Editors of Consumer Reports Books. *The New Medicine Show*. Yonkers, N.Y.: Consumer Reports Books, 1989. A practical guide to common health problems and products.

F. Fernandez-Madrid. *Treating Arthritis: Medicine, Myth, and Magic*. New York: Plenum Press, 1989. Combines a fascinating history of arthritis quackery with insights about modern treatment.

K. Frazier (ed.). *The Hundredth Monkey and Other Paradigms of the Paranormal*. Buffalo: Prometheus Books, 1991. An updated anthology of articles originally published in the *Skeptical Inquirer*.

J. Fried. *Vitamin Politics*. Buffalo: Prometheus Books, 1984. A classic investigation of megavitamin therapy and its proponents.

M. Gauquelin. *Dreams and Illusions of Astrology*. Buffalo: Prometheus Books, 1979. A detailed account of the history and debunking of astrology.

H. Gelband et al. *Unconventional Cancer Treatments*. Washington, D.C.: U.S. Government Printing Office, 1990. A comprehensive report from the Office of Technology Assessment.

H. Gordon. *Channeling through the New Age: The Teachings of Shirley MacLaine and Other Gurus*. Buffalo: Prometheus Books, 1988. A critical look at mysticism, yoga, reincarnation, psychological techniques for "increased awareness," and other components of the "New Age" movement.

V. Herbert and S. Barrett. *Vitamins and "Health" Foods: The Great American Hustle*. Philadelphia: George F. Stickley Co., 1981. An investigative exposé of the "health food" industry.

P. Huber. *Galileo's Revenge: Junk Science in the Courtroom*. New York: Basic Books, 1991. Describes how professional "expert" witnesses have been permitted to bolster unfounded health claims in liability suits.

C. Marshall. *Vitamins and Minerals: Help or Harm?* Philadelphia: J.B. Lippincott Co., 1985. A comprehensive look at the sources, functions, benefits, dangers, and controversial aspects of vitamins and minerals.

G. Mirkin. *Getting Thin*. Boston: Little Brown, 1983. Weight-control facts and fads.

W. Nolen. *Healing: A Doctor in Search of a Miracle*. New York: Random House, 1974. A two-year study of prominent faith healers.

J.P. Payne et al. *Alternative Therapy*. London: British Medical Association, 1986. A detailed report on "alternative" therapies and how they can be scientifically evaluated.

C. Pepper et al.. *Quackery, A $10 Billion Scandal.* Washington, D.C.: U.S. Government Printing Office, May 31, 1984. Report of a four-year Congressional investigation of health frauds and quackery.

J. Randi. *The Faith Healers.* Buffalo: Prometheus Books, 1989. A devastating exposé of evangelistic faith healers and related subjects.

J. Raso. *Mystical Diets.* Buffalo: Prometheus Books, 1993. A fascinating exploration of food cults, their gurus, and offbeat nutrition practices.

_____ *Mystical Healing.* Buffalo: Prometheus Books, 1994. An exploration of unscientific physical, mental, and spiritual approaches to health and health care.

J. Renner. *Health Smarts.* Kansas City, Mo.: HealthFacts Publishing, Inc., 1990. Brief essays on consumer strategies, dubious products, and quack practices.

J. Sholes. *Give Me That Prime Time Religion.* New York: Hawthorne Books, 1979. An exposé of Oral Roberts.

W.A. Sibley. *Therapeutic Claims in Multiple Sclerosis.* New York: Demos Publications, 1992. An evaluation of more than one hundred methods that indicates which are promising and which appear worthless.

D. Stalker and C. Glymour (eds.). *Examining Holistic Medicine.* Buffalo: Prometheus Books, 1985. A devastating exposé of "holistic" propaganda and practices.

R. Steiner. *Don't Get Taken!* El Cerrito, Calif.: Wide Awake Books, 1989. Reveals how people get fooled by astrologers, mystics, psychics, faith healers, blood readers, pyramid schemes, and bunko artists.

F.J. Stare, V. Aronson, and S. Barrett. *Your Guide to Good Nutrition.* Buffalo: Prometheus Books, 1991. A discussion of dietary balance and avoidance of nutrition fads and frauds.

F.J. Stare and E.M. Whelan. *Panic in the Pantry.* Buffalo: Prometheus Books, 1992. An analysis of facts and fallacies related to the safety of America's food supply.

V. Tyler. *The Honest Herbal, Third Edition.* Binghamton, N.Y.: Haworth Press, 1993. A referenced evaluation of more than one hundred herbs and related substances.

E.M. Whelan. *Toxic Terror: The Truth behind the Cancer Scares.* Buffalo: Prometheus Books, 1993. An exposé of false claims that Americans are seriously endangered by chemicals in food, air, water, and other elements of our environment.

J. Yetiv. *Popular Nutritional Practices: A Scientific Appraisal.* San Carlos, Calif.: Popular Medicine Press, 1986. A referenced analysis of more than one hundred nutrition topics of current concern.

J.F. Zwicky, A.W. Hafner, S. Barrett, and W.T. Jarvis. *Reader's Guide to "Alternative" Health Methods.* Chicago: American Medical Association, 1992. An analysis of more than 1,000 reports on unproven, disproven, controversial, fraudulent, quack, and/or otherwise questionable approaches to solving health problems.

## History of Quackery

M. Christopher. *Mediums, Mystics & the Occult.* New York: Thomas Y. Crowell Co., 1975. A history of spiritualism and modern psychic frauds.

R. Deutsch. *The New Nuts Among the Berries.* Palo Alto, Calif.: Bull Publishing Co., 1977. How nutrition nonsense captured America.

M. Fishbein. *Fads and Quackery in Healing.* New York: Blue Ribbon Books, 1932. A comprehensive analysis of healing cults and "various other peculiar notions in the health field."

N. Gevitz (ed.). *Other Healers: Unorthodox Medicine in America.* Baltimore: The Johns Hopkins University Press, 1988. Essays on homeopathy, chiropractic, Christian Science, divine healing, folk medicine, osteopathy, the botanical movement, and the water-cure movement.

B. McNamara. *Step Right Up.* New York: Doubleday & Co., 1975. An illustrated history of the American medicine show.

J. Roth. *Health Purifiers and Their Enemies.* New York: Prodist, 1977. An overview of the "natural health" movement and its critics.

R.L. Smith. *At Your Own Risk.* New York: Pocket Books, 1969. A critical look at the history and shortcomings of chiropractic. (Available for $5 from LVCAHF, P.O. Box 1747, Allentown, PA 18105.)

R. Swan. *The Law's Response When Religious Beliefs Against Medical Care Impact on Children.* Sioux City, Iowa: CHILD, Inc., 1990. Traces the development of children's legal rights to medical care when parents have religious objections to it.

M. Twain. *Christian Science.* Buffalo: Prometheus Books, 1993. Mark Twain's caustic exposé of Christian Science and its founder.

J.H. Young. *American Health Quackery.* Princeton, N.J.: Princeton University Press, 1992. A collection of essays dealing with many aspects of quackery.

_____ *The Medical Messiahs.* Princeton, N.J.: Princeton University Press, 1992. A social history of health quackery in twentieth-century America.

_____ *The Toadstool Millionaires.* Princeton, N.J.: Princeton University Press, 1961. A social history of patent medicines in America before federal regulation.

## Reference Books on Scientific Health Care

C.B. Clayman (ed.). *The American Medical Association Encyclopedia of Medicine.* New York: Random House, 1989. A 1,184-page guide to over 5,000 medical terms, including symptoms, diseases, drugs, and treatments.

K. Butler and L. Rayner. *The New Handbook of Health and Preventive Medicine.* Buffalo: Prometheus Books, 1990. A guide to preventing and treating common health disorders.

J.W. Friedman and the editors of Consumer Reports Books. *Complete Guide to Dental Health.* Yonkers, N.Y.: Consumer Reports Books, 1991. Comprehensive discussion of the types and costs of dental care.

J.F. Fries. *Arthritis: A Comprehensive Guide to Understanding Your Arthritis.* Reading, Mass.: Addison-Wesley, 1990. Facts about the causes and treatment of arthritis.

V. Herbert, G.J. Subak-Sharpe, and D. Hammock (eds.). *The Mt. Sinai School of Medicine Complete Book of Nutrition.* New York: St. Martin's Press, 1990. A comprehensive sourcebook by a nationwide team of experts.

D.E. Larson (ed.). *The Mayo Clinic Family Health Book.* New York: William Morrow and Co., 1990. A comprehensive guide to health and medical care.

R.S. Lawrence et al. (eds). *Guide to Clinical Preventive Services.* Baltimore: Williams and Wilkins, 1989. A detailed assessment by the U.S. Preventive Services Task Force of 169 strategies for preventing and detecting health problems.

D.R. Stutz, B. Feder, and the editors of Consumer Reports Books. *The Savvy Patient.* Yonkers, N.Y.: Consumer Reports Books, 1990. How to be an active participant in your medical care.

United States Pharmacopeial Convention. *The Complete Drug Reference.* Yonkers, N.Y.: Consumer Reports Books, 1993. A comprehensive guide to more than 5,500 prescription and over-the-counter drugs. Updated annually.

D. Vickery and J.F. Fries. *Take Care of Yourself: Consumers' Guide to Medical Care.* Reading, Mass.: Addison-Wesley, 1990. A practical manual with many flow sheets to help decide when medical care is needed.

D.R. Zimmerman. *Zimmerman's Complete Guide to Nonprescription Drugs.* Detroit: Visible Ink Press, 1993. Thorough evaluation of products and ingredients, based mainly on the findings of FDA expert panels.

## Newsletters

*Children's Healthcare Is a Legal Duty, Inc.,* Box 2604, Sioux City, IA 51106. Reports on medical neglect of children due to religious or cult beliefs.

*Consumer Reports on Health,* Box 36356, Boulder, CO 80322. Presents detailed reports on health strategies, with occasional reports on quackery.

*Diet Busine$$ Bulletin,* 181 S. Franklin Ave., Suite 608, Valley Stream, N.Y., 11580. Quarterly report on hard-to-get information about the products, services, and economics of the commercial weight-loss industry.

*Harvard Health Letter,* P.O. Box 420300, Palm Coast, FL 32142. Features superb analyses of controversial issues, particularly those involving recent research.

*Johns Hopkins Medical Letter, Health after 50,* P.O. Box 420179, Palm Coast, FL 32142. Solid information on basic health strategies.

*Lahey Clinic Health Letter,* P.O. Box 541, Burlington, MA 01805. Solid information on basic health strategies.

*Lawrence Review of Natural Products,* Facts and Comparisons, 111 West Port Plaza, Suite 423, St. Louis, MO 63146. Authoritative monthly monographs on herbs and other naturally occurring products.

*Mayo Clinic Health Letter,* P.O. Box 53889, Boulder, CO 80322. Solid, practical information with occasional reports on quackery.

*Mirkin Report,* Box 6608, Silver Spring, MD 20916. Excellent summaries of news on fitness, nutrition, and health.

*NCAHF Newsletter,* P.O. Box 1276, Loma Linda, CA 92354. Covers a wide variety of events related to quackery and health frauds.

*Nutrition Forum,* P.O. Box 1747, Allentown, PA 18105. Features in-depth reports and undercover investigations related to quackery and health frauds.

*Probe,* Box 1321, Cathedral Station, New York, NY 10025. David Zimmerman's investigative newsletter on science, media, policy, and health.

*Tufts University Diet and Nutrition Letter,* P.O. Box 57857, Boulder, CO 80322. Solid, practical information, with occasional reports related to quackery.

*University of California at Berkeley Wellness Letter,* P.O. Box 420148, Palm Coast, FL 32142. Practical advice with frequent exposure of fads and fallacies.

## Magazines

*Consumer Reports,* P.O. Box 53029, Boulder, CO 80322. Covers a moderate number of topics related to health and nutrition.

*FDA Consumer,* Superintendent of Documents, P.O. Box 371954, Pittsburgh, PA 15250. Covers nutrition, food safety, drugs, and other medical topics.

*Obesity and Health,* Route 2, Box 905, Hettinger, ND 58639. Covers research, frauds, and other topics related to weight control.

*Priorities,* American Council on Science and Health, 1995 Broadway, New York, NY 10023. Focuses on controversies involving life-style, environmental chemicals, and quackery.

*Skeptical Inquirer,* CSICOP, Box 703, Buffalo, NY 14226. Features critical analyses of paranormal claims.

# Index

Food faddism, 77–82
*Food Guide Pyramid*, 24
Food group system, 24, 31, 32
Food processing, effect on nutrient status, 33
Foods, Plus, Inc., 373–374
For Your Health Pharmacy, 380
Forer, Bertram, 60
Foundation for Alternative Cancer Therapy (FACT), 97
Foundation for Homeopathic Education and Research, 196
Foundation for the Advancement of Innovative Medicine (FAIM), 412–413
Fox, Margaret and Kate, 64
Frank, Dr. Benjamin, 392
Franklin, Benjamin, 326
Franklin, Robert, 374
Fredericks, Carlton, 80, 371, 373–375, 383
Freireich, Dr. Emil J, 9
Fried, John J., 14–15
Friedlander, Dr. Edward, 96
Frigard, L. Ted, 176
Frogley, Ronald, 169
Fry, T.C., 240
FTC; see Federal Trade Commission (FTC)
*FTC News Notes*, 478

Gaby, Dr. Alan, 379
Gadget quackery, 321–335
  Amalgameter, 315
  and Albert Abrams; *see* Abrams, Dr. Albert
  and arthritis, 102–103
  and Drown, Ruth, 55, 327–328
  electrodiagnostic devices; *see* Electrodiagnostic devices
  eye-related, 353, 354
  Spectrochrome, 321–323
Galileo ploy, 12
*Galileo's Revenge*, 147
Gardner, Martin, 440

Garlic, 221
General Nutrition Corporation (GNC), 288
Genetic engineering of foods, 75, 77–78
"Geraldo," show, 375, 376
Gerard, John, 216, 218
Gerber, Dr. Michael, 387, 401–402
Gerovital H3 (GH3), 134
Gerson, Charlotte, 87
Gerson, Dr. Max, 87
Gerson diet, 87–88
*Getting Well Again*, 96
Ghadiali, Dinshah P., 321–323
Gingko, 224
Ginseng, 218, 222
"Glandulars," 30
Glucomannan, 392
Glymour, Dr. Clark, 357–358
Glyoxylide, 27, 93
Gonzales, Dr. Nicholas, 93
Gordon, Dr. Garry, 402
Graham, Sylvester, 78, 237
Grant, W.V., 345
Grape cure, 87
Great Earth International, 152
*Great Medical Monopoly Wars, The*, 411
Green, Chad, 409
Green, Dr. Saul, 91
Greene, Dr. Charles S., 310
Grieve, Maud, 213–214
Griffin, Merv, TV show, 117, 375
Grisham, Dr. J. David, 352
Group therapy, 425
"Growth-hormone releasers," 119, 122
Guess, Dr. George A., 197
Gunther, Max, 447
Gymnema sylvestre, 122

Hackett, Clara A., 350
Hahnemann, Dr. Samuel, 13, 191–192
Hair analysis, 37, 186, 312, 419
Hair vitamins, 10
Hall, Dorothy, 214